Heroin Addiction: Theory, Research and Treatment *by Jerome J. Platt and Christina Labate*

Children's Rights and the Mental Health Profession *edited by Gerald P. Koocher*

The Role of the Father in Child Development *edited by Michael E. Lamb*

Handbook of Behavioral Assessment *edited by Anthony R. Ciminero, Karen S. Calhoun, and Henry E. Adams*

Counseling and Psychotherapy: A Behavioral Approach *by E. Lakin Phillips*

Dimensions of Personality *edited by Harvey London and John E. Exner, Jr.*

The Mental Health Industry: A Cultural Phenomenon *by Peter A. Magaro, Robert Gripp, David McDowell, and Ivan W. Miller III*

Nonverbal Communication: The State of the Art *by Robert G. Harper, Arthur N. Wiens, and Joseph D. Matarazzo*

Alcoholism and Treatment *by David J. Armor, J. Michael Polich, and Harriet B. Stambul*

A Biodevelopmental Approach to Clinical Child Psychology: Cognitive Controls and Cognitive Control Theory *by Sebastiano Santostefano*

Handbook of Infant Development *edited by Joy D. Osofsky*

Understanding the Rape Victim: A Synthesis of Research Findings *by Sedelle Katz and Mary Ann Mazur*

Childhood Pathology and Later Adjustment: The Question of Prediction *by Loretta K. Cass and Carolyn B. Thomas*

Intelligent Testing with the WISC-R *by Alan S. Kaufman*

Adaptation in Schizophrenia: The Theory of Segmental Set *by David Shakow*

Psychotherapy: An Eclectic Approach *by Sol L. Garfield*

Handbook of Minimal Brain Dysfunctions *edited by Herbert E. Rie and Ellen D. Rie*

Handbook of Behavioral Interventions: A Clinical Guide *edited by Alan Goldstein and Edna B. Foa*

Art Psychotherapy *by Harriet Wadeson*

Handbook of Adolescent Psychology *edited by Joseph Adelson*

Psychotherapy Supervision: Theory, Research and Practice *edited by Allen K. Hess*

Psychology and Psychiatry in Courts and Corrections: Controversy and Change *by Ellsworth A. Fersch, Jr.*

Restricted Environmental Stimulation: Research and Clinical Applications *by Peter Suedfeld*

Personal Construct Psychology: Psychotherapy and Personality *edited by Alvin W. Landfield and Larry M. Leitner*

Mothers, Grandmothers, and Daughters: Personality and Child Care in Three-Generation Families *by Bertram J. Cohler and Henry U. Grunebaum*

Further Explorations in Personality *edited by A.I. Rabin, Joel Aronoff, Andrew M. Barclay, and Robert A. Zucker*

Hypnosis and Relaxation: Modern Verification of an Old Equation *by William E. Edmonston, Jr.*

Handbook of Clinical Behavior Therapy *edited by Samuel M. Turner, Karen S. Calhoun, and Henry E. Adams*

Handbook of Clinical Neuropsychology *edited by Susan B. Filskov and Thomas J. Boll*

The Course of Alcoholism: Four Years After Treatment *by J. Michael Polich, David J. Armor, and Harriet B. Braiker*

Handbook of Innovative Psychotherapies *edited by Raymond J. Corsini*

The Role of the Father in Child Development (Second Edition) *edited by Michael E. Lamb*

Behavioral Medicine: Clinical Applications *by Susan S. Pinkerton, Howard Hughes, and W.W. Wenrich*

(*continued on back*)

GAME PLAY

OTHER BOOKS BY CHARLES E. SCHAEFER

How to Talk to Children about Really Important Things, 1984

Family Therapy Techniques for Problem Behaviors of Children and Teenagers (with J. Briesmeister and M. Fitton), 1984

Group Therapies for Children and Youth (with L. Johnson and J. Wherry), 1983

Handbook of Play Therapy (with K. O'Connor), 1983

How to Influence Children (Rev. Ed.), 1982

How to Help Children with Common Problems (with H. Millman), 1981

Therapies for School Behavior Problems (with H. Millman and J. Cohen), 1980

Therapies for Psychosomatic Disorders in Children (with H. Millman and G. Levine), 1979

Childhood Encopresis and Enuresis, 1979

Therapies for Children: A Handbook of Effective Treatments for Problem Behaviors (with H. Millman), 1977

Therapeutic Use of Child's Play, 1976

Developing Creativity in Children, 1973

Becoming Somebody: Creative Activities for Preschool Children, 1973

Young Voices: The Poetry of Children, 1970

GAME PLAY
Therapeutic Use
of Childhood Games

Edited by

Charles E. Schaefer
The Children's Village
Dobbs Ferry, New York

Steven E. Reid
The Hallen School
Mamaroneck, New York

A WILEY-INTERSCIENCE PUBLICATION

JOHN WILEY & SONS

New York • Chichester • Brisbane • Toronto • Singapore

Library of Congress Cataloging-in-Publication Data:

Main entry under title:

Game play.

  (Wiley series on personality processes)
  "A Wiley-Interscience publication."
  Includes indexes.
  1. Play therapy. 2. Child psychotherapy.
I. Schaefer, Charles E. II. Reid, Steven E.
III. Series.

RJ505.P6G36   1986   616.89'165   85-22663
ISBN 0-471-81972-7

Printed in the United States of America

10 9 8 7 6 5 4 3 2 1

List of Contributors

STEWART BEDFORD, PH.D., Clinical Psychologist, Chico, California

CONNIE BEHRENS, A.C.S.W., Psychiatric Social Worker, Charlotte, North Carolina

BERTHOLD BERG, PH.D., Associate Professor, Department of Psychology, University of Dayton, Dayton, Ohio

IRVING N. BERLIN, M.D., Professor of Psychiatry and Pediatrics, Director, Division of Child and Adolescent Psychiatry and the Children's Psychiatric Hospital, The University of New Mexico School of Medicine, Albuquerque, New Mexico

ELAINE A. BLECHMAN, PH.D., Department of Psychiatry, Albert Einstein College of Medicine/Montefiore Hospital Center, Bronx, New York

JAMES N. BOW, PH.D., Staff Psychologist, Children's Center of Wayne County, Michigan, Detroit, Michigan

BILLIE F. CORDER, ED.D., Co-Director, Psychological Services, Child Psychiatry Training Program, Dorothea Dix Hospital, Raleigh, North Carolina

BARBARA EDMONSON, ED.D., Habilitation Consultant, Chico, California

YAKOV M. EPSTEIN, PH.D., Department of Psychology, Rutgers—The State University, New Brunswick, New Jersey

DIANE E. FREY, PH.D., Professor, Department of Counseling, Wright State University, Dayton, Ohio

RICHARD A. GARDNER, M.D., Clinical Professor of Child Psychiatry, Columbia University, College of Physicians and Surgeons, New York, New York

TERRY E. GOLDBERG, PH.D., Director of Psychological Services, Aurora Hospital-Osteopathic, Detroit, Michigan

RICHARD MARK KAGAN, PH.D., Director of Research and Quality Assurance, Parsons Child and Family Center, Albany, New York

MICHAEL J. MCENROE, M.A., Research Associate, Behavior Therapy Program, Department of Psychiatry, Albert Einstein College of Medicine/Montefiore Hospital Center, Bronx, New York

NEVALYN NEVIL, M.A., Consultant, Social Habilitation Associates, Columbus, Ohio

CLAIRE RABIN, PH.D., School of Social Work, Tel Aviv University, Tel Aviv, Israel

ROBERT S. SCHACHTER, PH.D., Clinical Psychologist, New York, New York

SHRAGA SEROK, PH.D., Senior Lecturer, Department of Social Work, Ben-Gurion University of the Negev, Beer Sheva Department of Psychotherapy, School of Medicine, Tel Aviv University, Tel Aviv, Israel

ARTHUR J. SWANSON, PH.D., Supervising Psychologist, The Children's Village, Dobbs Ferry, New York

Series Preface

This series of books is addressed to behavioral scientists interested in the nature of human personality. Its scope should prove pertinent to personality theorists and researchers as well as to clinicians concerned with applying an understanding of personality processes to the amelioration of emotional difficulties in living. To this end, the series provides a scholarly integration of theoretical formulations, empirical data, and practical recommendations.

Six major aspects of studying and learning about human personality can be designated: personality theory, personality structure and dynamics, personality development, personality assessment, personality change, and personality adjustment. In exploring these aspects of personality, the books in the series discuss a number of distinct but related subject areas: the nature and implications of various theories of personality; personality characteristics that account for consistencies and variations in human behavior; the emergence of personality processes in children and adolescents; the use of interviewing and testing procedures to evaluate individual differences in personality; efforts to modify personality styles through psychotherapy, counseling, behavior therapy, and other methods of influence; and patterns of abnormal personality functioning that impair individual competence.

IRVING B. WEINER

University of Denver
Denver, Colorado

Preface

Since the days of the Pharaohs, games have been played avidly by young and old, rich and poor. No fewer than four board games were found in the tomb of King Tutankhamen, who died in 1352 B.C. The Greek philosophers Aristotle and Plato wrote about the importance of games in fostering learning and development in children. Plato recommended that "in teaching children, train them by a kind of game and you will be able to see more clearly the natural bent of each." Clearly, games are not only enjoyable, but they help children develop physically, cognitively, emotionally, and socially.

Despite the enduring and ubiquitous appeal of games, there was no mention of formal games in the early literature on play therapy. Even today, most therapists associate play therapy with the clinical use of sensory-motor and pretend play with young children. Few clinicians are aware of the therapeutic potential of games for school-age children and teenagers. The purpose of this book is to present a "state-of-the-art" overview of the therapeutic use of formal games with youth. To this end, experts in the field were asked to write original chapters describing their particular approaches to game play. These contributions are grouped into four major sections: communication games, problem-solving games, ego-enhancing games, and socialization games.

Just about every game, commercial or otherwise, has been used as a therapeutic medium. Some therapists use games as the central focus of their intervention, while others employ them as adjuncts to the therapeutic process, such as a way of engaging resistant children in meaningful interactions. The "action-oriented" nature of games is well suited to the lifestyle of children. More and more therapists are realizing that by "making a game out of it"—whether it be learning how to make friends or learning how to be a better problem solver—you can teach children more effectively.

Civilization depends on people interacting according to rules and a sense of fair play. To be an effective game player, you must also adhere to the rules of the game and be a good sport. What better way to teach children how to be civilized and well adjusted than to teach them how to be better game players?

This book should be of interest to all professionals who work with children, including psychologists (clinical, school, and counseling), social workers, psychiatrists, psychiatric nurses, child-care workers and child-life specialists.

CHARLES E. SCHAEFER
STEVEN E. REID

Dobbs Ferry, New York
Mamaroneck, New York
April 1986

Contents

GAME PLAY

INTRODUCTION

The Psychology of Play and Games

The purpose of this chapter is to give a brief overview of the psychology of play and games. Concepts with particular relevance to therapeutic work with children are emphasized.

DEFINITIONS

The terms "play" and "games" have somewhat different meanings in the play therapy literature. Although not easily defined, play is generally seen as a spontaneous activity that has no particular purpose and is motivated only by a desire for fun (Csikszentmihalyi, 1976; Erikson, 1950; Garvey, 1977). Play is a pleasurable, naturally occurring behavior found in both animal and human life (Beach, 1945; Huizinga, 1950; Hutt, 1970; Plant, 1979). Furthermore, play often involves a distortion of reality, a pretense. Pretend play has an "as if" quality that allows for expression of emotions which would not ordinarily be permitted in "real life." Yet reality is so interwoven with play that it is often difficult to judge whether children at play are pretending or not. Krasner (1976) observes that children often check with their playmates to find out if something in play was "for real":

(A, a boy, sits down on the stool with the circular glass in the seat.)

A: I have to tinkle. I have to go to the bathroom.

B: Do you really?

A: Pretend. I got to sit down. I'm tired. (p. 11)

Play also has an unrestricted, unstructured quality. Although all play involves some structure, such as limits on behavior imposed by adults or by the children themselves, it is not a confining structure; it allows for the

1

generation of novel and creative behavior (Garvey, 1977). The free "flow" of play renders play behavior highly variable across situations and children (Csikszentmihalyi, 1975, 1976).

What is the distinction between play and games? In the literature on the subject, the term "games" usually refers to formal, organized games with rules, such as hopscotch, *Monopoly*, and baseball, to name only a few of countless known games. Game playing is an activity that shares at least two of the basic elements of play: both are meant to be fun and provide a context for fantasy experience. However, when playing an organized game, children must abide by the relatively fixed set of rules. All games have rules which ordinarily do not vary across situations or children (Opie and Opie, 1976). Rules inform players about the roles they will play, the limits and expectations for behavior, and how the game works. As a result, the range and scope of game behavior is much more restricted and formalized than it is in play.

Games are further defined as almost always involving a contest. Avedon and Sutton-Smith (1971) define a formal game as "an exercise in voluntary control systems, in which there is a contest between powers, defined by rules, in order to produce a disequilibrial outcome (someone ends up a winner)." Some believe games are "models of power" (Sutton-Smith and Roberts, 1971) with which children and adults learn socially acceptable ways to succeed over others. Indeed, over the last 25 years, games and gaming have become a central metaphor as well as an important research tool for the study of social conflict. The competition inherent in games provides a useful analogy to naturally occurring conflicts of interest in business, political, and interpersonal interactions (Schlenker and Bonoma, 1978).

While competition appears to be a basic part of games, it can be minimized or even eliminated from some games. Schelling (1960) describes "pure coordination situations" which have been devised for the study of conflict resolution. In these games, the outcome of all players are perfectly positively correlated and the players must only cooperate to profit. However, it has been observed that when competition is removed participants are less involved and derive less enjoyment from the game (Holmes, 1964; Rapoport, 1966; Steele and Tedeschi, 1967). Rather than to minimize conflict, most games are designed to provide competition within a mutually acceptable framework. This permits high levels of friendliness and cooperation to coexist with overt competitive attitudes.

The emphasis on outcome (i.e., winning or losing) associated with game-playing contrasts with the lack of goals so apparent in the play of younger children. In play, victory can be merely a state of mind achieved through fantasy. Play lacks the sense of personal challenge implied by competitive game-playing. To compete means that each child should apply their skills in an attempt to win the game. Meeks (1970) observes that latency-age children often show a more serious, even strained approach to organized games than younger children show toward play.

In this vein, it is clear that games demand much more of children in terms of ego processing than does play. Children playing a game must have enough impulse control, frustration tolerance, and reality testing to accept limits on their behavior and follow the rigid rules of the game. A certain amount of persistence, attention, and concentration to task is necessary to follow a game to its conclusion. Furthermore, even the simplest of games requires greater cognitive ability than does play. To illustrate, in order to play War, one of the most basic card games, children must know primary numbers and understand the numerical concept of greater/lesser. Many games which involve strategy tap organized, planful, and logical thinking, as well as problem-solving ability.

The other key element common to most if not all games is interpersonal interaction. Games typically involve the interaction between two or more players. Furthermore, in most games, the actions of the participants are interdependent. This means that the outcome of the game depends on the interaction of the players, not on one player's actions alone. Game-playing is inherently more of a social activity than unstructured play, which can be carried on by two or more children with little interaction between them.

There are many games, of course, such as solitaire card games and video-computer games, which are played by one person. Throughout history, however, games have developed as social activities to be engaged in by at least two people. The social aspect of games is derived from the fact that, historically, games, particularly boardgames, have mirrored current events and popular culture. To illustrate, the first American boardgame, the *Mansion of Happiness*, was decidedly moralistic. The object of the game was to reach an ethereal mansion by not yielding to vice and temptation. A player landing on a space marked "idleness," for example, was sent back three spaces. This game was created in 1843 and reflected the moral standards of nineteenth century America. A host of games featuring "get rich quick" schemes were introduced during the Great Depression of the 1930s, including *Monopoly*, now the best-selling boardgame in history. These games offered the chance to fantasize about overcoming the economic hardships that pervaded American life during that time.

In summary, six aspects of games have been identified which provide their major defining characteristics. These characteristics provide a framework and working definition of games, especially as they contrast with play.

1.   Playing a game is an enjoyable activity.

2.   Games have an "as if" quality that separates them from real life and allows for fantasy experience.

3.   Rules exist or are created that define and restrict the behavior of the players and add organization and structure to the game.

4.   A contest is implied or explicit in games, in that players compete either with each other or with themselves in order to win the game.

5.   Games, by virtue of their structured, competitive makeup pose a challenge to the participants. At the lowest level, the challenge is to play with other people in a self-controlled, cooperative fashion. More complex games require more in terms of emotional control, intellect, and social skills.

6.   Game-playing usually involves interaction between two or more players.

TYPES OF GAMES

Games can be classified according to what determines who wins. The classification scheme developed by Sutton-Smith and Roberts (1971) is widely used in game research. These authors distinguish three types of games: (1) games of physical skill, in which the outcome is determined by the players' motor activities, (2) games of strategy, in which cognitive skill determines the outcome, and (3) games of chance, in which the outcome is accidental. Each category is discussed below with emphasis on their potential for use in therapy.

Games of Physical Skill

This category can be further divided into gross- and fine-motor games. The former include many childhood games such as relay races, tag, simple ball games, and so forth. One need only be a casual observer of children at play to see them create these types of games spontaneously. Fine-motor games include darts, *Tiddly winks*, *Pic-up stix*, *Operation*, and so forth. The advantages of physical games for the purpose of therapy are: (1) they have simple, easily explained rules, (2) physical motion can provide a cathartic release of energy for many children, and (3) the action-orientation of these games lends them for therapeutic use for behavior problems such as hyperactivity and impulsivity. The primary disadvantage of these games is that they are hard to perform in an office, especially gross-motor games. Another problem with physical games is that they often encourage acting out, instead of verbalization, of feelings and emotions.

Games of Strategy

Games whose outcomes depend primarily on cognitive skill include number and word games, tic-tac-toe, *Connect four*, Chinese checkers, checkers, chess, among many others. These games can usually be played by two people in an office setting. They also permit informal observation of the child's intellectual strengths and weaknesses. Another advantage of strategy games is that they permit expression of aggression without the physical arousal associated with physical games. Complex strategy games, however, such as chess or *Stratego*, are often time-consuming, intellectually draining affairs which leave little time or energy for therapeutic work.

Games of Chance

These include bingo, roulette, a few card games (e.g. War), *Candyland* and *Chutes & Ladders* boardgames, and others. Pure chance games, except for adult gambling, tend to be on a simple level and are therefore useful as an introduction to game-playing. Another therapeutic advantage of chance games is that they neutralize the adult's superiority in intellect, skill, and experience. On the other hand, children often quickly lose interest in chance games because of the lack of strategy or skill involved.

Most games involve a combination of any two or three of the elements of luck, physical skill, and strategy. Baseball involves all three, and poker involves chance and strategy. Games created specifically for therapy have been categorized on the basis of amount of rules and type of activity (cognitive, behavioral, or both) (Rabin, 1983; Varenhorst, 1973). As the number of new therapeutic games increases, it becomes possible to classify with respect to the therapeutic objective or emphasis of the game. In this book, chapters are divided according to the relative therapeutic emphasis of the game(s) described, yielding four categories: communication, problem solving, ego-enhancement, and socialization. Therapists who are beginning game therapy can keep these typologies in mind, along with considerations of the child's developmental level and constraints of the therapy setting, in choosing a game or series of games to suit the therapeutic needs of the child.

PLAY, GAMES, AND HUMAN DEVELOPMENT

It is generally recognized that play behavior of children proceeds along developmental lines and can therefore be classified according to stages of development. Piaget (1962) identified three stages of cognitive development in play; sensory-motor play (two months to two years), fantasy play (two to seven years), and games with rules (seven to 11 years). In the first stage, the sensory-motor actions of the child and their repetition are primary. With fantasy or symbolic play, the child starts playing roles, for example, playing doctor or playing house. The ability to pretend, to use one thing to represent another, signifies a major advance in intellectual development. Rule games begin when the child's use of reasoning becomes logical and objective.

Peller (1954), in her classical paper on the psychoanalytical meaning of play, ties the preference for playing games to the reduction of oedipal preoccupations. Oedipal play, according to Peller, is characterized by idiosyncratic fantasy and magical thinking, both of which typify the mental life of the child in this psychosexual stage of development. Resolution of oedipal strivings is achieved through identification with an adult figure and is reflected in the child's shift in interest from fantasy play towards games that parallel life in the adult world. This is the first step toward the formation of autonomous personality functioning within the confines of prescribed social roles, a task which reappears throughout latency and adolescence.

In regard to social development, Parten (1932) studied social participation in the play of preschoolers. She found that as children develop, their social play becomes increasingly complex, proceeding through the stages of solitary, parallel, associative, and cooperative play. More recent studies on toddler peer relations by Ross and her colleagues (Goldman and Ross, 1978; Ross and Kay, 1980; Ross, 1982a, Ross, 1982b) indicate that cooperative interaction in play begins very young, as early as 22 months. As toddlers develop, so does their interest in and ability to play cooperative, rule-governed games.

The parallels from these models of play development are clear: Play is seen as progressing from egocentric bodily movements to symbolic play to more complex social interactions which gradually approximate real life social phenomena. Games with rules gradually become the preferred play activity as children emerge from toddlerhood and enter the school age years, and remain primary throughout late childhood and adolescence.

Another theme that runs through the literature on play development is that play and game-playing not only reflect developmental stages and changes, but function to promote and enhance the process of change. Play is believed to have an important role in such early developmental tasks as separation-individuation (Mahler, Pine, and Bergman, 1975), exploration of the environment (Druker, 1975), mastery of anxiety (Cramer, 1975), and achievement of object permanence (Pulaski, 1974). Much has been written about games and game-playing in the development of social behavior. Mead (1934) was among the first to recognize the importance of games in the socialization process. Through participation in games, the child was seen by Mead as learning to differentiate himself or herself from others and gain practice in basic communication skills. By following the rules constraining game behavior, the child learns about the power of society as the "generalized other," and that social behavior is seldom removed from public view and sanction.

A significant body of literature has since accumulated indicating that organized game-playing constitutes a critical socialization process (Boyd and Simon, 1971; Brim, 1968; Livingston, Fennessey, Coleman, Edwards, and Kidder, 1973; Stoll, Inber, and James, 1968; Sutton-Smith, 1967; 1971; Zigler and Child, 1956). A "mini-life" situation (Serok and Blum, 1983) is created within the context of a game that provides an opportunity to acquire new information, experiment with new roles and behaviors, and adapt to the demands of the game and norms of the collective. Further socialization experiences occur when rules are violated. Rule violators are generally stigmatized or must offer an apology, admission of guilt, or retribution in order to be permitted to remain in the game. In this way, children are sensitized to the aversive consequences of rule-violating behavior.

Games also provide an opportunity for children to deal with aggressive and competitive urges in a socially acceptable way. By their very nature, games arouse competitive feelings in children, but at the same time the rules of the game require that children compete within certain limited boundaries. Children often argue the interpretation of the rules and "fairness" of the contest. Also, group norms usually exist that dictate how winners should behave in relation to losers; that is, how to be a "good winner." In short, games are an exercise in controlled, adaptive expression of aggression (Redl and Wineman, 1951; Zigler and Child, 1956).

Redl (1958) emphasized the concepts of power and control as intrinsic in games. He argued that subjecting oneself to control or command by others is a central aspect of most games. Many games require that a leader be designated and that the other players follow the leader. Therefore, games provide an experimental situation for learning to deal with others in the real world who are more powerful than oneself. The opposite is also true, in that some games offer children and adolescents a chance to adopt leader roles and learn leadership skills. Follow-the-leader type games, of course, provide the clearest examples of games in which specific leadership and followship roles are designated.

That games serve an important socialization function is supported by the findings of research on cross-cultural aspects of game-playing. In general, this research has found that games are not just the creation of a few advanced civilizations. Game-playing is a nearly universal human activity; only a handful of the most primitive societies do not possess games (Sutton-Smith and Roberts, 1971). In many cultures, game-playing appears to presage social skills that are required later in life. For instance, only some cultures possess "central person games" (tag, hide and seek, red rover, etc.). Central person games are thought to represent the child's anxieties about exercising social independence. Research has shown that in cultures that possess these games, there exists a significantly greater general concern with independence training during childhood, as well as a greater tendency for the "adolescent" girl to go out from her own kin group to marry amongst relative strangers, than in those cultures not having these games (Sutton-Smith, 1961).

It is no accident that many games, especially those that have endured for many years, are thematically similar to real-life social situations. Games seem to develop naturally as tools for dealing with real concerns. Cross-cultural research has shown that games of chance predominate in cultures associated with environmental uncertainty and unpredictability (food supplies, climate, settlements, etc. are nonfixed) (Sutton-Smith and Roberts, 1971). In these cultures, games mimic the uncertainty of life. Similarly, cultures possessing games of strategy are at a higher level of cultural complexity in which strategic skills and logical thinking are rewarded.

It appears, then, that games are more than just a form of amusement. They appear to provide a vehicle for dealing with a variety of real-life situations and concerns. Furthermore, for children games serve a specific, important function in development, that of providing key socialization experiences throughout their school years. Games provide the opportunity for social learning in several specific ways: (1) communication with others, (2) respect of and obedience to rules, (3) self-discipline, (4) dealing with independence issues, (5) cooperation with others, (6) awareness of and responsiveness toward group norms and expectations, (7) socialized competition and controlled expression of aggression, and (8) dealing with issues of power and authority.

THERAPEUTIC INGREDIENTS OF GAMES

Play was introduced into child psychotherapy by psychoanalysts such as Anna Freud (1928), who used play to lure the child into therapy, to interest the child in therapy and the therapist, and by Klein (1932) to promote fantasy expression. These therapists described their use of familiar toys such as cars, dolls, and simple figures. Axline's (1947) pioneering work in play therapy emphasized fantasy-stimulation play and toy materials, although she did mention checkers as something familiar that might help a shy child feel more comfortable in therapy. Loomis's (1957) article on the use of checkers in therapy marked the first serious discussion of the therapeutic value of organized games. Loomis emphasized the game as a vehicle for expression of resistance and unconscious conflict on the part of the child. The game of checkers was seen by Loomis to provide a safe, neutral context in which the normal adult-child boundaries of therapy are blurred somewhat, helping to relax the defenses of the child. This creates the conditions under which unconscious processes, especially those related to resistance to therapy, are readily transferred to the game situation.

Meeks (1970) and Beiser (1979) elaborated further on the use of games as a projective tool in psychoanalytic child psychotherapy. Beiser writes:

> The game is a projection of the relationship between the players to which each brings his own abilities, personality, and problems to bear. The child in treatment inevitably involves the therapist in his conflicts. If such struggles can be transferred to the game board, the therapist gets less angry, and the child less guilty. A very bright 6-year-old girl with poor peer relationships has started to play games with me, but we stopped because of her blatant cheating. There was a long period of testing both my interest in her and my superior physical powers. She taunted me with her powers, and openly said she was stronger than her mother. When I could prove she was not stronger than I without actually hurting her, she moved back to the game board. She asked me to start first in Chinese checkers to see how I won. We spent a long period developing her ability to play well and honestly, and I later received reports that she was able to use these skills in developing better peer relationships. (p. 487)

Meeks (1970) analyzed the meaning of cheating in games. He suggested that the central meaning of cheating is a compromise between a child's efforts to compete realistically and unresolved wishes for omnipotent control. Children who cheat at games rely on regression, that is, the return to magical devices and wishful thinking, when faced with personal inadequacy. The end result is "to perpetuate a weakened reality sense and to interfere with the development of coping abilities" (p. 276).

The use of games in therapy emerged from the psychoanalytical tradition of using a play medium to establish rapport and provide familiar, neutral stimuli onto which the child projects various aspects of his or her personality. The child's behavior and verbalizations during the game provide the basis for interpretations. With this approach, communication between child and therapist during the first phase of therapy often takes place within the metaphor of the game (Ekstein and Caruth, 1966). The eventual goal of psychoanalytical game therapy is to bring the child's unconscious conflicts, as expressed within the context of the game, into the arena of conscious awareness and verbal expression.

Since the early 1970s, there has been a dramatic rise in interest in the therapeutic possibilities of game-playing. With the increasing number of publications on the topic has come the recognition that games are widely used by child psychotherapists. It has also become clear that games have many advantages for therapy and that therapists emphasize particular aspects of games to meet the needs of their clients. The current trend is toward greater specialization; that is, the development of original games for specific therapeutic purposes. The following describe some of the more prominent therapeutic facets of games.

Diagnosis

As mentioned, the earliest clinical applications of games focused on their projective value. Valuable diagnostic information can be gleaned from observing how the child plays the game. For example, a passive/dependent child will constantly ask for help or advice or may lose on purpose to please the therapist; an obsessional child may get so wrapped up with rules that he or she loses sight of the goals of the game; a borderline child may get so involved with the fantasy aspects of the game that the original goals are forgotten. Gardner (1969) and Levinson (1976), however, caution that structured games, such as checkers, have limited value in directly eliciting fantasy. The structure and rules of these games invoke secondary (ego) processes, which work against the free expression of unconscious material. Furthermore, during a game, a substantial amount of time may be spent discussing rules, concentrating on strategy, or otherwise attending to the game situation. It appears that games are more valuable for examining a child's ego functioning than for uncovering unconscious conflicts. It should be mentioned, however, that games have been developed for the specific purpose of eliciting fantasy expression, such as the *Imagine!* game (Burks, 1978). The sense of safety and permissiveness that pervades the atmosphere of most games certainly lends them for use for this specific purpose.

Pleasure

Games are natural and enjoyable activities to children. Game-playing by itself, without therapeutic intervention, probably facilitates emotional growth. Pleasure, in moderation, is believed to be a potent medicine for preventing and alleviating psychological disturbance (Gardner, 1973). The field of recreational therapy is built on this premise.

Therapeutic Alliance

The "safety" of games refers to the feeling of comfort associated with what is familiar. Games are such an enjoyable part of children's lives that even the most resistant youth will usually participate in game therapy. Children usually begin therapy not of their own will but because of a decision made by their parents. They may not accept the premise that they have a psychological problem. Children with poor ego-strength may feel intense pressure being alone with an adult in the confines of a therapy office. Games can help children feel more comfortable and engage them in the therapeutic process.

Self-Expression

An important aspect of games is their separation from reality. The phrase, "it's just a game," is a familiar but psychologically powerful cue for loosening of restraints and relaxing of defenses. Capell (1968) observes that the intense affective involvement that commonly accompanies game-playing results in expression of feelings, thoughts, and attitudes that ordinarily would not be disclosed.

Ego-Enhancement

The competitive nature of games may create anxiety in children. Issues concerning competition, self-esteem, power and helplessness, and risk-taking may come to the fore in a game. The game provides an opportunity for the child in treatment to confront, work through, and gain mastery over uncomfortable feelings. Impulsive children, for example, can learn and practice self-control and frustration tolerance just by taking turns or by modifying their own responses in order to improve their game performance. Numerous opportunities arise during a game for the therapist to make suggestions and provide guidance, encouragement, and positive reinforcement. In a pretend situation, children are more willing to experiment with new behaviors, and direction given by authority figures is experienced as less "painful."

Cognitive

Cognitive skills, such as concentration, memory, anticipating consequences of one's behavior, reflectivity, and creative problem solving, can
be developed through game play. Over the last 15 years, games have
found a place in classroom instruction and remedial education because
learning these cognitive skills comes easier when the activity is experienced as enjoyable.

Socialization

As discussed in the previous section, there are many opportunities for social learning through game play. Games may have particular relevance
for conduct-disordered and delinquent youth, whose problems are
thought to stem from a failure in the socialization process (Redl and
Wineman, 1951; Zigler and Child, 1956). Games offer the opportunity to
experience positive peer pressure and acceptance of authority in a
nonthreatening atmosphere. Delinquents are also described as resistant to
traditional treatment approaches, so games might be helpful in drawing
these youths into therapy.

As a final note on the therapeutic aspects of games, the following recommendations, based on those presented by Beiser (1979) on adapting
game play to the therapy-office situation, are offered.

1.   Offer games that are suitable for two people or small groups.
This eliminates most team sports and some common childhood games
but includes most boardgames.

2.   The game must be suitable to the space available.

3.   The game equipment should not encourage the infliction of personal injury or property damage. Soft sponge balls, safety darts, and so
forth can be substituted.

4.   The game length should fit into the therapy hour. Most children
in therapy are unable to concentrate for longer games such as *Monopoly* or chess. Playing a game several times within the hour allows for
immediate application of what was learned from the previous game.

5.   There should be a variety of games with different complexities,
to allow for regression or progression, as the child may need. The vari-

ety should also satisfy different skills and preferences, as well as explore a variety of psychological issues.

6.   The therapist should be familiar with the rules and goals of the game and should get some enjoyment out of playing them. A game can acquire oppositional value if the therapist thoroughly dislikes playing it.

REFERENCES

Avedon, E.M. and Sutton-Smith, B. (1971). *The study of games*. New York: Wiley.

Axline, V. (1947). *Play therapy*. Boston: Houghton Mifflin.

Beach, F. (1945) Current concepts of play in animals. *American Naturalist, 79*, 523–541.

Beiser, H.R. (1979). Formal games in diagnosis and therapy. *Journal of Child Psychiatry, 18*, 480–490.

Boyd, N.L. and Simon, P. (Eds.) (1971). *Play and game theory in group work*. Chicago: University of Illinois at Chicago Circle.

Brim, O.G. (1968). *Socialization after childhood: Two essays*. New York: Wiley.

Burks, H.F. (1978). *Psychological meanings of the Imagine! game*. Huntington Beach, CA: Arden.

Capell, M. (1968). Passive mastery of helplessness in games. *American Imago, 25*, 309–330.

Cramer, P. (1975). The development of play and fantasy in boys and girls: Empirical studies. *Psychoanalysis and Contemporary Science, 4*, 529–567.

Csikszentmihalyi, M. (1975). Play and intrinsic rewards. *Journal of Humanistic Psychology, 15*, 41–63.

Csikszentmihalyi, M. (1976). What play says about behavior. *Ontario Psychologist, 8*, 5–11.

Druker, J. (1975). Toddler play: Some comments on its functions in the developmental process. *Psychoanalysis and Contemporary Science, 4*, 479–527.

Ekstein, R. and Caruth, E. (1966). Interpretation within the metaphor: Further considerations. In R. Ekstein (Ed.), *Children of time and space, of action and impulse*. New York: Appleton-Century-Crofts.

Erikson, E. (1950). *Childhood and society*. New York: Norton.

Freud, A. (1928). *Introduction to the technique of child analysis*. Translated by L.P. Clark. New York: Nervous and Mental Disease Publishing.

Gardner, R.A. (1969). The game of checkers as a diagnostic and therapeutic tool in child psychotherapy. *Acta Paedopsychiatrica, 38*, 142–152.

Gardner, R.A. (1973). *Understanding children*. New York: Aronson.

Garvey, C. (1977). *Play*. Cambridge, MA. Harvard University Press.

Goldman, B.D. and Ross, H.S. (1978). Social skills in action: An anlaysis of early peer games. In J. Glick & K.A. Clarke-Stewart (Eds.), *The development of social understanding*. New York: Gardner.

Holmes, D.J. (1964). *The adolescent in psychotherapy*. Boston: Little, Brown.

Huizinga, J. (1950). *Homo ludens: A study of the play element in culture*. New York: Roy.

Hutt, C. (1970). Specific and diverse exploration. In H. Reese & L. Lipsitt (Eds.), *Advances in child development and behavior*, New York: Academic.

Klein, M. (1932). *The psycho-analysis of children*. London: Hogarth.

Krasner, W. (1976). *Children's play and social speech*. Department of Health, Education, and Welfare: National Institute of Mental Health, Maryland.

Levinson, B.M. (1976). The use of checkers in therapy. In C. Schaefer (Ed.), *The therapeutic use of child's play*. New York: Aronson.

Livingston, S.A., Fennessey, G.M., Coleman, J.S., Edwards, K.J., and Kidder, S.J. (1973). *The Hopkins Game Program*. Baltimore: Johns Hopkins Press.

Loomis, E.A. (1957). The use of checkers in handling certain resistances in child therapy and child anlaysis. *Journal of the American Psychoanalytical Association, 5*, 130–135.

Mahler, M., Pine, F., and Bergman, A. (1975). *The psychological birth of the human infant: Symbiosis and individuation*. New York: Basic.

Mead, G.H. (1934). *Mind, self, and society*. Chicago: University of Chicago Press.

Meeks, J. (1970). Children who cheat at games. *Journal of Child Psychiatry, 9*, 157–174.

Opie, I. and Opie, P. (1976). Street games: Counting out and chasing. In J.S. Bruner (Ed.), *Play—Its role in development and evolution*. New York: Basic.

Parten, M.B. (1932). Social participation among preschool children. *Journal of Abnormal and Social Psychology, 27*, 243–269.

Peller, L.E. (1954). Libidinal development as reflected in play. *Psychoanalysis*, *3*, 3–11.

Piaget, J. (1962). *Play, dreams, and imitation in childhood*. New York: Norton.

Plant. E. (1979). Play and adaptation. *The Psychoanalytic Study of the Child*, *34*, 217–232.

Pulaski, M. (1974). The importance of ludic symbolism in cognitive development. In J. Magary, M. Poulson, and G. Lubin (Eds.), *Proceedings of the third annual UAP conference: Piagetian theory and the helping professions*. Los Angeles: University of Southern California Press.

Rabin, C. (1983). *Towards the use and development of games for social work practice*. Unpublished manuscript.

Rapoport, A. (1966). *Two-person game theory: The essential ideas*. Ann Arbor: University of Michigan Press.

Redl, F. (1958). The impact of game ingredients on children's play behavior. *Proceedings of the Fourth Conference on Group Processes*, *4*, 33–81.

Redl, F. and Wineman, D. (1951). *Children who hate*. New York: Free Press.

Ross, H.S. (1982). The establishment of social games among toddlers. *Developmental Psychology*, *18*, 509–518. (a)

Ross, H.S. (1982). Toddler peer relations: Differentiation of games and conflicts. *Canadian Journal of Behavioral Science*, *14*, 364–379. (b)

Ross, H.S. and Kay, D.A. (1980). The origins of social games. In K. Rubin (Ed.), *Children's play*. San Francisco: Jossey-Bass.

Schelling, T.C. (1960). *The strategy of conflict*. New York: Oxford University Press.

Schlenker, B.R. and Bonoma, T.V. (1978). Fun and games: The validity of games for the study of conflict. *Journal of Conflict Resolution*, *22*, 7–38.

Serok, S. and Blum, A. (1983). Therapeutic uses of games. *Residential Group Care and Treatment*, *1*, 3–14.

Steele, M.W. and Tedeschi, J.T. (1967). Matrix indices and strategy choices in mixed-motive games. *Journal of Conflict Resolution*, *11*, 198–205.

Stoll, C.T., Inber, M., and James, S.F. (1968). *Game experiences and socialization: An exploration of sex differences*. Baltimore: Johns Hopkins Press.

Sutton-Smith, B. (1961). Cross-cultural study of children's games. *American Philosophical Society Yearbook*, 426–429.

Sutton-Smith, B. (1967). The role of play in cognitive development. *Young Children*, *6*, 361–370.

Sutton-Smith, B. (1971). Play, games, and controls. In J.P. Scott (Ed.), *Social control*. Chicago: University of Chicago Press.

Sutton-Smith, B. and Roberts, J.M. (1971). The cross-cultural and psychological study of games. *International Review of Sport Sociology*, *6*, 79–87.

Varenhorst, B.B. (1973). Game theory, simulations, and group counseling. *Educational Technology*, *13*, 40–43.

Zigler, E. and Child, I.L. (1956). Socialization. In G. Lindzey and E. Aronson (Eds.), *Handbook of social psychology*. Reading, MA: Addison-Wesley.

ONE

Communication Games

This part of the book focuses on the therapeutic uses of games for promoting self-expression and communication. Communication between the therapist and client is considered by many to be the backbone of psychotherapy. Many if not most children in therapy, however, are reluctant to disclose their feelings, attitudes, and thoughts, and few readily accept the premise that such self-expression will have eventual beneficial effects for them. Furthermore, therapists of different theoretical orientations differ in terms of the type and style of communication they consider to be therapeutic. The chapters in this part cover a wide range of applications of games to facilitate self-expression, reflecting not only the variety of types of therapeutic communication, but the flexibility and adaptability of games to various theoretical approaches and therapeutic objectives. Among the types of communication elicited through game play are expression of fantasy and unconscious material, disclosure of conscious feelings, thoughts, and attitudes, active listening, providing feedback to others, nonverbal emotional expression, and problem solving.

With most communication games, there is a relative emphasis on their pretend, "as if" quality, and on the fun and pleasure involved in playing. Most of these games deemphasize competition, winning or losing, and the challenge to outperform other players. The result is to create a nonthreatening, permissive atmosphere that encourages self-expression. To further diminish anxiety about self-disclosure, many communication games are designed to channel thoughts and feelings through a "third person." Talking on a feeling level about someone else gives the child practice in self-expression and is a step toward acknowledging and sharing one's own feelings.

CHAPTER 1

Communication Boardgames with Children

DIANE E. FREY

While traditional forms of therapy are effective with many children, there are some children who find it difficult, for various reasons, to respond to traditional approaches that require self-disclosing to the therapist in a one-to-one relationship or a group therapy setting. Children are acquainted with boardgames, such as *Candyland*, *Monopoly*, *Clue*, and so forth, and usually have a positive association with such games. Even the most reticent and negative child will usually play a game with the therapist, since such play is not necessarily viewed as being self-disclosing by the client and is usually seen as more pleasant than sitting in silence and receiving direct confrontation from the therapist.

The majority of communication boardgames are noncompetitive, thus eliminating some cheating behaviors which often are an outgrowth of competitive games. Lack of competition puts the focus on the content of the game rather than the goal of winning. In the minority of communication boardgames where competition does exist, the value seems to be in enticing the child to respond and making the game very similar to nontherapy games. In the noncompetitive games, the play can continue for as long as the therapist and/or child agree to do so. This flexibility allows the therapist to continue play for as long as it is therapeutic—an advantage competitive boardgames do not have.

Communication boardgames enable children to project aspects of self, both known and unknown to the child. Often these projections involve the presenting problem which was the cause for referral and additional areas of clients concern which were not the initial focus of the therapist. This gives the therapist a plethora of information about the child.

It is also easy to involve the child's family in game play while in the therapy session and/or in the child's home. (Only the *Talking*, *Feeling*,

Doing Game cautions against nonprofessional involvement with the play.)

Boardgames provide both the child and the therapist with flexibility and variety for use with a multiplicity of childhood disorders. Whatever theoretical orientation the therapist has can be easily integrated into most communication boardgames. Other play therapy techniques can be used with boardgame play. For example, puppets, human or animal figures, clay, finger puppets, and so forth can be used in conjunction with or in addition to, the therapist's or child's response.

The age range of most boardgames is from about five to adulthood. Younger children can often play these games if the therapist reads the cards to the child and adapts the vocabulary level. Young adolescents will also play the games, since they are not seen as immature if introduced in the correct context. Adults can also play without inhibition. Boardgames also provide a modality for preventative, developmental, and remedial forms of therapy.

Due to the flexibility of responding in boardgames the therapist can focus on cognitive, affective, and/or behavioral dynamics of the child, depending on the presenting problem. For example, if the referral was primarily due to nonadaptive behavior, such as shoplifting, much discussion can focus on behavior. If the presenting problem is on appropriate anger management, the focus can be primarily on the affective component. The goal, of course, is to help the child become more aware of all of three domains and how they influence each other.

DESCRIPTION OF COMMUNICATION BOARD GAMES

Among the most commonly used communication boardgames are the *Ungame* (Zakich, 1975), *Reunion* (Zakich and Monroe, 1979), *Imagine* (Burks, 1978), *Social Security* (Burten, 1976), *Talking, Feeling, Doing Game* (Gardner, 1973), *Scrabble for Juniors*, (Gardner, 1975), *Board of Objects Game* (Gardner, 1975), *Tisket, Taskit* (Kritzberg, 1975), *Talking/Listening Game* (Shadle and Graham, 1980), *Self Esteem Game* (Creative Health Services, 1983), *Changing Family Game* (Berg, 1982), *Family Contract Games* (Blechman, 1974), *Transactional Awareness Games* (Oden, 1976), and *Rational Emotive Game* (Zitsman, 1984). These games fall into three general categories: those with a focus on increasing interpersonal communication skills, those with a focus on specific concerns of a specialized population, such as children of divorce, and those with a focus on communicating to children a particular theory of psychotherapy, such as, transactional analysis.

Interpersonal Communication Games

The *Ungame* is appropriate for ages 5 to 105. It is a noncompetitive game which encourages the exploration of attitudes, feelings, motives, and values. Two to six players can play the game, which comes with several decks of cards: yellow cards for lighthearted fun, white cards for deeper understanding, blank cards on which the child or the therapist can write his or her own question, blue cards written by students throughout the United States, pink cards designed to enrich family communication, green cards submitted by marriage counselors and psychologists, orange cards submitted by ministers, and red cards which are Spanish bilingual cards. The following is a representative sampling of the cards: "What would you do if you had a 'Magic Wand'?," "What is something that 'bugs' you?," "What kind of animal would you like to be, and where would you like to live?," "Name two famous people you'd like to have for parents," and "What would you do if you were invisible?" There are also "tell it like it is" spaces on the game board which encourage the player to self-disclose or ask the other player a question. The game proceeds until the therapist and/or the child decide to stop.

Reunion is a game appropriate for ages eight to adult. It is also a noncompetitive game which focuses on childhood relations, feelings, visual imagery and perceptions, and empathic understanding. It is appropriate for two to six players. Children might be asked to remember a time when they were frightened or the best day they ever had. The expression of affect comes from cards which ask the child to tell which picture he or she feels most like now. Visual imagery cards might ask the child to relax and picture a story in his or her mind, such as winning a $90,000 sweepstakes. The child is then asked to share what has been visualized. When a player draws an "interest" card he or she is requested to ask someone to write the answer to a given question, then the player guesses what answer was chosen. As in the *Ungame*, play continues until the therapist and/or the child decide to stop.

In *Imagine* the age range is 6 to 100 + . The focus is on understanding emotions, attitudes, and needs. Other game objectives include enhancing creativity and self-expression. The game is noncompetitive and encourages self-disclosure and expression through mythological symbols which hold conscious and unconscious meanings. The little pig can represent foolishness, troll—anger, candy house—greed, and amazing telephone —the need to be close to someone. A representative sampling of the cards includes, "Pretend you could take a ride on the flying horse. What happened?," "Pretend you are peeking into the candy house. What do you see?," "Pretend you are the little mouse. What would the wise wizard say to you if you asked him how to be braver?," "If someone called you up on the amazing telephone who would it be?," and "If you fall down the wonderful well what would you find?" Play continues in the same manner as in the previously mentioned games.

Social Security is appropriate for ages 6 to 106. The focus of the game is in six major areas: "ownership" of problems, feelings exploration, problem solving, adaptation to change(s), conflict management, and values exploration. In addition to these six areas, players are also given the opportunity to fantasize and express whatever is on their mind by landing on other spaces on the game board. Sample cards include: "What was the most recent important change in your life?," "You are at a dance and everyone is having fun. You are alone and don't know anyone there. What two things would you do to improve the situation?," "What are two things you can do when you have a problem?," "Do you agree or disagree? Why? 'Tell a child often enough that he is a brat and he will certainly become a brat?'," "Just using your mouth, show how someone might look if he was worried," "At what age do you think children are old enough to date?," "For thirty seconds, name different things that you might do or say if you were feeling silly," and "Show how you might stand if you were feeling super good." Some cards are presented in Figure 1.1. This game is also noncompetitive and continues until therapist and/or client decide to stop.

The *Talking/Listening Game* is appropriate for children ages 6 to 12. It can be played by two to six players, played individually, 2 to 12 players in partners or up to 30 players by dividing the group into six teams. The main focus of the game is improving interpersonal communication through enhanced listening and confronting skills, problem solving, positive feedback, problem ownership, and environmental changes. A sample of the cards includes: "You want your mother to visit your scout troop

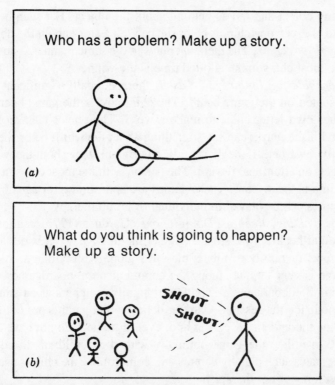

Figure 1.1.   Two game cards from *Social Security*. Reprinted with permission from "Social Security," © 1978 by the UnGame Company. (a) Who has a problem? Make up a story. (b) What do you think is going to happen? Make up a story.

meeting at 4:00 on Tuesday, but she has to pick up your little brother at the day-care center at 4:00. Tell (1) what each person wants or needs and (2) at least three possible solutions to the conflict," "Tell who needs to take responsibility for this problem—Your friend who sits next to you forgot to study for the test and now wants to copy your paper," and "Tell how you feel when someone gives you a compliment." The game is also noncompetitive and is played for as long as desired.

In *Tiskit, Taskit*, the *Talking, Feeling, Doing Game*, and the *Board of Objects Game* there is a competitive focus. In *Tiskit* and the *Board of Objects Game* a board of 64 squares is filled with small figurines such as zoo animals, small cars, trucks, family members, common objects, such as a toy knife, lipstick, trophy, and so forth. The child can select from the board any object and tell something about the object. For such behavior the child is given one chip; if he or she can tell a story about the object he or she gets two chips. The therapist plays in the same manner. The person with the most chips in the allotted time is the winner.

In *Scrabble for Juniors* and *Taskit*, therapeutically significant words are presented on the game board. The child covers the game board with his or her own letter chips to make a word. The player then receives a chip, and if the player can say something about the word, he or she is additionally rewarded. If the player tells an original story about the word, he or she gets an additional reward. The person with the most chips in the allotted time is the winner. These games are appropriate for ages 6 to 11. Both games can be played in individual or group therapy.

In the *Talking, Feeling, Doing Game*, Gardner (1973) cautions that *only* mental health professionals should play this game. It is not advised that parents or family members play this game with children. As such, this game is very unique among the communication boardgames. While other games encourage participation by family members as an adjunct to therapy outside the session, Gardner believes that parents are not trained to provide therapeutic responses and, even if trained, do not have the objectivity to utilize the game optimally with their children. In addition, Gardner states such play by parents will compromise the child's use of the game with his or her therapist.

This game is appropriate for children ages 7 to 12. The game cards can be read to young children (ages four to six) who will then actively participate. The game can be played by two to four players. The object of the game is to accummulate as many reward chips as possible after all players have reached the finish point. This is done by responding to cards which cover the cognitive, affective, and behavioral aspects of the child. Through the child's responding, underlying psychological processes are discovered. A representative sampling of the cards includes: "Make believe a piece of paper just blew in the window. Something is written on it. Make up what is said on the paper," "Name three things that could make a person happy," and "Make believe that something is happening that's very frightening. What is happening?"

Games for Specialized Populations

For children with low self-esteem, the *Self Esteem Game* can be very helpful. This game can be played by two to four players. Although the author does not state an age range, it appears to be appropriate for ages 8 to 12. The game can be played by families, and it is competitive in that there is a winner but cooperative in that the game is not over until all the players have reached the "well being" area of the game board. The most advanced player helps the player who is farthest behind. The focus of the game is on enhancing self-esteem by attending to individual behavior and interpersonal behavior with family, friends, and others. Sample game cards include: "A neat and clean appearance helps me feel good about myself. Move ahead 2." and "You don't finish things you start. Move back 2." The emphasis of these two cards is on the personal building blocks of self-esteem. The game focuses on coping options to help the child learn how to deal with intrapersonal and interpersonal setbacks.

The *Family Contract Game* is a boardgame in which players negotiate with each other in order to move around the board. Throughout the play, the therapist assists family members in developing a behavioral contract that is mutually satisfying and relevant to the stated problem. The focus is on the interdependence of the family and groups. This boardgame is noncompetitive and structured with a low threat level.

The *Changing Family Game* is a cognitive-behavioral boardgame to aid children in adjustment to divorce, visitation, single parent families, and blended families. The six areas are peer ridicule and avoidance, parental blame, maternal blame, self blame, fear of abandonment, and hopes of reunification. The cards to which the child responds are in four formats: advice cards that ask the child to advise a fictitious child with a divorce related problem, make believe cards that ask the child to respond as a mother, father or friend would to a divorce related situation, story-ending cards that ask the child to select the most appropriate solution from three or four alternatives, and pretend cards that ask the child to make up a unique divorce problem and offer a solution. "A Parent Separation Inventory" and a "Children's Separation Inventory" are provided to assist the therapist in determining the major areas of difficulty for the parent and the child. Examples of some cards include: "Bob has often gotten into trouble at school. Now Bob has been told by his parents that they will be getting a divorce and his father will be living in another city. Bob thinks that all of this must be punishment for his bad behavior at school. How is Bob feeling? What advice would you give to Bob" "Make up a problem that some boy or girl is having about a parent moving out. Try to make up a problem that you haven't heard before. What advice would you give this boy or girl," and "Arthur's father seems to think that his mother can do nothing right. He always seems to be criticizing her about one thing or another. How does Arthur feel? Pick the best ending to the story: (1) Arthur could join his father in criticizing his mother; (2) Arthur could talk with his father about his feelings, and (3) Arthur could begin criticizing his father."

There are also blank cards for this game. This boardgame can be played by two to six players and it is competitive, the players receiving chips for responding. Although there is no stated age range in the manual, it appears that the game is most appropriate for ages seven to adult. Parents, teachers, and other family members are encouraged to play the game also as an adjunct to therapy or in an educative manner themselves.

Games with Specific Theoretical Orientations

The Transactional Awareness Game (*TAG*) is a communication boardgame which can be played by one to six players. Its focus is on improving self-understanding and relationships through the use of feedback. The essential aspects of human transaction—power, warmth, acquiescence, and resistance—are woven into the game play. The players learn to identify various life scripts. The game is competitive; it is unique in that it is one of a few boardgames that is focused primarily on adolescents and adults, not younger children.

In the *Rational Emotive Game* children learn the difference between rational and emotional thinking through the game cards which present stories that demonstrate that beliefs are the underlying cause of emotions and actions. The game can be played by two to six players and the age range of the game is from age 6 to 11. Children win by thinking rationally and advancing themselves across the game board.

FUNCTIONS OF BOARDGAMES

Establish Rapport

Since boardgames are a familiar medium to children and since they are relatively nonthreatening they provide excellent opportunities for the therapist to establish rapport with the child client. By self-disclosing in response to game cards, the therapist becomes more human to the child.

The child is able to know the therapist better and the therapist, through empathic responding, communicates understanding to the child. By serving as a model for self-disclosure, the therapist can also encourage the child to become more expressive.

Diagnostic Value

Through the use of boardgames, the therapist can observe a variety of thoughts, feelings, and behaviors which the child client manifests. Among such areas which are often of diagnostic value to the therapist are behavior directed to the self, behavior directed to others, goal persistence, perceptions, verbal expression, affective expression, use of body, developmental level, relationship of the child to the therapist, and mode of communication. For example, therapists might encounter a child who hits himself or herself when he or she does not like the response he or she has given to a question from the boardgame, or a child might throw the game cards if he or she is frustrated. Children also might throw the dice at the therapist when angry or give up early if the game becomes too threatening. Through observing the child's perceptions of the world through his or her verbal and affective expression, the therapist can often begin to determine underlying causes of behavior. Some child clients have difficulty in continuing boardgame play for even short periods of time; they often move around the play therapy room from one play medium to another, continuously on the move. This use of the child's body can also be of diagnostic value to the therapists in assisting in diagnosing attention deficit problems. The developmental level of the child's play often can aid the therapist in discovering levels of intellectual functioning, emotional maturity, and/or regression. If the child client uses his or her turn to verbally attack the therapist, such behavior would lead to a very different assessment that if the child utilizes his or her turn to give positive feedback to the therapist. The mode of communication a child uses can also be of diagnostic value to the therapist: Some children respond to the boardgame tasks by using direct verbalization, some speak through puppets, finger puppets, or stuffed animals, some respond by using paper and pencil, others answer by using a play telephone or play typewriter. Some do not respond; this itself can be of diagnostic value. All these factors when analyzed and synthesized by the therapist can aid in facilitating a better understanding of the dynamics of the child.

Ego Enhancement

Throughout the boardgame play, there are numerous opportunities for the therapist to provide positive feedback to the child. In addition, the game play provides many chances for the child to gain a sense of mastery since boardgames are not difficult to play. Boardgame play is primarily experienced as pleasurable by the child. As such, this medium of play therapy can have a positive, motivating effect on children.

Catharsis

Psychodynamics which are, for some children, difficult to express directly are often expressed through communication boardgames. Such feelings as anger, resentment, frustration, jealousy, and envy can be safely expressed through the use of the boardgame. Thoughts and feelings of the client about the therapist can also be safely expressed through game play.

Sublimation

Through communication boardgames, the child client can rechannel impulses from forbidden outlets to the more creative outlet of the game. The child's sexual energy might be rechanneled into expressiveness through fantasy in a boardgame or the child's aggressive feelings might be rechanneled into a constructive activity in the game.

Reality Testing

The use of boardgames assists children in playing out various solutions to problems in a safe environment where reality testing can occur. The child has the opportunity to learn that the rules of the game are a depersonalized source of authority and are analogous to societal norms. The child also can learn about the rights and privileges of self in relation to the rights and privileges of others. The therapist can use boardgames to reinforce appropriate responses of the child if such an approach is consistent with the therapist's theoretical orientation. Communication boardgames can facilitate a generalization effect of such learning to the child's environment outside of therapy. As therapy progresses, the play therapist often directs his or her comments towards generalization of newly learned behavior(s).

Insight

Through communication boardgame play, behavioral patterns become more apparent to the child and therapist. Such increased self-awareness often results in changed behavior for the child. Insight is often developed by the child in response to the therapist's responses when it is the therapist's turn and/or is often developed by the child's response to his or her own comments. Such insight may occur spontaneously as when the child exclaims, "That's just like me!" or may occur over a period of time and in a more subtle way as when a child responds by giving an answer very similar to that of the therapist's answer given four sessions ago.

Progression in Therapy

The therapist can often acquire a sense of progress in therapy by observing differences in patterns of thoughts, feelings, and behaviors. These differences are easy to determine since structured games tend to elicit a somewhat restricted range of responses. Thus, game behavior is relatively consistent across sessions, so changes in behavior due to therapeutic growth or regression are readily apparent. It is often the case that a child might begin play with minimal responding or responding with intended inappropriate comments. Throughout the sessions the child's behavior becomes more responsive until, nearing termination, the child frequently is verbalizing and behaving with very appropriate responses, often ones articulated by the therapist in his or her turn at play.

Fantasy

The creative energies of children can easily be expressed in communication boardgames. When faced with a novel situation children often respond with curiosity. Such a situation often leads to innovation and exploration. Boardgames are sufficiently ambiguous stimuli to allow for all variety of responses, thus freeing a child's creativity. It is also not unusual for a child to want to change and adapt game rules or game boards. Such behavior can often be therapeutically valuable. The opportunity for free expression is, of course, very valuable to the child.

Group Play

Since communication boardgames can be easily played in individual or group therapy settings, their use is quite effective when focusing on the lessening of egocentrism, deepening children's empathy, fostering cooperative behavior, developing self-discipline, assisting in problem solving, and developing socialization skills. Group game play can facilitate such behaviors. The group could consist of other children in a similar age range or the child's family. Often in boardgame play, prepubertal children more readily accept feedback from same-age peers than from adult therapists.

Efficient Use of Time

As mentioned earlier, especially when dealing with difficult child clients in play therapy, the therapist can often make the most effective and efficient use of time through communication boardgames. Their structure and variety provide limitless opportunities for the therapist to creatively relate to the child in a therapeutic manner, which is time saving. Since referral sources, rightly or wrongly, frequently want to see behavior changed quickly, such games provide the opportunity to progress without years of therapy involvement.

Naturally, as the play therapist uses communication boardgames, he or she will notice some overlap of these functions of boardgames from child to child and within each child. This overlapping of functions might vary from session to session or even within a session, depending somewhat on the therapeutic goals.

CRITERIA FOR GAME SELECTION

Nickerson and O'Laughlin (1983) suggested the following criteria for the selection of games:

1. The game should be either familiar or easy to learn

2. The game should be appropriate for the individual or group in terms of age level and development

3. The game should have clear, inherent properties which are related to the therapeutic outcomes desired

TARGET POPULATIONS FOR BOARDGAMES

Resistant Children

Communication boardgames are especially effective for the resistant child. Some children will not self-disclose in therapy. This is often the case in court referrals or in instances when a child has been told by parents, teachers, or others not to disclose certain information as in the cases of child abuse, sexual molesting, and so forth. At times, children will self-disclose about some issues but not about others. For example, a child might disclose feelings of insecurity, inadequacy, and/or anxiety but will not discuss feelings of sexual curiosity. In such cases it is helpful for the therapist to be able to shift to communication boardgames from more traditional approaches. There are also children who are resistant to self-disclosure because of a generalized fear that such disclosure means they are weak or inadequate. Communication boardgames enable these children to self-disclose with lowered levels of anxiety.

Verbally Deficient Children

Some children do not have the ability to self-disclose in traditional therapeutic approaches. These children often lack the verbal skills which are necessary to communicate feelings; such children's feeling vocabulary is often limited to "happy," "sad," and "mad." Frequently, these are children who can discuss part of a situation but not all of it, as in the case of a child who can relate that he or she is anxious but cannot elaborate on the etiology of the anxiety or any associated feelings.

Psychologically Unaware Children

There are some children who have little idea of how they are feeling, what they are thinking, and/or what they are doing, thus rendering them unable to self disclose. It could be that the psychological dynamics of such children are mainly unconscious or that they are conscious to some extent but not to the degree which enables verbalization.

Some children lack awareness about the relationships of thoughts, feelings, and behaviors. For example, they might not understand how poor hygiene would lead to interpersonal problems. Consequently, they do not discuss such issues because to them they are not problematic. Or, in the case of some children of religious minorities, for example, total abstinence from films and dance might not be seen by them as deterrent to social interaction but rather as a strong religious conviction. Such children probably would not disclose their behavior in therapy because it is not perceived as being related to a socialization problem which they might be experiencing.

Denying Children

Often children do not own the presenting problem about which others have expressed concern. If the child is not bothered by having low grades in school, but his or her parents and teachers are bothered, the child will frequently be reluctant to discuss the problem, since he or she does not perceive this as a problem.

High levels of denial are often presented by children in therapy. For example, if a child denies he or she is urinating in class and on the bus, as reported by teachers and parents, and denies he or she is urinating in the therapist's office when indeed he or she is, it is unlikely that the child will discuss this behavior in a direct way. Communication boardgames provide a vital technique for therapists working with such children, since these children usually will discuss pertinent psychodynamics at varying levels through game play.

Self-Disclosing Children

Children who are adept at self disclosure in traditional one-to-one or group therapy approaches often can benefit from a lessening of anxiety through the use of communication boardgames. Such games provide a child with some variety in therapy and an interlude of lowered anxiety after which they can return to direct self expression again.

Inhibited Children

For varying reasons, some children are quite inhibited in and/or outside of therapy. The children have great difficulty in expressing themselves directly. They are usually much more successful at revealing themselves through boardgames where there is more structure and a greater definition of expectations of behavior.

PROCESS OF PLAY

In using communication boardgames, the play therapist, depending on theoretical orientation, might choose the specific game to be played himself or herself, allow the child to make the choice, take turns choosing games, or arrive at a mutual choice. Of primary importance in structuring the play should be the therapeutic goals for the child. If a child could benefit from increased empathic understanding, for example, *Reunion* would be an effective game. If a child denies a problem, then perhaps the therapist would choose *Social Security* or the *Talking/Listening Game*. If the therapist is using games to establish support then perhaps he or she would choose the *Ungame*, since it is more general than the others and, consequently, less threatening. Often therapists might play two or three games in a session. Some children automatically choose games with a content and format which will be facilitative for them, and then some clients studiously avoid any game which might have somewhat threatening content. Consequently, the factors influencing choice of game(s) to play include theoretical orientation of the play therapist, therapeutic goals for the child, dynamics of the child, dynamics of the child's family, therapist's skill, and knowledge of the game, and intended purpose of the therapy session (i.e., rapport building, catharsis).

Some therapists determine the length of playing time for the noncompetitive games themselves, others allow the child to play until he or she decides to stop, and still others mutually decide with the child when to stop play.

Play therapists whose theoretical concentration is congruent with more structure in play strategy often "stack the deck" of the game cards before the child arrives, thus facilitating more goal oriented play. The blank cards in some of the communication boardgames provide opportunities for the child and/or the therapist to write individualized situations for the specific presenting problem of the child. The cards can serve, of course, as a point of departure for further discussion. This type of interchange is often therapeutic and does not affect the integrity of the game.

In general, the process of play in communication boardgames involves the client realization of thoughts, feelings, and behaviors, therapist modeling of self-disclosure during his or her turn, therapist feedback to the child, increased client insight, adoption of alternate modes of coping, and generalization to the child's environment outside the therapy session.

Play therapists can utilize information about hemisphere dominance of the child and/or learning modalities (i.e., neurolinguistic programming) in an integrative way in boardgame play. For example, when playing with a child who is primarily a visual learner, the therapist might choose to respond using visual verbs and create or draw pictures for the child of the intended communication. On the other hand, when working with an auditory child, the play therapist might use auditory verbs and tell metaphors to the child through the game play. One advantage of boardgames is their flexibility. Therapists can use the techniques of confrontation, self-disclosure, interpretation, reflection of feeling, and so forth in a myriad of ways throughout the game play therapy. Limit setting in boardgame play is similar to that of other play approaches.

CASE ILLUSTRATION

Eleven-year-old Michael was referred for therapy by his mother and teachers. The presenting problem was acting out behavior of an aggressive nature at school and at home. Frequent fights occurred at school in the classroom and the playground. Michael was described by teachers as alienating himself from others. His mother, a single parent as the result of her husband's death two years prior, reported aggressive play at home toward toys, furniture, other children, and himself. This aggression was both verbal and physical.

On talking directly with the child, the therapist discovered a certain awareness level by the child about the behavior and a small degree of ownership of the problem. The child was unable to discuss the behavior further and had little insight about what was motivating such behavior.

Recognizing that therapy was not being advanced by traditional, direct, verbal responses, the therapist suggested playing the *Ungame*. Michael agreed. Michael's responses to the following cards were all related to grieving for his deceased father: "What would you do if you had a 'Magic Wand'?"—"Make my father come alive again." "If you could make a long distance telephone call, who would you call?"—"My father." "What would you do if you found $1000 in a vacant lot?" "Give it to my father so he would not have had to die." "Describe the 'ideal' father."—"My dad. He was the best." Although Michael responded in this manner, he still had no insight. When the therapist took a turn, she began to link together for Michael the psychodynamics of grieving and how they were being manifested in Michael's behavior—unresolved anger towards his father and the death experience. At this point, the game had been of diagnostic value to the therapist and of insight value to the client.

In the following sessions, the therapist stacked the deck with cards related to the child's psychodynamics—that is, "How do you look when you get angry?" "How do you feel when you are alone?" "What would you like to invent to make life better?" "Give three words to describe how you feel right now." "What do you think it's like after you die?" "What makes you feel frustrated?" "What is something that makes you feel angry?" "When was the last time you cried?" "What is the worst thing parents can do to children?" "Share a time when your feelings were hurt." "If you were told you only have one week to live—how would you spend it?" "Describe a happy family." Simultaneous discussion and boardgame play is inherent in all these boardgames. Carke (1972) stated that this is preferable to alternative discussion and play. Consequently, therapy proceeded through discussion through the boardgame play.

While client insight was increasing, the therapist responded to the "do your own thing" spaces by indicating adaptive behaviors to grieving and modeling therapeutic self-disclosure. ("Do your own thing" spaces afford the child and the therapist an opportunity to make a comment or ask a question.) The therapist also utilized the blank game cards to offer insight and model self-disclosure and provide alternatives which were more adaptive.

In subsequent sessions, the therapist continued play with the *Ungame* and also switched to the game, *Imagine*, using the same insight- and action-oriented approach. Since these communication games are very compatible with one another, they provide the client and therapist an opportunity for some variety, while still focusing on the necessary psychodynamics.

Following several sessions of boardgame play, the client began to more openly discuss his feelings and behaviors relative to death and dying issues without the use of the boardgame. Family therapy approaches followed, and the case was successfully terminated.

Play therapists can, of course, create boardgames themselves after developing an understanding of the uses, forms, structures, and purposes of such games. Such games could be individualized for child clients with specific concerns. For example, a five-year-old client with a dog phobia played a boardgame specifically individualized for her by her therapist in which the child could pretend she was various dogs responding to the playing card content. Through such play the therapist was able to discuss the sources of fear and how the child conceptualized dogs' motivations. The therapist could then respond in a manner more realistic to actual dog behavior and provide the client with appropriate coping skills. The play therapist could create the boardgame with a structure consistent with his or her theoretical orientation also.

SUMMARY AND CONCLUSIONS

The utilization of communication boardgames with children in play therapy is a contemporary development. The foundation of boardgame theory has been laid through clinical experience and professional dialogue. Boardgames can be utilized differently by therapists of varying theoretical orientations and adapted to meet a variety of dynamics of children. Such games represent a somewhat untapped modality which can be systematically used as a therapeutic tool. The games offer versatility, flexibility, and effectiveness. In using communication boardgames, therapists face an existing challenge and the promise of considerable reward. Future research on this play therapy modality should yield even more information to further assist young children in their growth.

REFERENCES

Berg, B. (1982). *The changing family game*. Dayton, OH: University of Dayton Press.

Blechman, E. (1974). The family contract game. *The Family Coordinator*, 269–281.

Burks, H. (1978). *Imagine*. Huntington Beach, CA: Arden.

Burten, R. (1976). *Social security*. Anaheim, CA: The Ungame Company.

Carke, D. (1972). *Principles of child psychotherapy*. Springfield, IL: Thomas.

Creative Health Services. (1983). *The Self Esteem Game*. South Bend, IN:

Gardner, R.A. (1973). *The Talking, Feeling, Doing Game*. Cresskill, NJ: Creative Therapeutics.

Gardner, R.A. (1975a). Board of objects game. In *Psychotherapeutic approaches to the resistant child*. New York: Aronson.

Gardner, R.A. (1975b). Scrabble for juniors. In *Psychotherapeutic approaches to the resistant child*. New York: Aronson.

Kritzberg, N. (1975). *The structured therapeutic game method of child anlaytic psychotherapy*. Hicksville, NY: Exposition.

Nickerson, E., and O'Laughlin, K. (1983). The therapeutic use of games. In C. Schaefer and K. O'Conner (Eds.), *Handbook of play therapy*. New York: Wiley.

Oden. T. (1976). *The transactional analysis game*. New York: Harper & Row.

Shadle, C. and Graham, J. (1981). *The talking/listening game*. San Luis Obispo, CA: Dandy Lion Press.

Zakich, R. (1975). *The Ungame*, Anaheim, CA: The Ungame Company.

Zakich, R. and Monroe, S. (1979). *Reunion*. Placentia, CA: The Ungame Company.

Zitsman, S. (1984). *The rational emotive game*. Dayton, OH: Unpublished manuscript, Wright State University.

CHAPTER 2

The Talking, Feeling, and Doing Game

RICHARD A. GARDNER

Many psychotherapeutic techniques have been devised to help children. Many rely heavily on the elicitation of self-created fantasies, but therapists have long experienced frustration in getting children to take a psychoanalytic stance and attempting to gain insight into the psychoanalytic meaning of their fantasies. Conn (1939, 1941a, 1941b, 1948, 1954) and Solomon (1938, 1940, 1951, 1955) dealt with the problem of children's unreceptivity to psychoanalytic inquiry by responding at the allegorical level. They held that one could impart important therapeutic messages by discussing the child's fantasy at the symbolic level. They were certainly receptive to the notion of helping children gain insight into their fantasies, but believed that important therapeutic changes could be brought about by discussing the fantasy at the symbolic level, for example, "Why did the fox bite the wolf's tail?" "Was there a better way the fox could have dealt with its anger toward the wolf than biting the wolf's tail?"

This author has also directed his attention to the question of how to utilize therapeutically the self-created fantasies of children who will tell stories, but who are unreceptive or unwilling to analyze them. The mutual storytelling technique (Gardner, 1971) deals with this problem by having the therapist create responding stories, using the child's own characters and setting, but introducing healthier modes of adaptation and resolution than those exhibited in the child's story. For children who are somewhat unreceptive to telling stories, the author has found that a series of games utilizing standard boardgame play and token reinforcement (1975a,b) proved useful in facilitating the creation of stories and other fantasy material of therapeutic value. However, there were still some children who, in spite of these games, were unwilling and/or too resistant to tell self-created stories freely or to provide other therapeutically useful fantasy material. It was for such children that the author developed the *Talking, Feeling, and Doing Game* (1973).

DESCRIPTION OF THE GAME

The *Talking, Feeling, and Doing Game* is similar in format and appearance to many of the typical board games with which most children are familiar. The game begins with the child and the therapist each placing their playing pieces at the *start* position. They alternate turns, throwing the dice and moving their playing pieces along a curved path of squares which utimately ends at the *finish* position. If the playing piece lands on a white square, the player takes a talking card; on a yellow square, a feeling card; and on a red square, a doing card. If the playing piece lands on a square marked *spin*, the player spins the spinner, which directs the player to move forward or backward or to gain or lose chips. In addition, there are go forward and go backward squares. The spinner and the latter squares are of little psychological significance. They merely add to the child's fun and thereby enhance the likelihood of involvement. It is the questions and directions on the talking, feeling, or doing cards, of course, that are of primary importance and the child is given a reward chip for each response provided. The first person to reach the *finish* position gets five extra reward chips. The winner is the person who has the most chips after both players have reached *finish*, or after the game has been interrupted because the session is over. Active competition for the acquisition of chips is discouraged; rather, the therapist plays at a slow pace and tries to use each response as a point of departure for a therapeutic interchange. Obviously, the greater the breadth and depth of such discussion, the greater the likelihood it will be of therapeutic value.

The core of the game, of course, are the questions and directions on each of the cards. As is implied by their titles, the talking cards direct the child to make comments that are primarily in the cognitive and intellectual realm. The feeling cards focus on emotional issues. And the doing cards involve some kind of physical activity and/or play acting. There are 104 cards in each stack. The questions in each category range from threatening to very nonthreatening (so that practically any child will be able to respond) to the moderately anxiety provoking. If the child responds (and the most liberal criteria are used—especially for the very inhibited child), a token reward chip is given from the "bank."

None of the cards directs the child into areas that would be as anxiety provoking as relating self-created stories or free fantasy expression. The main purpose of the low-anxiety cards is to ensure the child's providing a response and gaining a chip. These enhance the likelihood that the child will remain involved. Some typical low-anxiety questions: "What's your favorite flavor ice cream?" "What is your address?" "What present would you like to get for your next birthday?" "What is your lucky number? Why?" and "How do you feel when you stand close to someone whose breath smells because he hasn't brushed his teeth?" It is the questions which provoke moderate anxiety that are the most important and these make up over 90 percent of all the cards. Some typical questions: "Suppose two people were talking about you and they didn't know you were listening. What do you think you would hear them saying?" "A boy has something on his mind that he's afraid to tell his father. What is it that he's scared to talk about?" "Everybody in the class was laughing at a girl. What had happened?" "All the girls in the class were invited to a birthday party except one. How did she feel? Why wasn't she invited?" "What things come into your mind when you can't fall asleep?" "If a fly followed you around for a day, and could then talk about you, what would it say?" "If the walls of your house could talk, what would they say about your family?"

The child's responses are usually revealing of those psychological issues that are most important at the time. The questions cover the broad range of human experiences, and issues related to the responses are likely to be of relevance to the etiology of the child's psychological disturbance. One does well to view symptoms as the most superficial manifestations of underlying unresolved problems. The problems that are being handled inappropriately via symptom formation are generally the same problems with which all of us deal. Accordingly, the topics raised by the cards are likely to relate to issues that are at the very foundation of the psychopathological process. Each response should serve as a point of departure for therapeutic interchanges. The therapist does well to get "as much mileage" as possible from each response. Merely providing the child with a reward chip and then going on with the game defeats the whole purpose of this therapeutic instrument. However, the therapist should use his or her discretion when deciding how much discussion is indicated for each patient. The more resistant and defended child will generally not be able to tolerate an in-depth discussion as well as the child with greater ego-strength.

The therapist plays similarly to the child and also responds to the questions, which should be left randomized. The therapist's knowledge of the child's problems, as well as the responses that have been given to previous cards, can provide guidelines for his or her own responses. The game requires considerable judiciousness on the therapist's part regarding responses to his or her cards. The therapist must always be aware that a response should be selected that is in the child's best interests. Many of the cards ask personal questions about the therapist's life. This brings up an important therapeutic question regarding self-revelation. It is the author's belief that therapists who strictly withhold information about themselves certainly enjoy the advantage of getting more free associations from the patient—associations uncontaminated by the reality of the therapist's life. However, a price is paid for this benefit. I believe that it reduces the humanity of the therapeutic relationship and fosters unrealistic ideas about what other human beings are like. Elsewhere (1975) this author elaborated in detail on the question of the therapist's revelation versus nonrevelation. In accordance with this position, I answer each question honestly, even when a response involves the revelation of personal material. However, such divulgences are not made indiscriminately. Some personal experience is selected that will not only be relevant to the child, but will not compromise my own privacy and/or that of my family. I often find it useful to relate an experience that occurred at the time in my life when I was at the age at which the child is at the present time. This generally enhances the child's interest in my response, because children usually enjoy hearing about the childhood experiences of their parents and other significant figures.

It is rare that I do not answer a question. However, I give children the opportunity not to answer if they do not wish to. In such cases, I will often inform such children that failure to answer will result in their not getting a reward chip and thereby lessening the likelihood of winning the game. This can serve to motivate some children at least to try to respond to the card. It is not immediately appreciated by many therapists that the main determinant as to who wins the game is much more than luck than anything else. If each player were to answer each card, then the determinant as to who wins would be the dice. If a player gets a large number of high throws, then he or she will reach *finish* earlier and thereby acquire fewer chips. On the other hand, if a player gets a large number of low throws, then more chips will be acquired in the course of going from *start* to *finish*. Because high and low throws tend to average out for each player, the number of wins and losses also averages out over time.

CASE ILLUSTRATIONS

In this section, I present some of the common responses I give to some of the cards. The reader does well to appreciate that these are only examples and not my invariable replies. Each response is tailored to the particular needs of the specific child and his or her problems. These responses, however, are some of the more common ones that I provide.

Talking Cards

The *talking cards*, as the name implies, deal with cognitive, intellectual issues. They encourage the child to talk about his or her opinion on a particular issue. I am a strong proponent of the position that thoughts generally precede feelings. One's cognitive interpretation of an event is going to be an extremely important determinant of how one will react emotionally. If one interprets a stimulus to be dangerous, then one is going to respond with a feeling of fight or flight. If, however, one's view is changed and one learns that the stimulus is in no way dangerous, then the fight–flight emotional responses are likely to be reduced and even disappear. Many of the benefits that patients derive from treatment result from their having learned how to better deal with the inevitable problems of life with which we are all confronted. The *talking cards* help teach these lessons in better living.

It is important for the reader to appreciate that the following responses described are to be used as points of departure for discussion with the patient. They are not simply stated and then the dice rolled for the game to continue. Furthermore, although the responses I give are intellectual, my attempt is to engender emotional responses in order to enrich the efficacy of the conversation and add more clout to the therapeutic communications.

"IF YOU BECOME MAYOR OF CITY, WHAT WOULD YOU DO TO CHANGE THINGS?"For a child who is insensitive to the feelings of others and may need some help in this regard, I might respond: "If I became mayor of my city, I would do everything in my power to bring about the passage of two laws. One would prohibit smoking in public places and the other would fine people large amounts of money for letting their dogs crap in the streets. Let me tell you my reasons for saying this. I, personally, find cigarette smoking disgusting. I'm saying this because smoking causes cancer of the lungs. I'd say this even if smoking *cured* cancer of the lungs. I'm just saying it because I find smoking nauseating. I think that if anyone is stupid enough to smoke, that person should be required to do it privately, in his or her own home. Many people who smoke don't care about other people's feelings. As far as they're concerned, other people can choke or even croak on their smoke. They don't think about the feelings of the people who are suffering because of their smoking. Unfortunately, a lot of people don't speak up and say how the smoke bothers them. But more and more people are doing this.

The other law, about there being big fines for people who let their dogs crap on the streets, would be for the same purposes. People who let their dogs do this don't think about how disgusted others feel when they step in the dog shit. It's really a disgusting thing to have to wipe dog shit off your shoes. It's too bad there are so many people in this world who don't think about other people's feelings. What do you think about people who smoke and people who let their dogs crap on the streets?"

The major thrust of my responses here is to help an insensitive child appreciate how one's act can affect others and that those who don't think about how they are affecting others are generally scorned. Included also in my response was a message about self-assertion regarding nonsmokers in their relationships with smokers.

"A BOY WASN'T PICKED TO BE ON A TEAM. WHAT HAD HAPPENED?" For the child who shows low motivation in school or in other activities, I might respond: "No one was surprised that he wasn't picked. He just didn't take things too seriously or practice. The others were working hard and practicing, and while they were working hard and practicing they were thinking about the time when the coach would be picking kids for the team. Having this idea in their heads made them work harder. But this kid just didn't think about it. He thought that he could do nothing, or almost nothing, and that he would somehow get picked for the team. Well, the day came for the tryouts and you can imagine how surprised he was when the coach told him that he could not be on the team. He was not only surprised, he was sad. He realized that he was living in a dream world. Do you think he learned a lesson from this experience?"

"SUPPOSE TWO PEOPLE YOU KNEW WERE TALKING ABOUT YOU AND THEY DIDN'T KNOW YOU WERE LISTENING. WHAT DO YOU THINK YOU WOULD HEAR THEM SAYING?" Identification with the therapist and modeling oneself after him or her is an important part of the therapeutic process. This is very similar to the educational model in which the child learns, in part, because of identification with the teacher and the desire to gain the same gratifications that the teacher enjoys from learning. The therapist not only serves as a model for learning, but should be serving as a model for other desirable attributes as well, for example, healthy self-assertion, sensitivity to the feelings of others, feelings of benevolence toward those who are in pain, handling oneself with dignity, and honesty. This card can enable the therapist to provide examples of such traits. However, the therapist should select traits that are particularly relevant to the child's problems. Furthermore, the therapist must avoid presenting these with a flaunting or holier-than-thou attitude.

For a child with a lying problem, I might say: "I might hear the people saying that I'm the kind of a person who is direct and honest. Although people might disagree, at times, with what I've said, they would agree that I am direct about what my opinions are and don't pussyfoot about them. They know that when they ask me a question, they'll get an honest and direct answer with no hedging, beating-around-the-bush, or saying things that aren't true. I am not saying that they would say that I never lied in my whole life and that I never will, only that they are pretty confident that I'll be honest with them. You see, I believe that there is truth and wisdom to the old saying that 'honesty is the best policy.' If you tell a lie, you have to go around worrying that people will find out that you've lied. Also, lots of people feel bad about themselves when they lie, they feel guilty about it. And when people find out that you've lied, then they don't trust you even when you've told the truth. So these are the main reasons why I find it better to tell the truth, rather than to lie. What's your opinion on this subject?"

"WHAT IS THE WORST PROBLEM A PERSON CAN HAVE? WHY?" For children who are unreceptive to any kind of self-observation or self-inquiry, who are too inhibited to look into their own contributions to the problems for which they are being treated, I might respond: "There are many terrible problems people can have. Certainly having physical illness, especially if severe, is a terrible problem. However, if one is physically okay, there are still other kinds of problems that people can have. As a psychiatrist, I am interested in psychological problems. There are many kinds of psychological problems, some of which are very bad. I think that one of the worst kind of psychological problem is the one in which a person makes believe that there are no problems when there really are. That's a pretty lousy problem to have." I might at that point ask the patient why he or she thinks that making believe there are no problems when there really are is one of the worst problems a person can have. In the ensuing discussion, my main purpose would be to help the child appreciate that denial mechanisms prevent one from dealing with a problem, so it is likely to get worse. This could then serve as a good lead into the child's own problems which are being denied.

"DO YOU BELIEVE THAT PRAYING FOR SOMETHING WILL MAKE IT HAPPEN?" Most children, who are in therapy, are likely to engage in wishful thinking at times and believe that their problems will somehow go away by themselves. Unfortunately, it is probable that the vast majority of adults think along these lines as well. For such a child, I might say: "There are many people who believe that praying for something will make it happen. I, personally, do not believe that. I believe that if you want something to happen you have to *try* to make it happen. This doesn't mean that it will always happen if you try; it only means there's a better chance the thing will happen if you try to make it happen. I know, however, that there are many religious people who believe that praying for something will make that thing happen. But even those religious people generally say that 'God helps those who help themselves.' What is your opinion on this subject?" Of course, when providing this response, the therapist does well to take into consideration what the patient's family's religious beliefs are. It has been the author's experience that the vast majority of religious patients still subscribe to the 'God helps those who help themselves' principle. Accordingly, it is not likely that a response along the lines provided by the author is going to bring about significant philosophical differences between the therapist and the patient's family.

In the ensuing discussion, I might present the following question to the child: "Suppose two boys in the same class had a test the next day. One

studied for the test and the other watched television, but during the com-
mercials prayed to God that he would pass the test the next day. Which
kid do you think would get a better grade on the test? Do you think God
would help the boy who watched television get a good mark on the test?
Do you think God would put the answers in his head so that he would
pass the test anyway?"

"WHAT'S THE BEST STORY YOU EVER HEARD OR READ? WHY?" For the
child with poor academic motivation (a very common presenting problem), I might respond: "One of the best stories I ever read in my whole
life was one I read when I was a teenager. It was about the life of Thomas
Alva Edison. Do you know who Thomas Edison was?" At that point, I
would discuss Edison with the child and make sure that the child knows
what Edison's major contributions were. I would then continue: "As I'm
sure you will agree, Thomas Edison was one of the world's greatest in-
ventors. All of our lives were made better by Thomas Edison. I'm sure
you'll agree that the world is a much better place because of the electric
light. It must have been tough in the old days before they had electric
lights. They used to have to burn candles and use lanterns, and they used
to have a lot of fires. Also, they never got as much light from those things
as you can with an electric bulb. It also makes life happier to have phono-
graph records and now, of course, we have tapes, but they still work on a
similar principle and we have Thomas Edison to thank for that. The
whole world admires Thomas Edison and the whole world is grateful to
him. He can serve as an inspiration for the rest of us. Do you know what
the word *inspiration* means?" Here I will discuss with the child the meaning of the word inspiration in the hope that he or she will come to appreciate the gratifications that a person such as Edison can derive and the enhanced feeling of self-worth that such an individual enjoys. Most people
who have performed great deeds have done so, in part, because of some
model whom they are following. My hope here is to engender in the child
some of this desire.

"SOMEONE PASSES YOU A NOTE. WHAT DOES IT SAY?" For the child
who is unpopular in school, I might respond: "Dear Bill, we're forming a
secret club. We're going to have our first meeting behind the back door of
the school, right after school at 3 o'clock today. Then we're going to elect
a president, vice president, and secretary. We're only inviting a few peo-

ple, those whom we like best in the class. If anyone asks you about the club just tell them that it's a secret and if Tom or Bob asks about the club don't tell them anything at all. We don't want those guys in the club." I would then ask the child why he or she thinks that Tom and Bob weren't invited into the club? This may bring about a discussion of the child's own personality qualities that have contributed to his or her alienation. My attempt here also is to engender a certain amount of jealousy of those who are invited into the club. This jealousy may also motivate the child to look into his or her own qualities that have brought about the alienation.

"YOU'VE JUST SEEN YOUR FRIEND STEAL FROM A STORE. WHAT SHOULD YOU DO?" For a child who has a problem putting himself or herself in other people's position, I might say: "I would go over to my friend and tell her that she should return what she's stolen. I'd tell her that she should think about how badly the storekeeper must feel that his stuff was stolen. I'd ask her how she would feel if someone stole things from her. I'd try to help my friend put herself in the storekeeper's position. If I was able to do that, perhaps then she would feel sorry for the storekeeper and then return what she had stolen. What do you think of that?"

For the child who does steal, I might respond: "I would say to my friend, 'You know, some people have seen you do that. I don't think you're going to get away with it. I think you're going to get caught. I've seen you do it and others saw it also. I think you may get reported. Even if you don't you're going to have to walk around scared that someone is going to tell and then people will find out. Do you think it's really worth it to walk around scared all the time worrying about being found out. Also, if you are found out people are not only going to be angry at you, but you may get punished. If I were the man who owned the store and found out what you've done, I'd at least call your parents and I might even call the police.' I would hope that after my friend heard that she'd return the thing that she stole and then would realize that it really doesn't pay to steal things. Do you know what the old saying, 'Crime doesn't pay' means?"

"SAY ANYTHING YOU WANT. YOU DO NOT GET A CHIP IF YOU SAY NOTHING AT ALL." This card, of course, provides the therapist with significant freedom regarding what to say. There are indeed a greater universe of possible responses to this card than to many of the others. The

Talking, Feeling, and Doing Game is very much a verbal-projective game and this card can be compared to the blank card on the Thematic Apperception Test (Murray, 1936). For the child who is afraid to enter new and strange situations, to do new and different things, I might respond: "Do you know that many people don't realize that both the brave person and the coward are basically very similar. Both the brave person and the coward are usually afraid at first of the new and even scary thing. However, the difference between the brave person and the coward is that the brave person *does* the scary thing, whereas the coward runs away from it. The brave person also has a lump in his or her throat at the scary time, but he or she doesn't let it get the best of him or her. The brave person swallows the lump in his or her throat, grits his or her teeth, clenches his or her fist, and does the frightening thing because he or she knows it's important to do so. The brave person knows that if he or she doesn't, bad things will happen. The coward just runs away and then doesn't accomplish very much, if anything at all. How do you see yourself? Are you more like the brave person or are you more like the coward?"

For the child who cheats on tests in school, I might respond: "A boy used to cheat on a lot of tests. He felt good when he got a high mark and was relieved when he didn't get a low mark. He used to watch a lot of television at night and thought that everything would be all right if he continued to cheat on tests. However, he found himself not feeling so good when he would get a high mark. He knew in his own heart that he really didn't deserve it. And then the other kids used to watch him cheating and they would call him 'cheater.' This also made him feel bad about himself. Do you think that these things then made him change his mind about cheating?"

Feeling Cards

The *feeling cards* deal primarily with emotional and affective topics. They encourage children to express their feelings and this is particularly useful for children who are inhibited in this area. I consider it important for therapists to appreciate the therapeutic view that the mere expression of feelings is in itself salutary is somewhat naive. I believe the expression of feelings to be a good first step toward the alleviation of difficulties. The expression of feelings serves, among other things, to enhance one's efficiency in reaching certain goals. We fight harder when we are angry, we run faster when we are frightened, we mourn more effectively when we cry, we love more ardently when we are sexually excited, we eat more when we are hungry, and we sleep more when we are tired. These principles apply when feelings are expressed at low and moderate levels. However, when feelings are generated at a high level they may work differently. Anger, for example, when expressed in severe states of rage, may perpetuate itself even after the initial goal is reached. A murderer who stabs his or her victim to death may continue stabbing the dead body. Clearly, nothing new or further is being accomplished by such repeated stabbings. The same phenomenon relates to excessive drinking, eating, sleeping, and sexual indulgence. The satisfaction becomes an end in itself and goes beyond its initial purposes.

"EVERYBODY IN THE CLASS WAS LAUGHING AT A BOY. WHAT HAD HAPPENED?" For the child who is inattentive in the classroom, I might respond: "He wasn't listening to the teacher while she was teaching. Then, while he wasn't paying attention, the teacher called on him and asked him a question about what she had said. Instead of being honest and saying that he wasn't listening and that he didn't know the answer, he tried to guess. Well, as I'm sure you might imagine, he guessed wrong. In fact, he gave a very silly and stupid answer. It was such a foolish answer that everybody in the class started to laugh at him. He felt embarrassed. He was humiliated. He was sorry that he hadn't listened to what the teacher was saying. Do you think that he tried to pay more attention after that?"

Children with neurologically based learning disabilities often become class clowns. They recognize that they cannot gain the affection and esteem of their peers via the usual methods such as high academic standing, prowess in sports, talent at music or dance, or any other special skill that might warrant the admiration of their peers. One way of attempting to gain such a response is via clowning in the classroom. Unfortunately, they don't appreciate that they are much more likely to be laughed *at* than laughed *with*. To such a child, I might respond: "They were laughing at him because he was the class clown. He was always horsing around in the classroom and, even though the teachers would often get angry at him, he still continued to clown around. Some of the children would laugh, but others didn't think he was very funny. He thought this was making him popular, at least with some of the children. He didn't realize that they really didn't like him very much when he was clowning around that way.

They might have thought it was a good chance to have a little fun in the classroom, but they really didn't respect him. In spite of the fact that they laughed at him, they still didn't invite him to birthday parties or to join their after-school secret clubs. Do you think the boy finally realized what was happening?" Many children with neurologically based learning disabilities have difficulty differentiating between people who are laughing *at* them and people who are laughing *with* them. This is a manifestation of their cognitive impairment and it behooves the therapist to patiently attempt to help such children understand this kind of subtle differentiation.

"A BOY'S FRIEND LEAVES HIM TO PLAY WITH SOMEONE ELSE. HOW DOES THE BOY FEEL? WHY DID THE FRIEND LEAVE?" Some children have great difficulty sharing. They have difficulty putting themselves in the position of their peers and fail to recognize that the child with whom they refuse to share is likely to be alienated. Some of these children have neurologically based learning disabilities that interfere, on a cognitive level, with their capacity to project themselves into other people's position. Other children may have reached the developmental level where this is possible, but have psychological problems in the realm of egocentricism and narcissism that interfere with healthy functioning in this realm. For children in both of these categories, I might respond: "Bob invited Frank to play with him at his house. But Bob was selfish. He wouldn't share. Frank was his guest. He should have known that it's important to be courteous to a guest. He should have known that it's important to be nice to a guest. Anyway, Frank wanted to share Bob's toys with him and Bob refused. Also, Bob always wanted to decide which game they would play. Finally Frank said that if Bob wouldn't play nicely with him and share, he would leave and go play with someone else. Bob's mother overheard the boys talking and took Bob aside into another room. She didn't want to embarrass Bob in front of his friend Frank. She told Bob, while they were alone, that he wasn't playing nicely with his friend and that he wasn't thinking about how his friend felt. She told him that Frank would go home soon if he didn't start to share with him. She told him that Frank had another good friend, George, whom he could go play with it he wanted. What do you think happened? Do you think that Bob listened to his mother? Do you think that his mother was right or wrong in this case?"

Some children have a general "sourpuss" attitude. They tend to be unfriendly and expect others to make overtures to them. They don't reach out, and tend to display the hostilities that have originated in their homes onto their peers. For such children, I might respond: "Carol was having a lot of trouble at home. Her parents used to fight a lot and this made her very sad and irritable. Also, her mother and father didn't treat her well at times. But, instead of talking to her mother and father about the things that were bothering her, she just held all her thoughts and feelings inside herself. And she became a sourpuss kind of kid. She wasn't very friendly to other people and would be irritable with them. Accordingly, one day her friend Alice stopped playing with her and said, 'You're no fun to be with. You're not very friendly. I'm going to play with Linda.' And so Alice went away and played with Linda. How do you think Carol felt when this happened? What do you think she should have done?"

"ON THE LAST DAY OF SCHOOL A GIRL LEARNED THAT SHE WOULD HAVE TO REPEAT THE SAME GRADE. WHAT HAD HAPPENED?" There are many children whose presenting problem relates to their failure to appreciate the consequences of their academic negligence. They float along as if there will be no consequences to their failure to fulfill their school commitments. With such children, I might respond: "Betty had goofed off all year. Whenever her teacher would warn her that she might not get promoted into the third grade, she ignored her. And when her mother and father got upset and told her that her report cards were terrible and that she had better start studying harder, she again made believe that there was no problem. She didn't think they were serious. She couldn't imagine herself not being promoted to the third grade. Anyway, on the last day of school, you can imagine how amazed she was when her report card said that she would have to repeat the same grade. Although she was embarrassed to cry in front of the other boys and girls, she couldn't hold back her tears. And this made her feel even worse because she was crying in front of the other children. Some of the children were mean and even made fun of her. Others understood how badly she felt and told her how sorry they were that she was not being promoted. What do you think happened to her the next year? Do you think that she still continued to goof off in school?"

The author fully recognizes that his responses to many of the questions in the *Talking, Feeling, and Doing Game* are relatively "superficial" from the psychoanalytic point of view. The author, a psychoanalyst himself, is fully aware of this fact. However, he believes that psychoanalysts in general are not fully appreciative of the role of conscious control in the treatment of psychogenic disorders. In addition, he is not against an analytic-type inquiry and will on occasion use the child's responses as a point of departure for such investigation. However, he appreciates, as well, that most children under the age of 10 or 11, who are of average intelligence, are not cognitively capable of meaningful psychoanalytic inquiry. They have not reached Piaget's level of formal operations, the level at which the child is able to cognitively separate an entity from the symbol which denotes it and recognize the relationship between the two. Meaningful psychoanalytic inquiry requires such appreciation. Furthermore, even with analytic patients, much of the treatment involves learning better how to deal with the everyday problems of life and utilizing new techniques that may not have been part of the patient's original repertoire. And the learning of such techniques does not necessarily have to take place in the context of an analytic inquiry; it can be derived in part from more direct advice and recommendations by the therapist. This need not produce infantilization and exaggerated dependency on the patient's part.

"A BOY WAS SCARED TO MAKE A TELEPHONE CALL. WHAT WAS HE AFRAID OF?" Whereas the *Mutual Storytelling Technique* and other derivative games that involve a child's fantasies are useful to the age of 11 or 12, the *Talking, Feeling, and Doing Game* can be played meaningfully with the average child up to age 15 or 16. Children begin to recognize in the prepubertal years that their fantasies are quite revealing of their innermost thoughts and feelings and may then become defensive about such revelations. The *Talking, Feeling, and Doing Game*, however, because it does not generally delve so deeply, is less threatening and can be easily utilized through the mid-teens. For the teenager who exhibits the usual anxiety about calling up a girlfriend, I might respond: "He was thinking of calling up this girl in his class whom he liked. He wanted to ask her to go out with him. But he was scared. He was afraid that she would turn him down. He even went to the telephone and dialed her number and then hung up before it rang. Later on, he let the telephone ring but then hung up before anyone had a chance to answer. On another day, he called again and was even glad when no one answered, even though he *really* wanted to go out with the girl. What was worse, was that he thought that he was somehow very strange, different, or weak for having such feelings. He didn't realize that it was normal to have such fears. When he learned that it was normal, he felt better about being afraid. However, he was still afraid. He learned also that it's important to push through one's fears and do the scary thing anyway. He remembered the old saying, 'Nothing ventured, nothing gained.' And so he called her again. What do you think happened?" The child's response will generally be in one or two categories: "The girl is receptive or the girl is not." If receptive, I emphasize the joy of the success and how willing one should be to tolerate fears in the service of enjoying certain gratifications. If the answer is in the negative, I emphasize the fact that there are other girls out there whom the boy could call and reassure the child in the course of the conversation that there is likely to be someone out there who will be receptive.

"WHAT IS THE WORST THING YOU CAN SAY TO ANYONE?" For the child who is inhibited in the expression of anger and self-assertion, I might respond: "I think one of the worst things you can say to anyone is: 'I wish you were dead.' Of course, a wish cannot make a thing happen. However, most people would say that this is a pretty nasty thing to say to someone. I think it's important to know that thoughts like this come into most people's minds, even toward people they love most in the world— like mothers and fathers. It's normal to have such thoughts once in a while, even toward someone you love very much. This is especially true when that person does something that gets you very angry. Some kids think that it's a terrible thing to have such a thought. I have a different opinion. I think, that it's important not to say *everything* that comes into your mind when you're angry at somebody. That can cause a lot of trouble. Accordingly, when people have thoughts like that when they are angry, they do better to use words that are more polite than the ones that come into their minds. They should say things like, 'That's making me very angry,' or 'What you're doing is very mean and I don't like it one bit!' Then, if they talk calmly about the thing that's bothering them, it's more likely that they will solve the problem. What do you think about what I've said?"

"WHAT'S THE HAPPIEST THING THAT EVER HAPPENED TO YOU?" For the child who had little academic curiosity or motivation in the classroom and who gets little joy from learning, I might respond: "One of the happiest things that ever happened to me was the day I graduated from medical school. I was about 25-years-old at the time and it was the end of many years of hard work in school. I really felt very good about myself. I was very proud of myself and my parents and relatives were very proud of me also. I really felt *great* that day. Although that happened many years ago, I still remember the day clearly. Some of the work in medical school was very interesting, but some of it I didn't like too much. I knew I wanted to be a psychiatrist and so wasn't interested too much when they taught about how to help people with broken bones or rashes. However, I knew it was important to learn those things also if I wanted to be a doctor. And I also found that they weren't so boring as I had first thought. Anyway, all the hard work was certainly worth it and I have not been sorry to this day that I had to work so hard in medical school. What do you think about what I've said?"

We speak often of the importance of the therapist-patient relationship in therapy. However, the factors that contribute to the development of a good relationship in this area have not been well delineated. This question can be used to help foster a good patient-therapist relationship with a response such as: "I've had many happy days in my life. Three of the happiest were the three days on which each of my children were born. Of course, that happened many years ago, but I still remember the days clearly. I was so happy on each of those days that I cried. They were tears of joy. I still have those warm feelings when I see little babies. It's hard for me not to touch them and sometimes I'll even ask the mother to let me hold the baby so I can cuddle and kiss the child. Although my children, like all children, may give me trouble at times, they also give me great pleasures. And the pleasures are certainly greater than the pains." My hope here is that the child's relationship with me might improve (admittedly in a small way) by the recognition that children produce warm responses in me. The response conveys the notion that I have the capacity for such pleasure with children in general and this response is not simply confined to my own children.

"A BOY HAS SOMETHING ON HIS MIND THAT HE'S AFRAID TO TELL HIS FATHER. WHAT IS IT THAT HE'S SCARED TO TALK ABOUT?" For the child whose parents are divorced, who finds himself in the middle of loyalty conflict, I might provide this response: "He was scared to tell his father that he didn't agree with him. He didn't think that all of the terrible things that his father was telling him about his mother were true. However, be-

cause he was scared that his father would be angry at him if he told him
that he didn't agree with him, he didn't say anything at first. He was
scared that if he told his father how he really felt that he might even see
less of his father. After all, his father had left the house when he separated from his mother and that made him feel very lonely. Anyway, his
father then began to ask him a lot of other questions just to see if he
agreed or disagreed with his father. Then the boy made a *big* mistake. He
told his father that he agreed with him and then he started to make up bad
things about his mother that really weren't true. Because his father was so
angry at his mother, his father believed every one of these lies. And the
father then went and told the mother what the boy had said about her and
this, of course, made the mother get very upset at him because she knew
that the boy was lying. Then he told his mother that he really hadn't said
those things to his father and this made the situation even worse. What do
you think about what this boy did?" In the ensuing conversation, I would
try to get across the point that whatever discomforts the boy might suffer
as a result of his being honest with his father—even if he were to say that
he didn't want to get involved and criticize one parent to the other—he
would be much better off than handling the situation by lying and telling
each parent what he thought that parent wanted to hear from him at that
time.

"WHAT IS THE THING ABOUT YOURSELF THAT YOU DISLIKE THE MOST?
WHY?" Many children with feelings of low self-worth are intolerant of
any deficiencies within themselves. On becoming aware of even the
smallest deficiencies, they may denigrate themselves and consider themselves generally unworthy. This reaction, in part, stems from inordinately
high standards about what a person should really be like. Sometimes, significant figures in their environment portray themselves as being perfect,
or almost perfect, and the child, of course, can never completely measure
up to such individuals. In other situations, significant figures may place
inordinate demands on the child for perfection in a wide variety of areas.
Not being able to live up to these standards the child starts to loathe himself or herself. For such a child, I might respond: "I, like everyone else in
the world, am a mixture of good and bad things. There are many things
I'm very good at but there are also many things I am very poor at. I don't
think there's one big thing that I dislike the most in myself, but of all the
things about myself that I can think of that I dislike I would say that the

one that bothers me the most is that sometimes I work too hard and take things too seriously. Of course, it's important to work hard in life if you want to accomplish anything, but it's also important to enjoy oneself and to relax and have fun. Both are important. Did you ever hear the saying 'All work and no play makes Jack a dull boy?' What do you think it means?" I might then use this question as a point of departure for helping the child appreciate that balance in life is important, not only in terms of work and play but also in terms of accepting the fact that each person has both assets and liabilities. One of the elements that plays a role in successful treatment is identification with the therapist. Here, I am attempting to serve as a model of someone who can accept both assets and liabilities within himself and can comfortably reveal both under proper circumstances. My hope here is that the patient will then become more comfortable admitting his or her own deficiencies, both to himself or herself and to others. This can be useful in lessening feelings of self-loathing.

"WHEN WAS THE LAST TIME YOU CRIED? WHAT DID YOU CRY ABOUT?" This can be a particularly useful question for children with emotional inhibition problems. It is reasonable to say that individuals do not generally suffer with isolated inhibitions in the expression of single emotions; rather, such inhibitions tend to spread so that a person with such difficulties is generally inhibited in expressing a variety of emotions. Accordingly, any easing up that the therapist is able to accomplish in one area of emotional expression is likely to spread into others as well. For such a child I might respond: "I'm the kind of a person who tends to choke up in certain movies. I remember seeing a movie recently in which a person whom I admired very much died near the end of the movie. It was very sad. Lots of the people in the movie theatre were crying. Even though I knew that it wasn't real and that it was only a movie, I still felt bad—not only for the person who died but for the friends and relatives who were crying at the funeral. Some people think that boys and men shouldn't cry. What do you think about that?" If the child's response in any way suggests that he or she is an adherent to the notion that it is unmanly for a boy or man to cry, I try to dispel that idea. Then I'd likely enter into a discussion of the purpose of crying. Here, I first try to elicit from the patient his or her answers to that question. By the end of the discussion, I make sure that we have at least dealt with the cathartic value of crying as well as its value in communicating to another person one's frustrations, disappointments, resentments, and so on.

"A GIRL HEARD HER MOTHER AND FATHER FIGHTING. WHAT WERE THEY FIGHTING ABOUT? HOW DID SHE FEEL WHILE SHE WAS LISTENING TO THEM?" For the girl who has been doing poorly academically and who has been living in a dream world regarding the consequences of her poor school performance, I might provide this answer: "Well, the mother and father had spoken to the principal that day. She told them that she was thinking about not promoting their daughter into the fifth grade because she had done very poorly that year. She told them both that she and the teacher had warned the girl that if she didn't shape up, she would get left back. She told them that that didn't seem to help and that their daughter ignored these warnings. Now she was wondering whether it might be a good lesson for their daughter to repeat the fourth grade. She asked the mother and father for their opinions and told them that, although the final decision was going to be the school's, she was going to take into consideration their thoughts and feelings on the subject. The reason why they were fighting was that the father felt sorry for his daughter and said that he wanted her to go on to the fifth grade because she would feel so bad seeing all her friends being promoted when she had to remain in the fourth grade and be with all the younger kids. The mother, however, said that she certainly felt sorry for her daughter, but she thought it would be a bad idea to promote her if she wasn't ready to do fifth grade work and that her daughter would probably be embarrassed going there every day not being able to keep up with the others.

First, the girl was amazed when she learned that they were thinking of leaving her back. She really hadn't taken all the warnings seriously and really didn't think that they would do such a thing. Now she was shocked to learn that the people at school really meant business and that there was a strong possibility that she would have to repeat the fourth grade. She was really sorry then that she had goofed off all year and then began to cry. The mother and father, who didn't know she was listening, heard her crying and then came out of the room. She begged them to tell the principal to promote her and she promised that she would start trying very hard to do good work. What do you think happened?" In the ensuing discussion, I generally cover three options: (1) the child has to repeat the fourth grade, (2) the child is promoted into the fifth grade, and (3) the child is promoted on probation with the understanding that she will attend summer school and her work will be reviewed after two months in the fifth grade to see whether or not she should return to the fourth.

"A BOY WAS LAUGHING. WHAT WAS HE LAUGHING ABOUT?" For a child with little academic curiosity and motivation, I might provide this response: "This boy was not only laughing, but he was cheering. He was just jumping up and down with joy. He had just gotten his eighth grade report card and learned that he had gotten into three honors classes in the ninth grade. He was very happy. He had worked very hard in order to make the honors classes and had hoped that he might make one or two of them. But he didn't think that he would get into all three. He was very proud of himself and couldn't wait to get home and tell his parents. His teacher had written a note on the report card that said 'Robert, I am very proud of you. Good luck in high school.' He was also very happy because he knew that, when he would apply to college, having been in three honors classes would look very good on his record and this would help him get into the college of his choice. And so he ran home from school laughing and singing all the way. It was really a happy day for him. What do you think about what I said about that boy?"

At this point, the reader may be wondering why so many of my responses relate to academic performance in school. Although I must admit a possible bias on my part regarding my commitment to academics, I believe that the high frequency of responses related to academic performance is related to the fact that the overwhelming majority of children who are referred to me have problems in the area of academic achievement. In fact, I would say that the most common reason why a child is referred to me is because he or she is not performing up to expectations in the academic and/or behavioral realm in the classroom.

"TELL ABOUT AN ACT OF KINDNESS." For the egocentric child, the child who has trouble putting himself or herself in another person's position, I might respond: "A good example of an act of kindness would be visiting someone who is sick in the hospital and giving up a fun thing that you'd prefer to do. Let's say that a boy in a class was in an automobile accident, injured his leg, and had to be in the hospital for six weeks. Even though his mother and father visited him often, he was still very lonely. His really good friends were those who were willing to give up fun things like playing baseball, or watching their favorite television programs, or just hanging around and relaxing, and instead went to visit him in the hospital. He was very grateful when they came to see him. And they felt good about themselves for their sacrifices. Visiting the friend was an act of kindness. Do you know what the word sacrifice means?" In the ensuing discussion, I would try to help the egocentric child appreciate the feelings of loneliness suffered by the hospitalized child. I would also try to engender in the child the feelings of self-satisfaction and enhanced self-worth that comes from benevolent acts.

"WHAT DO YOU THINK ABOUT A GIRL WHO SOMETIMES PLAYS WITH OR RUBS HER VAGINA WHEN SHE'S ALONE?" As the reader can certainly appreciate, the kinds of questions found in the *Talking, Feeling, and Doing Game* are not the traditional *Monopoly*-type questions. Many younger children, even those who may not even have any incipient sexual inhibition problems, may not be familiar with the concept of masturbation. Others may be but are likely to have taken on certain prevalent social attitudes regarding its being a shameful or harmful practice. For these children, I might respond: "I think that that girl is perfectly normal if she does it in private. Most teenage girls do that and many girls do it when they're younger as well. There is nothing wrong with it. It is generally considered very poor manners, however, to do that in public. Most people consider that to be a private thing. What is your personal opinion on this subject?" My aim here, of course, is to lessen any inhibitions a child may have regarding masturbation and to plant the seeds for a more balanced attitude toward the practice in the future if the child has no experience or knowledge of the practice.

"WAS THERE EVER A PERSON WHOM YOU WISHED TO BE DEAD? IF SO, WHO WAS THAT PERSON? WHY DID YOU WISH THAT PERSON TO BE DEAD?" This question can be particularly useful for children with antisocial behavior disorders who have little sensitivity to the pains they inflict on others. For such a child, I might respond: "During my childhood and early teens there lived a man in Germany named Adolph Hitler. He was a madman. He was insane. He was the leader of Germany during World War II and was personally responsible for the deaths of millions of people. He was one of the greatest criminals in the history of the world. He used to murder people whose opinions, skin color, or religion differed from his. He not only had them shot but he gassed them to death and burned their bodies in ovens. Millions of people died this way. When I was a boy, I used to wish that he would die. I wished that someone would kill him. I hoped then that maybe all this crazy murdering would stop. To this day, I and many other people in the world feel sorry for the millions of people he killed and all the millions of friends and relatives that also suffered because of his murders. Even though the war ended in 1945, there are still millions of people who are suffering because of the terrible things Adolph Hitler did. These are the people who were put in his prisons and concentration camps and escaped, or were fortunate enough not to have been killed. And these are also the people who are the friends, relatives, children, and grandchildren of those who died there. He was a very cruel man. I really hated him, and I often wished he would die or be killed. Finally, in 1945, he committed suicide. He knew he would soon be caught and executed for his terrible crimes." My hope here, by elaborating on Hitler's atrocities, is to engender in the antisocial child a feeling for the pain that criminal behavior causes others. It is important for the reader to appreciate that when responding to *feeling cards* the therapist does well to try to dramatize as much as possible his or her responses in order to bring about a kind of resonating emotional response in the patient. To engender these feelings in the child who is out of touch with them or who has not experienced them to a significant degree is one of the goals of treatment.

"WHAT'S THE WORST FEELING A PERSON CAN HAVE?" Most children in treatment are not moving along life's path. They have been diverted into pathological roads and are not gaining the gratifications of life that they might otherwise be enjoying. Children with academic problems are not learning and so are not likely to derive the benefits they would otherwise enjoy from an adequate educational experience. Children with behavioral problems are compromising significantly their capacity to form meaningful and satisfactory human relationships and this too is a significant deprivation in their lives. And there are a wide variety of other problems which individuals become obsessive over and dwell on, often with conscious control, and deprive themselves thereby of the healthier gratifications that life has to offer. For such children, I might respond: "I believe one of the worst feelings a person can have is to know that one is going to die very soon. All of us must someday die and most people hope that they will live a long and full life. If, however, one is going to die soon and if, in addition, one has wasted a lot of one's life, then the feeling that one is going to die soon is made even worse. It's sad enough to know that you have to die. But it's even sadder to know that you wasted a lot of your life and it's now to be over and you're not going to have another chance. How do you feel about *your* life yourself? Do you think that you're wasting your life? Do you think that if you continue living your life as you are that you'll be sorry some day that you didn't do things better for yourself?" The younger the child, the less the likelihood that he or she will be able to project himself or herself into the future and think about the questions I have asked. However, there are children who are capable of doing so and can do so meaningfully if the therapist is able to facilitate an introspective and somewhat philosophical conversation. My hope here is that the painful feelings engendered by the prospect that one is wasting one's life will serve to motivate the child to reduce the wasteful psychopathological behaviors and preoccupations.

"WHAT DO YOU THINK IS THE MOST BEAUTIFUL THING IN THE WHOLE WORLD? WHY?" Healthy pleasure is well viewed to be a general antidote for just about all forms of psychogenic psychopathology. When one is enjoying oneself in a healthy way, one is at that time not suffering the psychological pain attendant to psychiatric disorder. In addition, the pleasurable feelings are esteem enhancing. Because feelings of low self-worth are often involved in bringing about psychopathological reactions, any experience that can enhance self-worth can be salutary. And aesthetic pleasures are in this category. Accordingly, anything a therapist can do to enhance a child's appreciation of beauty is likely to be therapeutic. In the service of this goal, I might respond: "Watching a beautiful sunset, whether it be from the top of a mountain or at the seashore is to me one of the most beautiful things in the world. It makes me feel relaxed and happy to be alive. Sometimes I will read poetry while watching such a scene. And the poems also make me think of beautiful things that help me appreciate how beautiful the world can be if one is willing to stop and enjoy them. Sometimes I will bring along a tape recorder and play a tape of some calm, beautiful music while watching such a scene. This is indeed one of the great pleasures of life." Again, children are generally less self-conscious about these pleasures and probably less cognitively aware of them. Certainly, they more often enjoy things without conscious recognition and this may be an advantage they have over adults.

Doing Cards

The *doing cards*, as their name implies, deal with actions. As is true of the *talking cards* and *feeling cards* there are a few cards in each stack that are of little, if any, psychological significance. These can be answered by just about any child ("What's your favorite flavor ice cream?" and "With your finger make a circle in the air?") and ensure that even the most resistant and obstructionistic child is likely to obtain a reward chip. The remaining cards involve some physical activity and, of course, deal with activities that are likely to touch on important psychological issues. There is a fun element in many of these cards that can make the session more enjoyable and this, of course, can serve to counterbalance some of the less pleasurable aspects of treatment—aspects that are likely to reduce even the more highly motivated child's motivation for therapy. Some involve role modeling which in itself can be therapeutic. It is important, however, for the reader to appreciate that the author is not in agreement with those who place great emphasis on physical activity as a therapeutic modality per se. Rather, he believes that it plays only a limited role in the therapeutic process. In accordance with this position, he most often uses the *doing cards* as a point of departure for therapeutic interchanges that are directly relevant to the child's problems. And this is the approach that is utilized in the following examples.

"YOU'RE STANDING IN LINE TO BUY SOMETHING AND A CHILD PUSHES IN FRONT OF YOU. SHOW WHAT YOU WOULD DO." For the child with an antisocial behavior disorder, I might respond: "Let's say I'm a kid and I'm standing here in line and some kid pushes himself in front of me. A part of me might want to push him away and even hit him. But another part of me knows that that wouldn't be such a good idea. I might get into trouble or he might hit me back and then I might get hurt. So the first thing I would do would be to say something to him like, 'Hey, I was here first. Why don't you go back to the end of the line and wait your turn like everybody else.' If that didn't work I might threaten to call some person like a parent, teacher, or someone else around who is in charge. But sometimes there are no other people around to call, so I might just say that it's not worth all the trouble and that all it's causing me is the loss of another minute or two. If, however, the person starts to push me, then I might fight back. But that would be the last thing I would try. Some people might think that I'm 'chicken' for not hitting him in the first place. I don't agree with them. I think that hitting should be the last thing you should do, not the first. I don't think that people who hit first are particularly wise or brave; rather, I think they're kind of stupid." As is obvious here, I am trying to educate the antisocial child to the more civilized option that individuals have learned to use in order to bring about a more relaxed and less threatening society. These options may not have been part of the antisocial child's repertoire. Whatever the underlying factors there are in such a child's antisocial behavior (and these, of course, must be dealt with in the treatment), such education is also a part of the therapy.

"WHAT IS THE WORST KIND OF JOB A PERSON CAN HAVE? WHY? MAKE BELIEVE YOU'RE DOING THAT JOB." This question can be useful for children who are compromising their lives via academic underachievement or behavioral problems in the classroom which are interfering with their learning. For such a child, I might respond: "There are all kinds of lousy jobs in this world. And there are all kinds of good jobs. Most people agree that the harder you work to learn a job, the more likely you'll get one of the more desirable and better jobs. I think one of the worst jobs a person can have is to clean toilets. I'm sure you'll agree that it's a very smelly job cleaning out toilet bowls in which are other people's wee-wee and doo-doo. You have to get down on your knees and not only clean the toilet but clean all around on the floor, which is also usually pretty filthy. I'm sure that most, if not all, of the people who have such a job wish that they could be doing something better. I'm sure many of them are sorry that they goofed off in school, or even quit when they possibly could have stayed—which is usually when they were teenagers. Now it's too late. They may have families to support and it may be very difficult for them to go back to school." The hope here is, obviously, that the plight of these people will engender in these children some appreciation of what they are doing to themselves by their impaired commitment to school work and motivate them to try harder to overcome their difficulties.

"MAKE BELIEVE YOU'RE DOING SOMETHING THAT'S SMART TO DO. WHY IS IT SMART TO DO THAT THING?" Many children with neurologically based learning disabilities exhibit a significant problem in impulsivity. Probably the impulsivity for these patients has a neurologic basic. There are children with psychogenic problems, however, who are also impulsive. Regardless of the etiology for such children I might respond: "One of the smartest things a person can do is think in advance about consequences. Do you know what *consequences* mean?" For the child who is not familiar with the meaning of the word, I might respond: "Consequences are the things that happen when you do something. For example, if you hit your sister, the consequences may be that your mother will send you to your room. If you do well in school, the consequence will be that you will get a good report card. Anyway, one of the smartest things a person can do is to think about what will happen in the future after one does something. Many people don't think about consequences. They don't think about what's going to happen later on after they do something. They just think about what's going to happen now. And that's a bad idea. That causes a lot of trouble.

Now I'm going to make believe that I'm playing a game with someone and I'm losing. Because I feel bad that I'm losing I'm thinking of cheating. But then I remind myself that if I cheat I might be caught. Then the consequence will be that the person won't want to play that game with me anymore. Or, I think about the fact that even if I'm not caught I won't feel good about myself for having cheated. So, after thinking about the consequences, I decide not to cheat. And I think that's a smart thing to do. How are you when it comes to thinking about the consequences of the things that you do?"

My purpose here, obviously, is to instill in the child a sense of the importance of thinking in advance. Impairments in this area are not confined to children. In fact, I would go so far as to say that there is hardly an adult (including the author) who doesn't regret at times not having thought about consequences.

"MAKE BELIEVE YOU'RE SMOKING A CIGARETTE. WHAT DO YOU THINK ABOUT PEOPLE WHO SMOKE?" My response here is for every patient, regardless of the reason for coming to treatment: "First, in order to get a chip, I'm going to have to make believe I'm smoking. Boy, is this tough. (Cough, cough, cough.) This is very hard to do. It's really painful to get this chip. I hate smoking. In fact, I never smoked in my whole life. It's hard for me to understand how people would want to do such a disgusting thing. It really burns my mouth, throat, and lungs. You know, of course, that smoking can give you lung cancer and a lot of other diseases as well. But I would say what I'm saying even if smoking cured lung cancer. It's a disgusting and a dangerous habit. It nauseates me. Sometimes, when I smell smoke, I feel like vomiting. Some people who smoke think that everyone else can get sick from it but that they won't. You can imagine how surprised they are when they come down with one of those terrible diseases that comes from smoking. Some people who smoke think that others should breathe in their smoke and not say anything. I always tell smokers that it bothers me. We nonsmokers have to stick up for our rights. We can't let people smoke in our faces and let them think that they can get away with it. We have to say something or do something about it. Even kids have to speak up if adults smoke and they don't like the smoke. What do you think about what I've said." My response here does not simply direct itself to the health hazards of smoking. Rather, I also comment on self-assertion.

For some children, especially those who are in the preteen or early teen period, I might also say: "I think that one of the reasons why people start smoking is that they think that it makes them look like bigshots. They think that they're more like grown-ups when they have a cigarette in their mouths. Many boys think that girls will like them more if they smoke because the girls will be impressed with how grown-up they look. And many girls smoke because they think that boys will think the same thing. Many kids think it's sexy to smoke. I don't think so. To me it's just the opposite. I once saw a sign that said, 'Kissing a Smoker Is Like Licking a Dirty Ashtray' and I agree with that. I don't think it's sexy at all.

Some kids really don't like smoking but they think that if they don't get used to it that they'll be different from the others and that the other kids will look on them as babies. Those kids may spend long hours practicing smoking in order to get over the disgust they have for the habit. I think they're really stupid to do this. I think that they would be braver to say that it's a disgusting and terrible habit and that even if they are the only one not doing it, they're not going to do such a stupid thing. That's real bravery." My comments here, of course, direct themselves to some of the major psychodynamic factors involved in the early phases of smoking addiction. My hope here is that my comments will be of preventive value in reducing the likelihood of the child's ultimately becoming habituated.

"MAKE BELIEVE YOU'RE DOING SOMETHING THAT WOULD MAKE A PERSON FEEL SAD." For a child with an antisocial behavior disorder, I might respond: "Teasing and laughing at someone can make that person feel sad. Let's say that a boy is playing baseball and he strikes out and starts to cry. He is probably very sad that he struck out. However, he's probably even sadder now that he is crying in front of everyone. He's probably embarrassed that he's crying. In fact, I can see now that he's trying to hold back his tears because he's so ashamed of himself that he's crying in front of everyone. He's covering his eyes now and trying to make believe that he's really not crying, but everyone knows that he is. Then, if I were to tease him and call him a 'crybaby' or something like that, that would make him feel even sadder. But I don't have the heart to do that to him. So I'm not going to do it, even though I won't get a chip. I wouldn't want to do such a cruel thing." As the reader can appreciate, I attempt to engender feelings of sympathy for the victim of the antisocial child and introduce dramatic elements, repetition, and some exaggeration in order to get across my point.

"MAKE BELIEVE YOU'RE HAVING AN ARGUMENT WITH SOMEONE. WITH WHOM ARE YOU ARGUING? WHAT ARE YOU ARGUING ABOUT?" For the child with a neurologically based learning disability, who needs some lessons in social protocol and getting along better with others, or the egocentric child who does not appreciate his or her effect on others, I might respond: "I'm having an argument with a kid with whom I'm playing a game of checkers. She was starting to lose and then wanted to change the rules in the middle of the game. We both agreed that a person has to jump when he or she can and now she wants to change the rules and say that you don't have to jump if you don't want to. And then she's starting to lie and say that we never made that rule in the first place. So I'm telling her that I'm not going to play the game unless she goes by the original rules. I'll also tell her that if she wants to change the rules for the next game and play by different rules, I'll be happy to talk to her about that. However, if I agree to different rules, it will only be with the understanding that we will stick with those rules throughout that game. Anyway, I tell her that she has to make a decision: either she's going to play by the original rules or I won't play the game anymore. She gets angry at me and bangs her fist on the table. And that makes all the checkers jump up and down, so that we don't know anymore where they all were. And, of course, that ends the game. What do you think about what happened during that game?" The vignette lends itself well to a number of comments on the child's part regarding the feelings of other people, following the rules, obeying social protocol, and general cooperation.

"MAKE BELIEVE YOU'RE DOING SOMETHING THAT MAKES YOU FEEL VERY GOOD ABOUT YOURSELF? WHY DOES THAT THING MAKE YOU FEEL SO GOOD?" For the child who is an academic underachiever, I might provide the following response: "As you know, I like to write books. I have already given you one of the children's books that I've written. As I'm sure you can appreciate, writing a book takes a lot of work. It's a very hard job. Sometimes I may work over many years on one single book. However, when I finally finish, I really feel good about myself. I feel that I've accomplished a lot. Although I may be very tired over all the work I've put in to it, I'm very proud of what I've done. And then, when the final printed book comes out, that really makes me feel good about myself. I have what is called a 'sense of achievement.' Do you know what I mean when I say 'sense of achievement?'" After this is clarified, I might ask the child to tell me things that he or she has done that have provided him or her with similar feelings of accomplishment. My hope here, obviously, is to provide the child with some appreciation of the ego-enhancing feelings that one can enjoy after diligent commitment to a task.

"MAKE BELIEVE YOU'RE DOING SOMETHING THAT COULD MAKE YOUR TEACHER PROUD OF YOU. WHAT ARE YOU DOING? WHY WOULD THAT MAKE YOUR TEACHER PROUD OF YOU?" Again, for our old friend the academic underachiever, I might respond: "I'm making believe that I started off as one of the worst students in the class. Let's say that I got mainly Cs and Ds on my report card. The teacher has told me that I've been goofing off, horsing around, and that if this keeps up, I'm not going to get promoted at the end of the year. My parents also have been on my back and are very upset over my poor grades. Although at first I don't listen to what they're saying, after a while I realize that they all mean business and that I'm going to be in a lot of trouble if I don't start to shape up. So I decide to try harder and even stop watching a couple of television programs that I was hooked on. Then, over the months, I start getting better grades and by the end of the year the teacher gives me a special certificate that says that I showed the most improvement of all the children in the class. She says on the certificate that she's very proud of me. And I'm also very proud of myself." My responses here, of course, hope to engender some motivation in the child to enjoy similar feelings of accomplishment.

CONCLUSION

It is important for the therapist to appreciate that the responses provided to each of the selected cards are only representative of possible answers to the question. There is no such thing as a *standard* response to any of the cards. Each response must be tailored to the particular needs of the child and direct itself to the specific problems for which the child is being treated. Just as the responding story in the Mutual Storytelling Technique (Gardner, 1971) is specifically tailored to relate to the particular problems that the child is revealing in the story, the therapist's responses to the *Talking, Feeling, and Doing Game* cards should also be designed to the specific psychological needs of that particular child. My experience has been that the *Talking, Feeling, and Doing Game* is a particularly attractive therapeutic tool and will predictably involve the vast majority of resistant, uninhibited, and uncooperative children. Like all therapeutic modalities, it has its advantages and disadvantages. One of the main disadvantages of the *Talking, Feeling, and Doing Game* is that it may be *too* attractive to both the patient and the therapist. Accordingly, the therapist may thereby be deprived of the kind of deeper unconscious material that one obtains from projective play and storytelling. And the child then will be deprived of the therapeutic benefits that may result from this type of activity. Accordingly, I generally warn therapists not to be drawn into the temptation of using this game throughout the session and to do everything possible to balance the therapeutic activities with other modalities.

REFERENCES

Conn, J.H. (1939). The child reveals himself through play. *Mental Hygiene, 23*(1), 1–21.

Conn, J.H. (1941a). The timid, dependent child. *Journal of Pediatrics, 19*(1), 1–2.

Conn, J.H. (1941b). The treatment of fearful children. *American Journal of Orthopsychiatry, 11*(4), 744–751.

Conn, J.H. (1948). The play-interview as an investigative and therapeutic procedure. *The Nervous Child, 7*(3), 257–286.

Conn, J.H. (1954). Play interview therapy of castration fears. *American Journal of Orthopsychiatry, 25*(4), 747–754.

Gardner, R.A. (1971). *Therapeutic communication with children: The mutual storytelling technique*. New York: Aronson.

Gardner, R.A. (1973). *The Talking, Feeling, and Doing Game*. Cresskill, NJ: Creative Therapeutics.

Gardner, R.A. (1975a). *Psychotherapeutic approaches to the resistant child*. New York: Aronson.

Gardner, R.A. (1975b). Psychotherapeutic approaches to the resistant child (2 one-hour cassette tapes). Cresskill, N.J.: Creative Therapeutics.

Murray, H. (1936). *Thematic Apperception Test*. New York: The Psychological Corporation.

Solomon, J.C. (1938). Active play therapy. *American Journal of Orthopsychiatry, 8*(3), 479–498.

Solomon, J.C. (1940). Active play therapy: Further experiences. *American Journal of Orthopsychiatry, 10*(4), 763–781.

Solomon, J.C. (1951). Therapeutic use of play. In H.H. Anderson & G.L. Anderson (Eds.), *An introduction to projective techniques* (pp. 639–661). Englewood Cliffs, NJ: Prentice-Hall.

Solomon, J.C. (1955). Play technique and the integrative process. *American Journal of Orthopsychiatry, 25*(3), 591–600.

CHAPTER 3

Game Therapy for Children in Placement

RICHARD MARK KAGAN

This chapter addresses the dilemma of helping children in placement who desperately need a home and yet often seem to do everything in their power to be sent away from their families. These are severely disturbed children with long histories of aggressive or self-destructive behaviors who have frequently moved back and forth over the years between their families and foster homes, group care facilities, or psychiatric hospitals. For such children, separations and placements have led to intolerable feelings of loss and abandonment, overt denial of problems, and acting-out of conflicts. These children have often experienced such immense pain through repeated separations, physical abuse, neglect, and so on that they have cut off the normal grief process. Behaviorally, they provoke others—their parents, teachers, child-care workers, and clinicians—to reject them and confirm once again that everybody hates them. In this way, they gain a fleeting sense of mastery over their destiny while repeating tragic separations from the past. Effective treatment programs must assess the meaning of a child's behaviors in the context of interpersonal, family, and intrapsychic factors. It is essential to evaluate the impact of significant relationships on children's behaviors and utilize the potential of families for promoting growth and development. Therapeutic interventions for children in placement must address the needs of these children for consistent, nurturing family ties now and in the future. Games can be utilized within an integrated treatment program to: (1) engage resistant

The author would like to thank Nadia Finkelstein, Steven Sola, Shirley Schlosberg, Adele Pickar, Peter Watrous, Jan Silverman-Pollow, Kathy Raymond, and David Nevin for their help in the preparation of this manuscript and *Cast Adrift*.

children and their parents in therapy, (2) identify significant attachments and messages children have received, (3) facilitate expression of beliefs and feelings to significant others, (4) clarify discharge goals, for example, return home or adoption, and (5) make often covert behavioral patterns involving children and family members overt with identifiable consequences. Individualized games can help children and their families explore new models of interpreting their world which in turn can lead to more adaptive behaviors in and out of placement.

THEORETICAL FOUNDATIONS

Acting-Out Children and Their Families

Acting-out children typically display a very constricted range of behaviors characterized by a narrow perspective, little thought of the future, intense feelings of loss, and a reliance on aggression or running away to solve problems. From the child's perspective, acting-out behaviors generate excitement and can provide enticing feelings of control in a chaotic, abusive, or depressing environment. Acting-out children often feel a responsibility to maintain a fragile family balance through negative behaviors they have learned over the years (Ausloos, 1978). These behaviors may function to unite parents who are threatening divorce, energize a depressed parent, block an unwanted marriage by the youth's parent, elicit help for family members, or avoid the risks inherent in developing attachments with a prospective adoptive family.

When family conflicts and problems are unable to be resolved within the family, they frequently become acted out with community agents of control, for example, teachers, police, case workers, and so on. The penalties imposed on a child by a community often appear insignificant from a child's perspective in contrast to the necessity for protecting one's family, the excitement of stimulating powerful forces in the community, and the need to release intense feelings of anger and fear. Moreover, acting out can lead to additional counseling or financial services being provided to a child's family.

Placement of Acting-Out Youth

Even the threat of placement can elicit feelings of abandonment in children (Moss and Moss, 1984). A child will often experience placement as a message of being unloved and worthless. Children are likely to distrust their parents out of fear of further rejection and to hide their feelings behind a mask of indifference or belligerence (Moss and Moss, 1984).

Residential treatment centers for emotionally disturbed and acting-out children typically provide a group living environment in which adaptive social and academic behaviors can be learned and where parents can be helped to understand their child's difficulties and how they can better deal with them (Finkelstein, 1980). Community authorities, for example, county departments of social services, refer children to child care agencies to provide the structure, control, and nurturing environment that may be lacking in a child's home. A person in need of supervision (PINS) petition will likely be filed in Family Court with custody of the child transferred (temporarily) from the parents to the county department of social services.

Parents, however, often feel "put down" by contracts imposed by state authorities which essentially say: "You as a parent have failed. Now we 'professionals' will help your child." Parents who accept this implicit contract often "give up" and further distance themselves from their sons or daughters. Such children often carry the label of "identified patient" and come to represent the locus of a family's problems.

In other situations, parents may resist taking responsibility for their child's behaviors and may covertly support a child's continuing to act out within a child-care agency or foster home. This can help the family to regain their self-respect, since even the "professionals" are eventually proven unable to help such a difficult child. In such situations, progress is often slow, and families frequently end up labeled "hostile," "resistant," or "unworkable" (Finkelstein, 1980).

Despite the behavioral gains made during placement, a child may still face enormous pressures and conflicts in their family environment when they return home. The child may feel more detached from his or her parents and may be given increased power in the family as a result of his or her growing reputation as an "ungovernable," disturbed, and even a dangerous individual in the community.

Further incidents of acting out may occur, and the youth is likely to experience the inner terror of feeling disengaged from their family or having more power and responsibility than they can tolerate (Haley, 1973). Consequently, replacement in a psychiatric facility becomes highly probable. In fact, the recidivism rate of children returning from foster care systems to their families has been reported to be as high as 43.6 percent for youths aged 13 to 15 and 22.6 percent for children aged 10 to 12 (Block, 1981).

A Community Systems Perspective

The aggressive and self-destructive behaviors of acting-out children reflect the intense conflicts and feelings of anger, fear, and emptiness experienced by these children and their families. These behaviors will be experienced as dangers by "helping adults" in governmental or private agencies who then feel an obligation to impose stringent controls on the child (Ausloos, 1978) in order to protect the community, family, and often the child from further injury or harm. Such children will often be given a diagnostic label and will be placed in a treatment center, with responsibility for the child transferred from the parents to a governmental authority.

These are well-intentioned efforts to provide help and control for acting-out children. Nevertheless, these efforts frequently backfire by undermining families and the agencies which seek to serve them. Children, parents, and public and private agencies frequently become locked into dysfunctional relationships which serve to maintain children in powerful but dangerous roles.

Dysfunctional Roles that Maintain Problems

Game therapy must address the interactional systems that have led to a child's behavioral problems and placement. The responses of parents, public agency workers, private agency staff, and children often fit the classic triangle of: victim, rescuer, and persecutor (Karpman, 1968). The child or parents may be initially identified as a *victim* with the public agency or private agency operating as a *rescuer*. Blame for problems may be placed on any of the individuals or agencies involved, for example, the police, school officials, a negligent parent, or an aggressive child. At the same time, "victims" may be perceived as relatively helpless to resolve their problems without the assistance of professionals.

When the child is identified as the victim, parents are frequently blamed, and the youth is frequently seen as harmed or hampered by the environment of his or her parents' home with relatively little control over his or her behaviors. This frequently leads to public agency workers or staff of child care agencies telling parents to do things which are felt to be helpful to the child. Parents in turn often react with anger to these messages and by their mandated (e.g., court-ordered) involvement with public and private agency workers. Parents often become resentful of repetitive demands that they must do more when they, too, have suffered through years of physical abuse, neglect, and chronic instability in their relationships with their own parents, extended family, and spouses. Such parents often feel that their own needs are not being considered and that these personal problems and needs are overwhelming. As a result, they may resist making any substantial changes despite the pleas (or threats) of professionals.

In other situations, *parents* may be seen as *victims*, and the child (or other individuals) may be blamed for problems. The behavior of the child may be seen as unmanageable by anyone but professionals. In some cases, parents may be seen as physically or mentally disabled; and as a result, minimal expectations will be made of them. In such cases, it is not infrequent to find up to 10 agencies involved with a given family. Family members may be preoccupied with traveling from appointment to appointment with public or private agency workers. Often in such situations, diagnostic evaluations lead to recommendations for still more services to help such parents with their problems. This further supports parents in their role as victims who need an ever-increasing array of services. If parents do take more control, they may lose some of these social and financial services. Families thus experience a strong disincentive for change.

In other situations, a *child care agency* or psychiatric hospital may feel that it is a *victim* of uncooperative parents, aggressive children, unfair funding cutbacks, and repressive demands for accountability from governmental authorities. In such agencies, morale will frequently be poor with agency managers pressed into "freezing" positions, increasing caseloads, eliminating raises, or accepting questionable placements of youths in order to "fill beds."

When an acting-out child is involved in such an agency, he or she will likely repeat aggressive or self-destructive behaviors with staff members. The stress caused by an acting-out child (or their family) will often appear to be too much for the limited resources of the agency. As a result, the child will frequently be sent to another, more restrictive, institution. The child, parents, and staff will experience this last placement as another in a long series of failures.

Engaging Family Competence

Effective foster care, hospital, and residential treatment programs must assess the impact of community and family systems on maintaining problem behaviors. Triangles for relationships involving children, parents, practitioners, and state authorities become fixed through repetitive crises and efforts to determine (diagnose) a focused cause of current problems, that is, some person, thing, condition, or entity to blame. Triangular relationships, in effect, help families and professionals to avoid facing painful issues and consideration of each one's own participation in behavior patterns (Fogarty, 1977) that lead to a child's repeated placements. Intense fears of loss, abandonment, and past (or ongoing) violence can be diverted through well-intentioned efforts to address the isolated needs of an acting-out child (or parents).

A community systems approach involves a collaborative effort with public and private agency staff to utilize the power of a child's family to facilitate the growth and development of a severely disturbed and acting-out child. Triangular relationships are viewed as involving the overt (or covert) participation of parents, children, and often practitioners (Fogarty, 1977). At the same time, each person involved is considered to have some potential for changing their own behaviors within significant relationships.

Group care can be used as a context for engaging parental competence and freeing a child from a powerful but dangerous role in his or her family and community (Kagan, 1983). This involves bringing out behaviors on the part of family members and community agents that again and again demonstrate that the parents are in charge of their homes and lives (after Haley, 1973; Madanes, 1980). At the same time, children face realistic consequences for their behaviors (after Dreikurs & Soltz, 1964). Parents are considered to be equal partners engaged in a change process—rather than as victims or persecutors who professionals must change in order to save children from placement. At the same time, parents are helped to give children age-appropriate responsibilities (and consequences) in their homes.

The thrust of this approach is to help parents and children to avoid repetitive behaviors that may serve to maintain problems (after Watzlawick, Weakland, and Fisch, 1974). From a systems perspective, most problems are assumed to be caused by "habitual but ineffective cycles of behavior" in individuals and organizations (Blake and Mouton, 1976, p. 4). The child-care agency or psychiatric hospital may play a major role by helping children, parents, and governmental agencies to avoid being locked into dysfunctional roles, such as: the rescuer, victim, and persecutor.

Game Therapy for Children in Placement

Children have always used fantasy and creative processes to help them work through difficult problems and intense feelings. Family conflicts, rejection by parents, losses and deaths can be found in many classic children's stories, for example, Hansel and Gretel (Grimm, 1980). In group care, games can be used to help children communicate both verbally and nonverbally fears and resentments. Such "play" activities can provide the child in placement with an appropriate means for self-expression and self-help (Uhlig, Plumer, Galasy, Ballard, and Menley, 1977; Klein, 1975).

Therapeutic games provide an effective medium for engaging otherwise resistant children and can be utilized conjointly with parents (Gardner, 1975). Within the community systems perspective outlined, games can be used to identify in a concrete visual format some of the covert behavioral patterns repeated by a child in their homes and in placement. Triangular roles can become overt choices with clear consequences rather than the inevitable problems of helpless "victims" and unchangeable "persecutors."

Therapeutic messages which foster a child's (or parent's) confidence can be dramatized through a participatory (and enjoyable) process. Perspectives of children and families can be expanded to include multiple options. Games can help a child and his or her family see that they need not be trapped by problem behaviors (Gardner, 1975).

In therapeutic relationships, games can also be utilized by a therapist to show that professionals, too, have had problems and feelings, for example, anger, sadness, and so on, similar to those that may be troubling a child. Careful expression of the therapist's own deficiencies can raise a child's and parent's self-esteem (Gardner, 1975). This is especially effective with families who have been labeled negligent and have come to expect professionals to tell them to behave better or be better parents. Lectures and direct advice often lowers the self-esteem of clients (Gardner, 1975) and promotes distrust and resentment toward the therapist.

Games can also be an effective approach for helping children who must face the trauma of losing their parents. For children who have been (or are in the process) of being freed for adoption, games can provide permission and safety for experiencing and expressing feelings of rage, abandonment, fears, and grief. Games can also be used to engage such children in therapeutic processes designed to stop repetitive and antisocial behaviors that offer protection from dealing with painful losses but block the grief process (Kagan, 1980).

CASE ILLUSTRATION AND GAME DESCRIPTION

Cast Adrift

Cast Adrift was originally based on the feelings, belief, and behaviors of Cindy, a 12-year-old girl who had lost her biological mother as an infant and the foster family who raised her for 11 years. She had been surrendered as a child and placed in an emergency shelter and then a residential treatment program after her foster parents decided they could no longer manage her. In residential treatment, Cindy had an individualized educational program, art therapy, and activity group therapy. A life road map tracing her various "homes" and a life story (Jewett, 1978) illustrating her history was drawn up with her help. Gardner's mutual storytelling techniques (Gardner, 1971) were utilized in individual counseling along with other interventions. At the same time, efforts were made to find a prospective adoptive family.

Like many rejected children, Cindy had a very limited perspective on what she could do. She seemed to be almost continually "oozing with anger" toward her foster parents and everyone else who came near her. Beneath this anger, Cindy was extremely frightened of losing her foster family. However, in her view of the world, things were "crummy" and always would be. She couldn't trust anyone. She saw herself as a mean kid and thought she would always be a mean kid. Everybody hated her, and her problems were caused by everyone else.

As Cindy's foster family withdrew from contact, she became more and more distressed. She panicked at the thought of losing her foster parents and at the anticipation of reattachment to a new adoptive family. Cindy internalized messages she had received from her foster family on how terrible she was, her destiny of becoming a prostitute like her biological mother, and her culpability for past violence (suspected abuse) in the foster family. Her behaviors became more and more dangerous to herself and others; and she eventually had to be moved from the residential treatment center to a locked psychiatric ward.

Game Description

The following game was created to help Cindy to get a more positive outlook and more control over her behavior. The game stressed the difficulties of her situation, that is, rejection by her biological and foster parents and helped to normalize typical feelings of children experiencing loss and grief, for example, denial, rage, withdrawal, and depression. The game also diagrammed the typical results of Cindy's usual approaches to her problems. For instance, running away usually led to such outcomes as the loss of privileges or sickness. Sulking put her away from the fun others were having. Swearing, cursing, and hating everyone usually led to angry encounters and the loss of privileges. The game also emphasized the sense of going in circles which went along with Cindy's typical behavior. Finally, the game stressed that Cindy, her foster parents, and prospective adoptive families had some control over what happened. Beliefs and behaviors involved choices with predictable consequences.

Considering Cindy's rejections by her foster parents and lack of contact with them or her biological mother, the game was called "Cast Adrift." The game was played with players moving along the outside squares of the board by the throw of the dice (see Figure 3.1). Squares were designed to reflect common behaviors and feelings of children (like Cindy) in placement. Players moved from the first square marked "Feeling Hurt," to such crucial squares as "Parents (or Foster Parents) say Good-by (locked out)," to "Freed for Adoption," to "Begin to Live at New Home," to "Continue to Work out Problems with New Family." Players took turns throwing the dice and moving until one player made it to "Finish."

Along the way, players were rewarded (by moving ahead) for positive behaviors and suffered (moved backwards) for negative behaviors. For instance, a player could land in several detours. The "Trail of Heavy Hassles" typified a cycle of running away because "Who Cares?" and led through several consequences, such as "Detention" and "Sickness." "The

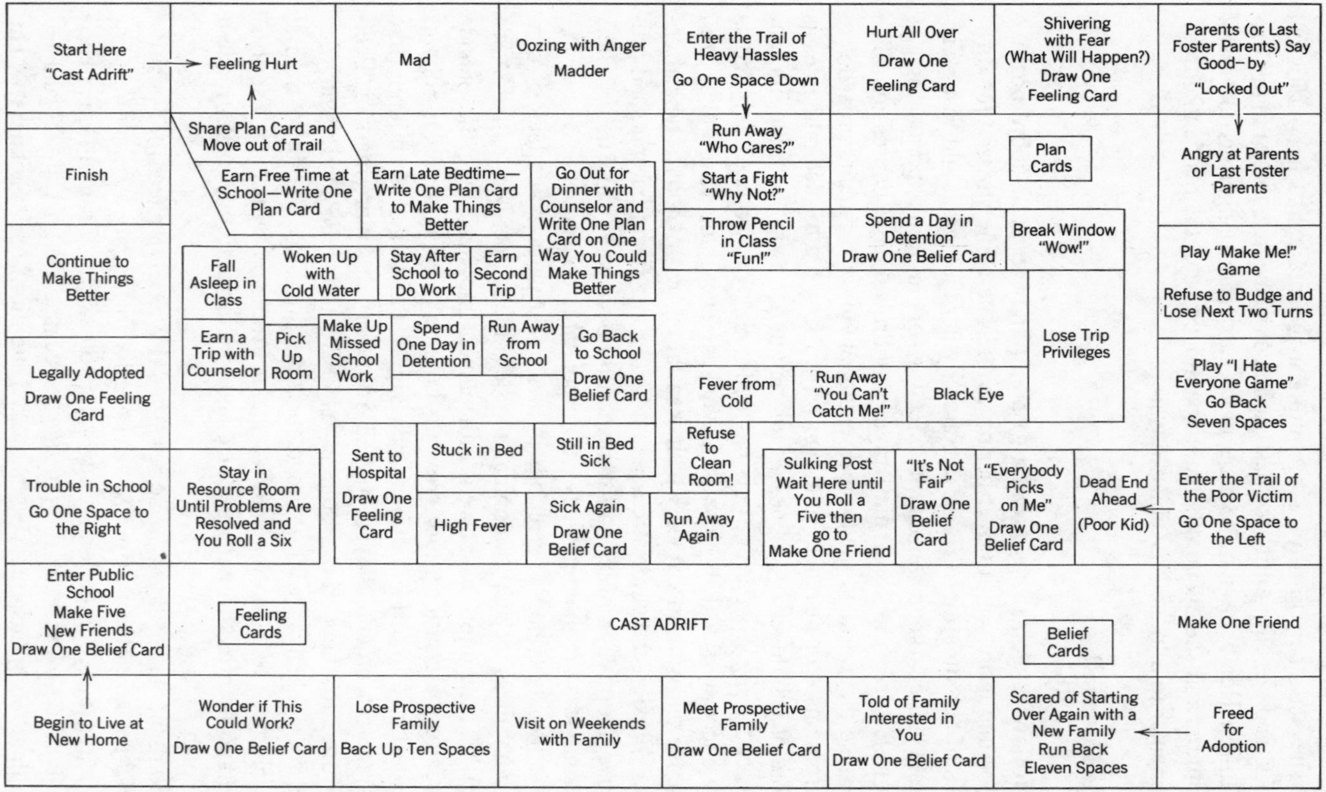

Figure 3.1. *Cast Adrift.* Reprinted with permission of Human Sciences Press from Kagan, R.M. (1982). Storytelling and game therapy for children in placement. *Child Care Quarterly, 11,* 280–290.

Trail" came back to the first square after a player earned privileges back and made a positive plan (on a plan card) to make one thing better in their life.

Consequences were set up to reflect children's typical reactions to realistic events in their lives. Landing on the "Make Me" game involved refusing to budge for two turns. The "I Hate Everyone" game moved a player back seven spaces to "Oozing with Anger." The "Trail of the Poor Victim" involved going to a "Sulking Post" after passing through squares marked "Dead End Ahead," "Everyone Picks on Me," and "It's Not Fair!" Players who landed on the "Sulking Post" had to wait there until they threw a five after which they moved directly to "Make One Friend."

When a player landed on "Scared of Starting Over with a New Family," he or she went back 11 spaces to "Oozing with Anger." Landing on "Losing a Prospective Family" moved a player back 10 spaces to "Angry at Parents or Last Foster Parent." "Trouble in School" could lead to "Staying in Resource Room Until Problems are Resolved and You Roll a Six."

On several squares, players had to draw belief cards which stated either a positive or a negative belief and gave a consequence. For example, a player might draw "It's Everybody Else's Fault!" and had to say this out loud and move back three spaces. Or a player might draw "I Can Figure This Game Out!" and was asked to keep thinking ahead as he or she moved ahead two spaces. The list of messages for belief cards is printed in Table 3.1.

On other squares, players had to draw feeling cards which stated a feeling and a positive or negative way of dealing with that feeling with a resulting consequence. For example, a player may draw "Feel sad and tell someone something that makes you feel sad. Say it softly . . . then move ahead two spaces." On the other hand, another feeling card read, "Feel sad but keep it all to yourself. Go for a long, lonely walk and miss your next turn." Messages from feeling cards are listed in Table 3.2.

"Cast Adrift" was specifically designed for Cindy. She was willing to make up her own stories and to play "Cast Adrift," but steadfastly refused to discuss any of the implications of the stories or games for her own situation. Her refusal to verbally discuss her situation was accepted; however, Cindy was repeatedly confronted by the dilemmas of characters (like herself) in stories and the frustrations of going around and around in circles on "The Trail of Heavy Hassles" in *Cast Adrift*. Use of this game

Table 3.1   Belief Cards

1. I am in charge of my life and I choose to move ahead four spaces.
2. I am a bad kid. Everybody hates me. Repeat two times and go back seven spaces.
3. Life is crummy and always will be! Say this two times as you go back two spaces.
4. I don't have to be perfect; I will just do my best. Move ahead four spaces.
5. I can be good or bad. It's up to me. Move ahead three spaces.
6. I don't need to get people to hate me. I can make friends and make it in a new family. Say this as you move ahead four spaces.
7. I can figure this game out! Keep thinking ahead as you move ahead four spaces.
8. I can't trust anybody! Repeat two times and go back four spaces.
9. It's everybody else's fault! Say this again and move back three spaces.
10. I know two good things that I am able to do. Name two things you can do and move ahead five spaces.
11. I am a mean kid and always will be! Think about this as you go directly to "The Trail of Heavy Hassles."
12. I am proud of what I can do. Share something that you are proud of with another person and move ahead four spaces.
13. I know two good things that I am able to do. Name two things you can do and move ahead four spaces.
14. I can make it! Say this three times as you move ahead three spaces.

Source: Reprinted with permission of Human Sciences Press from Kagan, R.M. (1982). Storytelling and game therapy for children in placement. *Child Care Quarterly*, 11, p. 287.

and storytelling (Kagan, 1982) helped her to return within two weeks from a locked psychiatric ward of a general hospital to a residential treatment program. She was almost immediately introduced to a prospective adoptive parent and within six months was living in a potential adoptive home.

Use of *Cast Adrift*

Cast Adrift and other therapeutic games must be adapted to the abilities, needs, interests, and problems of each family. These techniques should

Table 3.2 Feeling Cards

1. Feel scared but don't tell anyone. Instead "run away" back three spaces.
2. Feel sad but keep it all to yourself. Go for a long, lonely walk and miss your next turn.
3. Share with someone the saddest thing that happened in your life and as you do move ahead four spaces. What happened?
4. "I can let myself feel scared without running away from my feelings." Instead of running away, move ahead three spaces.
5. Tell someone about one of the angriest times in your life and move ahead three spaces. What happened?
6. Tell someone about one of the happiest times in your life and move ahead three spaces. What happened?
7. Tell someone about one of the scariest times in your life and move ahead three spaces. What happened? What did you do?
8. Feel sad and tell someone something that makes you feel sad. Say it softly. Move ahead three spaces.
9. Feel scared and share something that scares you with one person. Move ahead three spaces.
10. Feel angry and show everybody by smashing your radio! Go directly to "The Trail of Heavy Hassles."
11. Feel angry and tell someone. I feel mad because _____. Move ahead four spaces.
12. Feel happy but don't ever let anyone know. Keep a straight face. Don't laugh and get ready to feel angry as you move back three spaces.
13. Feel angry and show everybody by setting someone else up to get angry at you. And as they get angry, move back two spaces.
14. "It's okay to feel sad. I can let myself be sad and still be okay." Think of one thing that makes you feel sad as you move ahead two spaces.

Source: Reprinted with permission of Human Sciences Press from Kagan, R.M. (1982). Storytelling and game therapy for children in placement. *Child Care Quarterly*, 11, p. 288.

not be used with psychotic children or children who do not have the capacity to deal with the anxiety created. For fairly secure and well-balanced youngsters, games may involve very realistic situations. For more anxious or resistant children, it may be necessary to use much more obscure and milder situations and consequences on the playing board, belief cards, and feeling cards. Belief and feeling cards can be carefully selected to utilize less threatening items (see Tables 3.1 and 3.2) or other items may be substituted, for example, adaptations can be made from Gardner's *Talking, Feeling and Doing Game* (Gardner, 1975). However, games should embody the important themes which affect the child and his or her family.

Cast Adrift was designed for use by skilled practitioners working individually with children or youth in day or residential group care settings. These techniques work best in *brief* individual sessions with children but can be utilized in small groups of two to four children who are fairly secure and well-balanced. Most children will quickly grasp elements of the game that apply to themselves and thus will have an opportunity to deal with personal issues. Individual sessions minimize the contagion effect of children's anxieties on each other.

Practitioners should have a solid understanding of the stages of grief, loss, and separation (Bowlby, 1960; Thomas, 1967), an introduction to developmental disturbances in childhood (e.g., Kessler, 1966; Wicks-Nelson and Israel, 1984), and a basic understanding of family systems (e.g., Nichols, 1984). These techniques must be used as part of a comprehensive team approach to helping a child deal with grief, loss, and reattachment within the context of his or her family.

Cast Adrift should not be used as an isolated intervention. Use of this (or other games) without addressing the child's family and interpersonal relationships could inadvertently serve to maintain a child (or parents) in dysfunctional roles. The intent of this game is to move beyond specific problem behaviors and address the meaning of these behaviors in the child's life.

Cast Adrift was intended for children who are being freed for adoption. For children in placement who have the goal of returning to their original families, a revised version can be substituted (see Figure 3.2). In this game, the last 11 squares have been altered to reflect a child's beginning visits home, weekend visits, and returning to their families. The title was also changed to *Heading Home*.

Cast Adrift or *Heading Home* can be introduced as games that have been used with other children. The child can be told that he or she will have an opportunity later, if desired, to make up his or her own game. Rules for the game include a time limit with the winner being the one who has advanced the farthest or reached the finish square in that amount of time—typically 30 to 40 minutes. A player is not required to express a

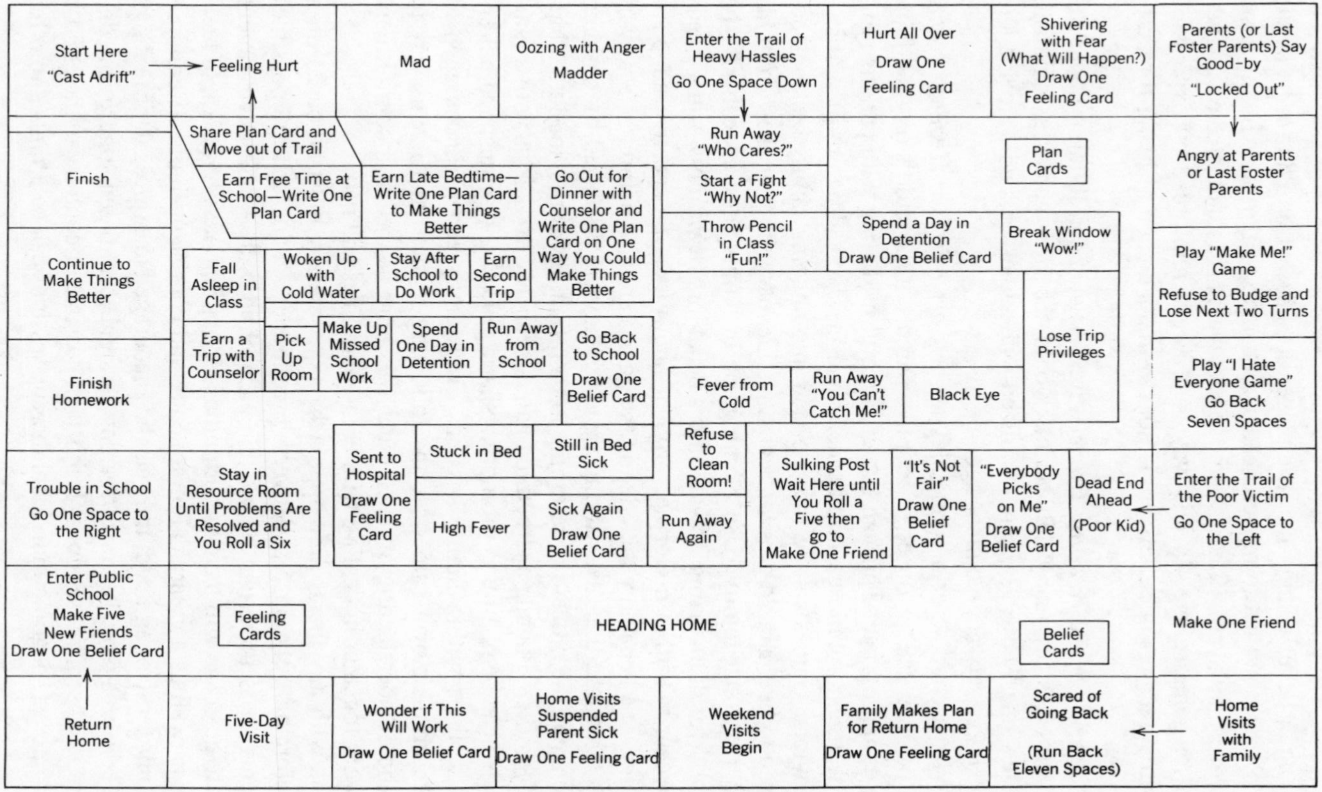

Figure 3.2. *Heading Home.*

feeling or belief at any time. If a player does not wish to do so, he or she simply does not get to move ahead as indicated on the card. In any case, however, a player will have to move backwards if so indicated on a given card or game square. In this way, a player is reinforced by expressing positive feelings or beliefs but is not put in a situation of being forced to change.

Cast Adrift and *Heading Home* were designed for children under the age of 14, since many adolescents would see such games as childish. These games, however, can be utilized with adolescents who are socially and cognitively at a younger age.

With a child's permission, playing of *Cast Adrift* or *Heading Home* can be done with prospective adoptive parents or the child's original family, as appropriate. This can be very helpful in sharing with parents typical feelings of children in placement and the cyclical nature of problem behaviors. Games can be incorporated into ongoing family sessions designed to help a child develop a positive identity within or apart from his or her original family. Use of the game in family sessions can also be helpful for dramatizing how a child's behaviors fit with his or her needs for security within his or her original family or a prospective adoptive family. The behaviors included in the games are also helpful as a way of predicting and thus detoxifying typical behaviors displayed by children who are in the process of returning to their families or moving into adoptive families. Playing a structured game, such as *Cast Adrift*, with a family also can be helpful in promoting sharing of otherwise unstated beliefs and feelings within family sessions. The family can be encouraged to make up their own game (see the following section) and in this way to promote understanding of each other's feelings as well as a commitment to work together in dealing with both good times and bad.

As with any therapeutic approach, game therapy must be based on a comfortable relationship between practitioner, child, and (if possible) parents. It is important to provide each child with a safe environment where he or she will have opportunities for appropriate ventilation of feelings as well as a great deal of structure and consistent limits. If children become tense or agitated, they can be encouraged to express their feelings and concerns directly to their parents or significant parent-figures in conjoint or subsequent sessions. If this is impossible or contrary to the child's best interest, ongoing individual therapy sessions can be arranged to offer the child a special time, place, and relationship within which he or she can express intense feelings and learn new behaviors.

Developing "My Game"

After *Cast Adrift* or *Heading Home* is played several times, it is especially useful to encourage a child to develop their own personal game. This can be done on blank game grids (see Figure 3.3.). It is helpful to encourage children to highlight important goals for themselves, such as adoption, and to put these in key places, such as the corners of the game board. Corner squares can thus be used to represent goals for the child in working through conflicts with their families. Side trails and special cards to be drawn can then be developed and many of the situations, feeling cards, and belief cards from *Cast Adrift* or *Heading Home* can be incorporated into a child's own game. It is important that a child's own game be relevant to their current interpersonal dilemma as well as to their internal feelings. For instance, a child coping with the loss of his or her parents will need to work through stages of the grief process (Bowlby, 1960; Thomas, 1967) including: denial, rage, anxiety, withdrawal, and reattachment. Each of these feelings and behaviors is tied to interpersonal relationships in the child's life. Denial and rage maintain a child's distance from both past and potential family relationships as well as from developing bonds to group care staff, therapists, or foster parents. Experiencing anxiety may allow the beginning of new relationships or the renegotiation of bonds to a child's family. Withdrawal reflects a child's need to experience feelings of emptiness (Fogarty, 1977) and also may serve to protect a child from the risks involved in renewing attachments or developing new attachments to another family. The child's personal game can reflect these feelings and interpersonal relationships. By so doing, the game can facilitate expression of painful feelings and thus reduce their intensity. At the same time, key squares on the game board (e.g., corners) come to represent a child's goals in terms of his or her family situation.

Use of games in this way provides a child with an opportunity to express his or her own perception of his or her behaviors and situation with an opportunity to work out better consequences for him or herself. A child's own game also can provide significant clues to important attachments, for example, to former foster parents that may continue to have a

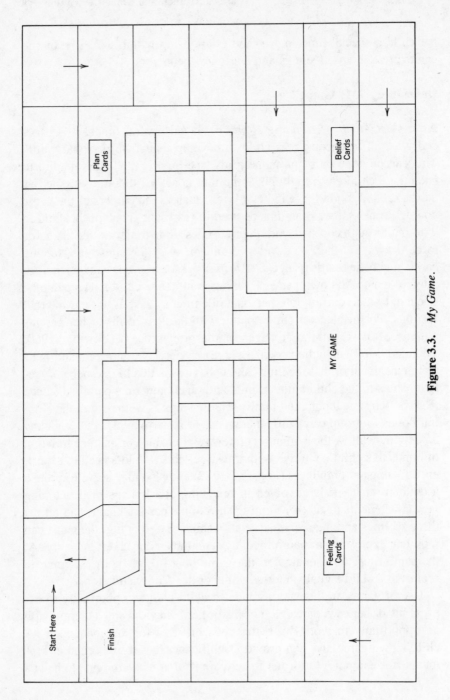

Figure 3.3. *My Game.*

90

great impact on the child's behaviors. Messages from parents (or foster parents, etc.) may also be revealed, for example, a parent's message that a child will grow up in a specific institution just as the parent once did. Children's own games typically reveal relationships which are causing them a great deal of trouble and visually dramatize their difficulties in working through feelings of grief and loss. Personal games can also clarify a child's goals, for example, to be adopted and his and her assessment of whether this is really possible.

SUMMARY AND CONCLUSIONS

Children in placement are frequently mired in repetitive cycles of denial and aggressive or self-destructive behaviors which reflect feelings of loss and intense rage following repeated losses, neglect, and/or abuse in their families. Returning to their families or moving into adoptive homes involves changes in their relationships with their family or families. This in turn involves changes in their perspectives on their world, and changes in their behaviors. Therapeutic games, such as *Cast Adrift* and *Heading Home*, can be valuable interventions for use along with family therapy, activity group therapies, and individualized educational programs as part of an integrated treatment program for families which addresses both interpersonal and intrapsychic needs. Games can be utilized to help these children to find (or renew) security and commitment within families which they can call their own.

Games can be effective tools in engaging resistant children into counseling relationships as well as in identifying significant attachments and conflicts in a child's life. Games can provide a child with permission to deal openly with some of the painful covert issues, for example, loss, grief, rejections, abuse, and so on that have led to ongoing aggressive or self-destructive behaviors. With some of these issues identified, therapists can then deal more effectively with a child's need to work on significant relationships with family members, or past parent figures, for example, foster parents, and so on. Children can use games such as "Cast Adrift" to experiment with a variety of adaptive and maladaptive beliefs and to see the results of various behaviors.

Games can dramatically illustrate the difficult situations of children in limbo. This can be very helpful in preparing prospective adoptive parents or in redefining a child's behaviors to his or her biological family so that change can occur (after Watzlawick, Weakland, & Fisch, 1974). Therapeutic games can also emphasize children's and families' many choices about their beliefs and their methods of dealing with feelings through overt behaviors. Family members can then experiment with new models of interpreting their world and also have an opportunity to share otherwise hidden feelings and beliefs. Painful conflicts may thus be dealt with through a concrete visual format, for example, the game board. As conflicts are addressed by the family, a child can be freed from his or her role as a "bad" or "crazy" youth. Dysfunctional roles, for example, victims, rescuers, persecutors, and so on are highlighted and parents engaged to develop competence in coping with their lives and in managing their children.

In summary, game therapy can be used to help families of children in placement to broaden and clarify their perspectives on their world. This involves illustrating how a child's and family's behaviors fit in with consequences. Game therapy makes *covert* beliefs, feelings, and behavioral cycles of a child and his or family *overt*. "Cast Adrift" and "Heading Home" presents a child's and family's situation in a visual and kinesthetic mode and highlights choices between alternatives of beliefs and behaviors. By presenting maladaptive behaviors in a way that a child or parent will find unacceptable (after Papp, 1981), family members will be inclined to experiment with more adaptive behaviors and to take responsibility for their choices. For the child in placement, game therapy can facilitate moving on with the terribly difficult task of coping with grief, return to the child's family, or reattachment to a new family (Kagan, 1982).

REFERENCES

Ausloos, G. (1978, October). *Delinquency and family dynamics*. Paper presented at the International Psycho-Education Seminar, Paris.

Blake, R.R. and Mouton, J.S. (1976). *Consultation*. Reading, MA: Addison-Wesley.

Block, N.M. (1981). Toward reducing recidivism in foster care. *Child Welfare*, *60*, 597–610.

Bowlby, J. (1960). Grief and mourning in infancy and early childhood. In R.S. Eissler, A. Freud, H. Hartmann, and M. Kris (Eds.), *Psychoanalytic Study of the Child*, Vol. 15, New York: International Universities Press.

Dreikurs, R. and Soltz, V. (1964). *Children: The challenge.* New York: Hawthorn.

Finkelstein, N.E. (1980). Family centered group care. *Child Welfare, 59,* 33–41.

Fogarty, T.F. (1977). Operating principles. *The Family, 5,* 35–42.

Gardner, R.A. (1971). *Therapeutic communication with children.* New York: Aronson.

Gardner, R.A. (1975). *Psychotherapeutic approaches to the resistant child.* New York: Aronson.

Grimm (1980). *The complete Grimm's fairy tales.* New York: Pantheon.

Haley, J. (1973). *Uncommon therapy, the psychiatric techniques of Milton H. Erickson, M.D.* New York: Norton.

Jewett, C. (1978). *Adopting the older child.* Harvard, MA: Harvard Common Press.

Kagan, R.M. (1980). Using redefinition and paradox with children in placement who provoke rejection. *Child Welfare, 59,* 551–559.

Kagan, R.M. (1982). Storytelling and game therapy for children in placement. *Child Care Quarterly, 11,* 280–290.

Kagan, R.M. (1983). Engaging family competence to prevent repetitive and lengthy institutionalization of acting-out youth. *Residential Group Care and Treatment, 1,* 55–70.

Karpman, S. (1968). Script drama analysis. *Transactional Analysis Bulletin, 26,* 39–43.

Kessler, J. (1966). *Psychopathology of childhood.* Englewood Cliffs, NJ: Prentice Hall.

Klein, A.F. (1975). *The professional child care worker. A guide to skills, knowledge, techniques, and attitudes.* New York: Association Press.

Madanes, C. (1980). *Strategic family therapy.* New York: McGraw-Hill.

Moss, S.Z. and Moss, M.S. (1984). Threat to place a child. *American Journal of Orthopsychiatry, 54,* 168–173.

Nichols, M. (1984). *Family therapy concepts and methods.* New York. Gardner.

Papp, P. (1981). Paradoxes. In S. Minuchin, & H.C. Fishman (Eds.), *Family therapy techniques.* Cambridge, MA: Harvard University Press.

Thomas, C.B. (1967). The resolution of object loss following foster home placement. *Smith College Studies in Social Work, 37,* 163–234.

Uhlig, R.H., Plumer, E.H., Galasy, J.R., Ballard, G., and Henley, H.C. (1977). *Basic training course for residential child care workers*. Washington, DC: Children's Bureau, Office of Child Development, Department of Health, Education and Welfare.

Watzlawick, P.W., Weakland, J.H., and Fisch, R. (1974). *Change*. New York: Norton.

Wicks-Nelson, R. and Israel, A.C. (1984). *Behavior disorders of childhood*. Englewood Cliffs, NJ: Prentice-Hall.

CHAPTER 4

Techniques of Kinetic Psychotherapy

ROBERT S. SCHACHTER

Kinetic psychotherapy (KPT) is a form of group therapy designed for children who have difficulty identifying and verbalizing feelings. As previously described (Schachter, 1974, 1984), it has been used to treat a range of adjustment difficulties and depression in children, and as a useful tool for family therapy (Schachter, 1978). This approach uses as its base a series of physical interactive games which are similar to sport games or recreational activities, such as the child's game of "dodgeball" or "keep-away." Each game is modified to facilitate interaction and mimic in "feeling tone" real-life situations. As the child plays, the therapist can observe behaviors which occur in life situations and can intervene by helping the child learn more adaptive coping mechanisms. He or she can also explore associations to psychodynamic material which underly the behavior.

In the game, three things occur. First, the child begins to experience certain emotional reactions. These appear to be projected into the game rather than being produced by it. Second, the child, by resorting to his or her particular manner of "coping," displays his or her characteristic response pattern to the therapist. Third, the participant associates to previous situations that had evoked similar feelings, thereby freeing associations and lessening defenses and anxiety.

During the activity, when a youngster begins to exhibit signs of anger, fear, joy, or sadness, the game is stopped and the group is used to help him or her to verbalize the feelings experienced and learn effective and acceptable means of responding to them. As a result of group feedback, the child can experiment with, and select from, alternative ways of coping with emotional reactions and thus gain mastery. Behavioral changes are noted with increasing verbalization, usually within a total treatment time of six to nine months.

An interpersonal group discussion follows the activity period. This approach has proven to be effective with youngsters who are nonpsychotic but have a range of symptomatic problems ranging from being overly aggressive and bullying to being overly passive and scapegoated. Also, children who have secondary overlay to learning problems appear to benefit.

The goals of KPT are similar to those of traditional approaches with children. These are to help the child experience catharsis, insight, enhanced self-esteem, testing of reality, and development of mechanisms for sublimating, coping, organizing, and dealing with situations in school interactions in order to achieve behavioral change with peers, family, and school personnel. Additional goals are: to encourage the individual to take responsibility for him or herself and the consequences of his or her actions, to encourage him or her to become aware of how and what he or she is feeling and how he or she is responding to these, and to encourage active rather than passive dealings with life situations. The use of physical activity appears to have an effect of lowering anxiety and defenses while providing a shared activity. Because every action in the game is undeniable and characteristic of real-life behavior, a child can be confronted with the consequences of his or her actions by the group, and therefore must take responsibility for the act.

Theoretical Bases

Theoretically, KPT incorporates the principles of three schools of thought—existentialism, behaviorism, and psychoanalysis. With the KPT approach, the psychodynamics of the individual child is constantly considered in understanding his or her actions. The defenses are completely respected at all times, the therapist *never* pushing past them to provoke catharsis or any other psychological phenomenon.

The existential focus lies in regarding behavior in the therapy session as characteristic of behavior in life. In KPT, the child can be helped to function more effectively in the world by being helped to become aware of his or her feelings and learn a range of responses more adaptive than those he or she presently uses. A primary reason for the rapidly occurring behavioral changes is the opportunity to test and experience new behavior patterns through interaction with other children. An outlet for specific emotions through activities is provided by KPT, which also helps the child learn and experience new mechanisms for dealing with those emotions. The result is the child's discovery that he or she will be able to face and cope with real situations about which he or she is angry, sad, or happy, the next time they arise in life.

Behaviorist theory explains the persistence of the new behavioral patterns which are reinforced by the therapist and members of the group. By helping the child experience a range of proadaptive behaviors, discrimination learning allows the child to select those which are responded to by the group. A child who initially is passive and given to "whining" will be responded to more positively by peers when he or she asserts him or herself in an appropriate manner. Likewise, the child who behaves more responsibly at home will be treated more positively by the parents. Because these responses are gratifying, the child continues the behavior that evokes them. Adjunctive family therapy is useful here to integrate communication skills learned in the group into the family setting.

Psychoanalytic theory is considered in assessing the individual's defensive structure as well as helping him or her broaden his or her repertoire of ego skills. Since the major focus in KPT is to help the youngster adapt more effectively, it is considered an ego therapy.

KPT Compared to Other Group Therapy Approaches

Slavson (Slavson, 1952; Slavson & Schiffer, 1975) pioneered the field of activity group therapy for latency-aged children. While carefully considering the psychodynamics of the individual and the group, he used arts and crafts, woodworking, and other creative activities to provide a base on which children can freely act out their characteristic role responses in life. Participants learn alternative styles from one another while the therapist is a totally accepting bystander. A refreshment period follows the activity.

Ginott (1961, 1965) used an abundance of toys and a playroom as media for his play-group therapy with children. He differs from Slavson in advocating the setting of firm limits. His basic view is that children will modify their behavior in exchange for adult acceptance.

Axline (1947) applied nondirective therapy to groups of youngsters. By reflecting back statements made by the children, the therapist provides an atmosphere of complete acceptance, while limits are set as they appear appropriate. Toys and the playroom are the primary media.

The group play therapy techniques previously described offer opportunities for the projection of feelings onto fantasy situations, played out with dolls, toys, and other tools. Thus, hostility toward a rivalrous sibling may be projected and displaced onto toys, dolls, and puppets, permitting the child to experience catharsis without feeling threatened. Opportunities also exist for strengthening other ego functions.

These approaches have proved to be extremely valuable and effective techniques in child psychotherapy. As a major tool KPT similarly utilizes the child's projections, but differs from other forms of group play-therapy in that the projections are directed onto real life, interactive game experiences rather than onto fantasy situations. Once latency is entered, reality and learning the skills of dealing with reality become the focus of development, with less use of fantasy than at an earlier age. The KPT games used are designed to permit displacement, sublimation, catharsis, esteem-enhancement, and learning of ego-skills in general, and appear to fit the needs of the latency-aged child. The benefit of this approach, if the child can tolerate the experience, is that emotional responses in a real-life situation can be worked through to resolution. As a result, the skills acquired in a KPT session can be directly tested and used in the outside environment; in turn, positive feedback from the "real-life" arena helps encourage and perpetuate the child's progress.

Another obvious advantage is that the therapist can observe the youngster's responses and interactions with other children, as they normally occur in school and at home. This author has found that most nonpsychotic children easily tolerate intensity levels reached in KPT, because the games used simulate those played during recess or gym periods at school.

Because a child is never forced past his or her defenses, the child can always control his or her affective participation and set his or her own therapeutic pace. When the child feels trusting and safe enough to express his or her feelings, he or she is taught the skills to do so.

THE GROUPS

The groups consist of four to six participants and are carefully constructed to allow a balance of personality types. An average group consists of two aggressive children, two passive ones, and two neutral children, as prescribed by Slavson (Slavson, 1952; Slavson & Schiffer, 1975). In this way, a modeling procedure occurs, whereby a passive child can learn more aggressive behavior from an aggressive one and vice versa. Each member is carefully evaluated before placement, and the groups are formed on a open-ended basis. The average length of treatment is usually six to nine months.

THE ACTIVITIES OF KPT

The activities may arouse a range of emotional responses experienced in real-life situations. *Keepaway* is a modified game similar to the prank of taking another's hat and keeping it away from him or her. Another type of game, *Freeze Tag*, provides a base for feelings of comradeship and sharing: An antagonist, usually the therapist, attempts to tag the participants with a soft plastic ball; when they are hit, they must "freeze" until a team member tags them by hand, thus freeing them. In this activity, a child can request and obtain help as well as give it. Aggressive games are also included, such as *Bombardment* in which the participants throw harmless soft plastic balls at each other, while another entails fending for oneself; in the latter variation there is no place to hide and feelings of isolation often surface.

A fascinating element of this process appears to be that the games do not manufacture the feelings, but as mentioned previously, serve as a screen onto which those that the child is carrying with him or her can be projected. Thus, five different youngsters may have five different reactions to the same game. In *Freeze Tag*, for example, one child may get angry, another may feel exhilarated, and experience a sense of belonging, while yet another may feel isolated and lonely. Usually, emotions most recently experienced outside the group situation will emerge in a game. As the child is taught how these can be dealt with in the game setting, he or she develops the ability to talk about the outside situations and his or her responses to them, and can learn more effective ways of dealing with them. This is a relatively rapid process. The first month of treatment is usually characterized by the participants testing limits, exploring each other and the game situation, and getting acquainted with the therapist. Alternative means of expression, primarily the skills of verbalizing emotions, are acquired during the second and third months.

The following case illustration shows the more or less rapidly changing response pattern in KPT.

Case Illustration

Two separate interactions between the same two children occurring at two different stages in treatment are described. The first interaction occurred after Steven, the primary participant, had been treated for one month. The second episode took place three months after the start of therapy.

Steven is one of a group of six 11-year-old boys meeting once weekly for 1½ hours. He had been referred by his school administration because of consistently aggressive behavior toward other children and defiance toward his teacher. His parents are recently divorced and he misses his father who no longer lives with him.

When admitted to therapy, Steven had been angry about his home situation and did not know what to do with his anger. Comprehensive evaluation revealed that this represented an "acting out" response to a depression which had emerged at the time of his parent's separation two years earlier. The primary goal of treatment was to help him learn to express anger in a constructive manner and to complete the grieving process for the loss of his accustomed family unit.

Session Four at One Month of Treatment.

The game *Team Bombardment* is being played. Its rules require that players at opposite sides of the room throw balls at each other and that, when a participant is hit five times, he is "out." This procedure is followed until all members of one team are "out." The game involves interdependancy among team members as well as individual competition.

Steven and Mark are on opposite teams; both are vigorously involved in the game, ducking, weaving and throwing balls. While Steven is bending down to recover a ball, Mark catches him off-guard and hits him. Steven stands up grimacing and begins to run toward Mark with raised fists as if to hit him. This type of behavior is Steven's typical response whenever he becomes angry at other children. The following interaction occurs:

THERAPIST: "Time out! Everybody stop. Steven wait a minute. You can't hit here! If you want, you can tell him what you feel."

STEVEN: "I'll get him, I'll get him! He hit me when I wasn't looking."

THERAPIST: "I know, but you can't hit here. That's one of the rules. Do you want to tell him how you feel and try to work it out?"

STEVEN: "No."

THERAPIST: "That's okay. You don't have to if you don't want to. There are other things you can do besides hit, however."

At this point, it is apparent to the therapist that Steven is resistant to verbalizing the feeling, and so he does not push the situation. When possible, the therapist wants to encourage a direct interaction between participants; however, in this case this is not advisable. Therefore, the therapist calls for a rest and begins a group discussion around the situation. From the beginning of treatment, the children are advised that half the time is spent playing and the other half is spent talking and the therapist can call talking times whenever he or she wants to, but these will not exceed 50 percent of the time. With latency aged children and younger, this issue is usually accepted. In any case, at this point in the group, the therapist wants to explore with the group what options are available when someone feels the way Steven must feel. It may be noted that the therapist has not attempted to tell Steven what he is feeling but gives the group a chance to explore the issue. If this is not discussed, Steven will probably attempt to hit Mark at a later time. Here, however, Steven is given a chance to vicariously ventilate some of the anger as well as begin to learn an alternative to his usual style of dealing with this situation which generally gets him in trouble.

THERAPIST: "How do you think Steven feels? Have any of you ever felt that way?"

GROUP MEMBERS: "He probably is mad. I felt that way today in school. . . ."

The discussion would go on without demanding direct participation of Steven. Mark would have a chance to speak about how the interaction affected him, while Steven would see that other children get angry also and that this feeling does not have to be dangerous.

Depending on the involvement of the group in discussing the issue of anger, the discussion may continue or another game might be played.

Generally, at the beginning phase of treatment, discussions are short, lasting 5 to 15 minutes. The same procedure of stopping the action is invoked any time it appears that a participant is experiencing a feeling. The result is to encourage the expression of these, and to help the children become familiar with emotions and learn to express them. As they gain mastery in this area, the participants appear to feel comfortable in stopping and do so spontaneously.

Session Twelve at Three Months.

Another game called *Keepaway* is being played. In this activity, a ball is passed around a circle of participants while it is kept away from the one who is in the middle. When the person in the middle gets the ball, the person who touched it last goes to the middle. The game continues until each has had a turn in the center. Soon after the game begins, Steven is in the middle of the circle, and another boy is teasing him with the ball, poking it at him and then taking it away. Steven starts to grimace.

THERAPIST: "Time out. Steven, what's going on?"

STEVEN: "He made me mad."

THERAPIST: "Do you want to tell him?" (setting up a direct confrontation between the boys)

STEVEN: (to other members of group) "You made me mad."

THERAPIST: "Would you tell him a little louder?"

STEVEN: "You made me MAD."

THERAPIST: "Okay, tell him once more, really loud."

STEVEN: "YOU MADE ME MAD!"

(At this point Steven is shouting and appears completely connected with the affect. The effect is one of catharsis. He was ready to experience this; otherwise, he would not have reached this level of intensity, even with encouragement.)

THERAPIST: (to other boy) "Do you know what he's mad about?"

OTHER BOY: "No."

THERAPIST: "Would you ask him?"

OTHER BOY: "What are you mad about?"

STEVEN: "You're poking the ball at me. That's not fair!"

OTHER BOY: "So, that's part of the game."

(This youngster is a child who has a problem with teasing other children, and is using his characteristic response in this situation.)

THERAPIST: "Well, can you understand why that would get Steven mad?"

OTHER BOY: "Yes."

THERAPIST: "Did you want to get him mad?"

OTHER BOY: "No."

THERAPIST: "So if you know that this gets him mad, is there anything you can do differently?"

OTHER BOY: "Yes, I can stop teasing him."

THERAPIST: "Are you willing to do that?"

OTHER BOY: "Yes."

THERAPIST: (to Steven) "What do you feel now?"

STEVEN: "I feel okay."

THERAPIST: (to other boy) "What were you trying to say by teasing Steven?"

OTHER BOY: "I don't know . . . that I wanted to get the ball more."

THERAPIST: "I see. Well, let's see if there's another way to ask for that without getting him mad. Does anybody have ideas about that?"

GROUP MEMBERS: "Maybe, he could just say, 'pass the ball to me or something'"

THERAPIST: "If he said that, would you pass him the ball?"

GROUP MEMBERS: "Yes."

THERAPIST: (to other boy) "Would you be willing to try that?"

OTHER BOY: "Yes."

THERAPIST: "Okay, let's keep playing."

The teasing behavior on the part of the other boy is a statement. His manner of expressing it, however, alienates Steven. By allowing Steven to confront him, the other boy is immediately faced with the consequences of his behavior, while allowing him to learn more adaptive responses. The game continues and after another 5 or 10 minutes, a group discussion is begun.

THERAPIST: "What kind of feelings did people have in the game?"

STEVEN: "I was mad."

THERAPIST: "When else do you feel mad like that? You said it was not fair."

STEVEN: "I felt that way today. My mother yelled at me for knocking over a glass of milk. I didn't even do it, and she wouldn't listen to me. My little brother did it."

THERAPIST: "You got blamed for something you didn't do?"

STEVEN: "Yeah. That happens all the time, it's not fair and it gets me mad . . . real mad."

THERAPIST: "What do you do when you're mad like that?"

STEVEN: "I try to get my mother mad , or I break something."

THERAPIST: "Does this happen to anyone else in the group?"

OTHER MEMBERS: "Yes . . . "

The discussion goes on with members sharing their experiences and talking about alternative ways of handling situations like the one Steven described.

Discussion

This session is significant in several ways. It is the first meeting in which Steven is able to verbalize a feeling with appropriate affect. Previously he would stop before he reached the level of intensity described previously. Second, a direct interaction is established between Steven and the other boy. Steven could verbalize his anger and experientially find that neither he nor the other child is destroyed. Third, he is then able to talk about the situation which had been bothering him since early in the day, and he has an outlet for his pent-up emotions. Fourth, by discussing this with peers, he can find that he is not alone in this type of problem and can find alternative solutions. These issues of being treated unfairly were later addressed by him in a family therapy meeting. Meanwhile, the other boy mentioned has an opportunity to learn from peers a more adaptive way to say he wants to be included. He then has a chance to try their suggestions in the game until he finds a way that works best for him.

With Steven, learning to constructively express anger was a primary goal; however, by no means is this the only feeling explored in KPT. Joy, fear, sadness, and the full range of emotions are dealt with as they come up. Most sessions have a number of interactions similar to that described with each of the participants.

Steven's treatment lasted nine months and consisted of weekly KPT meetings with adjunctive family therapy twice monthly. At the time of termination, his behavior in school and at home had changed dramatically. His mother reported that he seemed happier, was playing every day with children, and talked about things that bothered him rather than act out his discontent. Grades in school improved significantly, and his teacher reported that he had not been engaged in a fight over the last month. Periodic (once a month or two months) family therapy continued for five months after the end of group treatment. Follow-up two years later indicated continued success.

The children who most appear to benefit from this approach are non-psychotic and range in behavior from being overly aggressive to being overly passive and scapegoated. Youngsters with adjustment reactions, behavior disorders, phobic reactions, immature and withdrawn behavior, or emotional overlay secondary to learning disabilities show impressive improvement as do normal children who need to learn basic verbal and social skills.

RESEARCH

Two studies have been undertaken to assess the effectiveness of KPT. The first was a nonexperimental, retroactive look at the patients treated over a two year period at a private clinic by the author. Of these 90 cases, approximately 80 percent showed remission of presenting problems with no substitution symptoms within a treatment time of nine months. Follow-up 1½ years later showed a 10 percent regression rate. Treatment consisted of weekly KPT sessions with monthly family therapy meetings. Since no control group was considered nor was the sample randomly selected, these results can only serve as a gross measure of the effectiveness of this treatment.

The second study was of orthodox experimental design involving elementary school-aged boys. A random sample of youngsters from three grades—first, third, and sixth—were randomly assigned to a no-treatment control group and an experimental group. The experimental group received six weeks of twice weekly KPT sessions in school. Pre- and posttesting was performed to assess differences due to treatment. Results of a teacher rating scale indicated that statistical significance was attained on a measure of self-esteem with the experimental showing higher self-esteem after the treatment period. Additionally, a cluster of behaviors characterized by "poor classroom behavior" showed improvement which approached statistical significance with the experimental groups. A behavioral observation indicated a positive change in poor lunchroom behavior in the experimental group. First graders showed greater gains than others.

SUMMARY AND CONCLUSIONS

The process of KPT has proven useful in helping children with a range of symptoms learn more adaptive behavioral responses. The technique consists of involving the participant in a series of games which resemble real-life situations, observing characteristic responses, and helping the child learn alternatives by means of a structured experiential situation. The activity period is followed by an interpersonal verbal interchange in which associations are freed up and defenses are lowered. Kinetic psychotherapy is not a psychotherapeutic panacea and obviously, not all cases are as clear cut as the example; however, from this illustration one can get a sense of a useful alternative approach to therapeutic work with children.

REFERENCES

Axline, V. (1947). *Play therapy*. Boston: Houghton Mifflin.

Ginnot, H. (1961). *Group psychotherapy with children*. New York: McGraw-Hill.

Ginnot, H. (1965). Group therapy with children. In G. Gazda (Ed.), *Basic approaches to group psychotherapy and group counseling*. Springfield, IL: Thomas.

Schachter, R.S. (1974). Kinetic psychotherapy in treatment of children. *American Journal of Psychotherapy*. 28, 430–437.

Schachter, R.S. (1978). Kinetic psychotherapy in the treatment of families. *Family Coordinator*. 283–288.

Schachter, R.S. (1984). Kinetic psychotherapy in the treatment of depression in latency age children. *International Journal of Group Psychotherapy, 34*(1), 83–91.

Slavson, S.R. (1952). *Child psychotherapy*. New York: Columbia.

Slavson, S.R. and Schiffer, M. (1975). *Group psychotherapies for children*. New York: International Universities Press.

T W O
Problem-Solving Games

Many popular games require strategy and logical decision-making. These types of games reward rational thinking by surrounding it in an atmosphere of enjoyment and challenge. Good strategy is usually met with improvement of a player's position, moving him or her closer to the goal of winning. Making a game of the process of logical thinking and problem-solving is the basic premise that underlies the games described in this section. In recent years, a number of original therapeutic games have been developed to help individuals deal with specific problems, such as divorce, dysfunctional family communication, academic underachievement, and hyperactivity. Other games have been developed, as presented in the chapters by Bedford and Behrens, that focus on improving general problem-solving skills.

Problem-solving games tend to be highly structured, cognitively oriented activities that nevertheless retain the basic elements of games: pleasure, competition, rules, challenge to perform well and win, pretense, and interpersonal interaction. The trend among newer games is to incorporate behavioral strategies to provide incentives for participation and involvement in the problem-solving process. While the chapters in this section describe therapeutic game-play for a limited range of psychological problems, it is evident that the games are flexible enough to be adapted to a wide range of problems and situations.

CHAPTER 5

The Changing Family Game: Cognitive-Behavioral Intervention for Children of Divorce

BERTHOLD BERG

Cognitive-behavioral modification has in recent years been among the most innovative psychotherapeutic interventions. It is an intervention strategy that recognizes that behavioral change often demands cognitive change; how we interpret events largely shapes our reaction to them. Also, practicing or rehearsing a new response to a problem situation prepares one to implement the behavior and further increases the probability that the behavior will meet with success.

Applications of these cognitive-behavioral principles to the problems of children are increasing. To cite only a few applications, cognitive-behavioral methods have been applied to problems of conduct disorders (DiGiuseppe, 1983), frustration tolerance (Knaus, 1983), impulsiveness (Kendall and Fischler, 1983), underachievement (Bard and Fisher, 1983), and anxieties, fears, and phobias (Grieger and Boyd, 1983) to name only a few.

The *Changing Family Game* (Berg, 1982) is an application of cognitive-behavioral principles in helping children cope with divorce. Utilizing a boardgame format, intervention entails both cognitive restructuring and behavioral rehearsal in the nontrivial pursuit of divorce related problem solving. Some 300 cards, representing divorce related problems in eight major areas, constitute the core of the game. In moving from start to finish, players respond to cards representing these problem areas and are awarded tokens for adequate responses.

DESCRIPTION OF THE GAME

The *Changing Family Game* represents the therapeutic culmination of the author's earlier work in assessing the problematical attitudes of children experiencing parental divorce. The children's separation inventory (included with the game) is itself the product of an earlier version (Berg, 1979; Kelly and Berg, 1978) and was found to be both reliable and valid as an instrument measuring children's divorce related problem attitudes (Berg, 1980; Kurdek and Berg, 1983).

It would be profitable to devote some space to the nature of these problem attitudes because they, in addition to problems associated with single parenting and visitation, form the core of the therapeutic intervention, that is, the game. A sample question from the questionnaire and a sample card from the game follows each of these descriptions.

Peer Ridicule and Avoidance

Children may view parental separation and divorce as a stigma that reflects on themselves. To feel oneself different from peers may constitute a significant source of stress. Children may therefore seek to hide the fact of separation or divorce from their peers, limiting their interaction with potentially supporting friends in fear lest the secret be discovered.

Question

I like talking to my friends as much now as I used to ... Yes   No

Card

Terry used to walk to school with one of his friends. Now he goes to school alone because he doesn't want to talk to his friend about his parents' divorce. How is Terry feeling? What advice would you give Terry?

Paternal Blame

A mature attitude toward divorce is that neither husband nor wife is alone entirely responsible for the events leading to separation; both parties in subtle or obvious ways contributed to marital disruption. It has been found that children very often—and often their parents as well—do not hold such a view, but tend to place blame exclusively on one parent. In instances of paternal blame, father is blamed for the divorce specifically and often seen as a "bad" person generally. Such an attitude can be expected to interfere with the father-child relationship and hamper identification with the father.

Question

When my family was unhappy it was usually because of something my father said or did .... Yes   No

Card

Sara knows that her father was the first person to talk to a lawyer about the divorce. That's why she knows that the divorce was entirely her father's fault. How is Sara feeling? What advice would you give her?

Maternal Blame

This attitude is the same as paternal blame, with the difference that the divorce is attributed to the mother along with a negative evaluation generally.

Question

If my mother were a nicer person my parents would still be living together .... Yes   No

Card

Nick is certain the divorce was entirely his mother's fault. Whenever his father would come home from work his mother would start to nag him. Finally Nick's father decided to move out of the house. How is Nick feeling? Pick the best ending to the story.

1. Nick talks to his father and asks if there is anything he can do to get back at his mother.

    2.   Nick talks to both his mother and father about his feelings and discovers the divorce was neither parent's fault, but happened because both were unhappy living together.

    3.   Nick refuses to talk to his mother and begins to misbehave at home.

    4.   Nick starts to do poorly at school to teach his mother a lesson.

Self Blame

Children sometimes feel that if they had been better behaved, or never born, their parents would still be living together. Children may perceive that their misbehavior led to marital arguments and ultimately to marital separation. While such an attitude is most prominent in the egocentric constructions of younger children, it is sometimes also seen in older children.

Question

My parents probably argue more when I'm with them than when I'm gone .... Yes   No

Card

Rick notices that very often his parents got into arguments with each other over his behavior. Then his parents got a divorce. He figures that it must have been his fault that his parents got a divorce. How is Rick feeling? Pick the best ending to the story.

    1.   He apologizes to his parents for his bad behavior and promises never to misbehave again if his parents get back together.

    2.   He blames his misbehavior on his sister and so tries to get his parents to blame her.

    3.   He decides to run away from home so his parents could get back together again.

    4.   He talks to his parents about how he feels and they tell him that they used to argue about almost everything, not just him, and that the divorce was not his fault.

Fear of Abandonment

Separation and divorce generally force children to reconcile themselves to life with one parent and occasional visits with the other. It is not usual for children to catastrophize such a situation, feeling that they may be on the verge of being orphaned since they now have only "one" parent, thus doubling the chances of being left alone in the event of death. Perhaps more prominent is the fear of psychological abandonment. Through the divorce, the child has learned that people can fall out of love and go their separate ways. If parents can stop loving each other, can they not also stop loving their children? The insecurity inherent in such an attitude can be expected to underlie substantial anxiety.

Question

I know there will always be someone to take care of me ....
Yes   No

Card

Heather's parents got divorced because her mother stopped loving her father. She wonders whether parents could also stop loving their children. What would happen then? How is Heather feeling? Suppose Heather said, "Mom, you stopped loving Dad. I'm worried that you might stop loving me too." What might her mother say?

Hopes of Reunification

Children may not be fully reconciled to the typical finality of divorce. They may come to hope fruitlessly that their parents will one day come back together again. Some may even feel that becoming sick, or getting into trouble, may hasten such a reconciliation. Such an attitude can only lead to pervasive disappointment, and seriously undermine the acceptance of any parent substitute who might otherwise be a source of support.

Question

My parents will probably see that they have made a mistake and get back together again .... Yes   No

Card

Almost whenever Judy and her mother are together Judy will ask, "When are you and Daddy getting back together again?" She figures that if she reminds her mother enough, she'll ask her father to come back. How is Judy feeling? Suppose Judy said, "Mom, what would I have to do to get you and Dad back together again?" What might her mother say?

Two other areas of adjustment problems are *single parenting* and *visitation*. The game allows children to address several problems associated with single parenting, such as learning to cope with diminished financial resources, lessened leisure time and increased responsibility, and discipline. Children can also address problems associated with visitation, such as cancellations and unpredictability, boredom, competition with stepsibs, and parental hostilities surrounding visitation. As with the problematical attitudes, children are encouraged to cope with these problems through cognitive restructuring and behavioral rehearsal. Examples of such cards follow.

Single Parenting Cards

There have been a lot of changes since Melissa's parents separated. The biggest change is that her mother now has to work full-time and isn't with Melissa as much as she used to be. How is Melissa feeling? Suppose she said, "Mom, I miss not spending as much time with you as I used to. Maybe you could quit work or something." What might Melissa's mother say?

Visitation Cards

Ed likes to visit with his father but his parents are something else when he gets picked up. The minute his father walks in the door his parents start calling each other names. How is Ed feeling? What advice would you give Ed?

The description of these various problem attitudes and situations related to divorce suggest some important features of the game. Foremost is the integration of assessment and intervention. The identification of problem attitudes as measured by the *Children's Separation Inventory* (norms are provided in the manual accompanying the instrument) allows the counselor to "stack the deck," placing at the top those cards that are more representative of the problem attitudes of the child(ren) playing the game (identification of single parenting and visitation issues is best made through information provided by the parent(s)). Other features of the game include: (1) variation in card format to facilitate either cognitive restructuring or behavioral rehearsal; (2) can be played by individuals aged five to adult; (3) can be played individually with the child or in groups of up to six players; (4) can be played with children and their parents conjointly; (5) can be played within strict time limits; (6) can be played with children whose parents have not separated, either to sensitize them to the problems of their peers or to prepare them for parental separation should it occur; (7) can be further individualized by typing unique problem situations on blank cards included with the game and adding these to the deck; (8) can be adapted to mother, father, or joint custody arrangements by selection of the appropriate cards; (9) can be used effectively with children reluctant to discuss divorce related concerns directly, as well as for children who need greater focus in divorce related problem solving; (10) can be played with maximum effectiveness by reference to the extensive manual accompanying the game; (11) can facilitate group discussion since all players are rewarded for listening and making unique contributions; (12) can be played over a period of sessions without loss of variety, and with the maintenance of continuity, through the use of over 300 different cards; and (13) can be used as the exclusive method of divorce intervention or in conjunction with other methods.

The design of the board and structure of the game is a recapitulation of the divorce process, beginning with marital problems as perceived by the child and ending with coping in blended families. The six circles successively entered depending on where the child's adjustment problems lie—are *Family Troubles, Told of Separation, Parent Moves Out, Life With Mother, Life With Father, Life With Different Families.* (See Figure 5.1.)

The six problem attitudes and the problems associated with single parenting and visitation are distributed (although not in all) among these six stages of the divorce cycle. The counselor can determine which circle(s) are to be entered both from the point of view of where the most salient problem attitude cards are located and the particular stage of the divorce

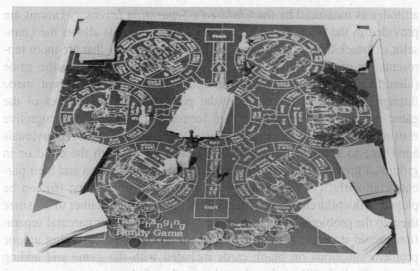

Figure 5.1. *The Changing Family Game.*

process that the child's family is at (although work in circles representing a previous stage might help the child to deal with some unresolved problems, or in working in a future stage, prepare for and perhaps prevent problems by working in a circle representing a stage not yet entered).

The inner circle, traversed throughout the game, contains cards dealing with questions unrelated to divorce in order to allow for humor and greater self-expression generally (e.g., Tell us something that happened to you that made you feel appreciated; Throw this card in the air. If it lands right side up take two chips of any color from the bank; and What is your favorite subject in school? Why?).

Players are awarded plastic tokens for their appropriate responses to the cards, as well as listening to and repeating or elaborating on the response of another player. The winner of the game is the player with the most tokens at the end of a designated time period, or when the first player reaches "finish."

Various rules of the game are intended to maximize the impact of the game. The rule that a player may not exit a circle until having accumulated a specific number of chips in the color appropriate to that circle assures maximum exposure to the issues associated with that area. The rule that the player, before exiting a circle, summarize some problems and solutions of the families at that stage of divorce process further maximizes integration of problems and solutions, and may further identify those issues most salient to the child. Other rules of the game are present to bring chance and strategic elements into the game (e.g., a player may win or lose chips to the bank with the spin of a spinner, give or take chips from a neighboring player by landing on a square so indicating, or by landing on a square already occupied). Strategic or competive elements (admittedly very minor from an adult's point of view) are also provided for in the rules; a player may select a chip of a particular color that will retard his or her opponent's, and enhance his or her own, race to the finish line. Seemingly minor details such as these have proven themselves through trial and error to foster considerable interest in playing the game over a period of time.

THERAPEUTIC GUIDELINES

The core therapeutic elements of the game as discussed earlier are behavioral rehearsal and cognitive restructuring. Behavioral rehearsal is embodied primarily in those cards that quote a child's response to a significant other, and asks the player to play out how the other might respond. It is expected that such an exercise is preparatory for a similar statement to an analogous situation in real life. Furthermore, the other's response—often through coaching and selective reinforcement from the counselor—is expected to be of a positive, sympathetic nature so as to lead to a positive expectation for the outcome.

Cognitive restructuring is facilitated primarily through the advice format cards. In advising a fictitious child of a better or more adaptive attitude toward a problem—again, through coaching and selective reinforcement of the adaptive elements of the child's initial response—it is expected that children will apply similar corrective attitudes toward problems of their own.

While it would be impossible to suggest "good" responses to each card of the game, some general therapeutic guidelines can be given (taken from the manual accompanying the game), as follows:

1. *Encourage an increase in divorce-related communication between parent and child.* Following divorce, many children are reluc-

tant to discuss divorce related concerns with their parents and thereby tend to have their misconceptions perpetuated. Seeking clarification would be a valuable therapeutic goal.

2.   *Encourage disengagement from parental conflict.*   Children are often asked to take sides against the other parent. This represents a "no win" situation for the child since to take sides only fosters guilt and anxiety. Children should be encouraged to see parental conflict as something they can do nothing to change and to disengage from it. The child should not attempt to cope with husband-wife issues generally, but limit himself or herself to parent-child issues.

3.   *Enable the child to recognize that his or her parents are themselves having to cope with much divorce related stress and are therefore often unable to act reasonably and/or attend fully to the child's needs.*

4.   *Encourage tolerance of individual reactions to the divorce.* Children are often angered or distressed that others, particularly siblings, have a different view than their own. People have a right to their individual opinion, based on their unique experiences.

5.   *A child's fears of abandonment should be addressed by stressing that a parent's love for a child is different than the kind of love adults have for each other.*   A parent's love for a child continues, even though it may be difficult to express around the time of divorce. Also, parents don't just leave their children on their own; there will always be someone to care for them.

6.   *A child's fear of peer ridicule and avoidance should be addressed by noting that divorce is a very common experience today.* Over a million children a year are affected by divorce. It is important to encourage an increase in interaction with peers rather than avoidance.

7.   *Children with hope of reunification should be encouraged to abandon such an idea.*   It is an attitude that significantly interferes with adjustment to changed living circumstances and the acceptance of other intimate relationships that parents may develop. In any case, children are

typically incapable of undoing their parents' choice to divorce, and to wish otherwise, or to act in ways thought to realize such a wish, can do nothing but assure the child's frustration.

8. *Children prone to self blame must come to learn that neither their presence nor behavior caused the divorce.* It is not uncommon for a child's misbehavior to lead to marital arguments. Where there are differences of opinion regarding childrearing, and where the marital relationship is not a good one, arguments are likely to erupt. But it is important to emphasize that it was not the child's behavior that was the cause of marital difficulties.

9. *Children must come to accept the fact that divorce is not necessarily a "bad" thing and that neither parent is exclusively responsible for it.* Maternal or paternal blame for the divorce is an attitude which interferes with the continued relationship with the blamed parent, and an attitude that carries with it the risk—because the child is the offspring of this "bad" parent—that the child will see him or herself as "bad." While it is true that divorce is rarely a mutual decision of the parents, it would be false to assign blame for the divorce based on the precipitating action of one parent. Divorce is typically the consequence of a poor spousal relationship of many years—to which both parties contributed and from which neither received sufficient reward—and not the result of one or several events which might appear most salient to the child. The child is typically not privy to all the events in the chain leading to divorce and is thus prone to erroneously attribute cause to that parent whose actions appeared most decisive. While most divorced parents come to see the divorce as a solution to a mutually unsatisfying relationship, many tend to blame the other parent exclusively and thus reinforce the child's blaming attitude. Such a blaming attitude among parents is not uncommon in the early months following separation, but tends to reflect their own anger and stress rather than reality.

Finally, it should be noted that the game serves as a stimulus for self-disclosure. While cognitive restructuring and behavioral rehearsal serve as important components of the game, the cards themselves often serve to stimulate revelations of similar real life problems. This is of course to be expected, given that the cards were selected for play largely because they bore such an analogous relationship to the child's actual circumstances. It is entirely appropriate to suspend play and to process this material (although the counselor should be alert to pressures from other players to "get on with the game").

CASE ILLUSTRATIONS

Peer Ridicule and Avoidance

Card

When Terry's friend found out that his parents had separated he asked what happened. Terry answered, "Leave me alone. I don't want to talk about it." How is Terry feeling? What advice could you give Terry?

CHILD: That it's a way to get your feelings out. And if you don't want to talk about it, it is your business.

COUNSELOR: So talking to his friend would be a way of getting his feelings out.

CHILD: Yeah.

COUNSELOR: But right now Terry doesn't want to talk about his feelings.

CHILD: Yeah.

COUNSELOR: Maybe Terry could let his friend know that he doesn't want to talk about his feelings now but might want to at another time.

Paternal Blame

Card

After an argument with his mother, Jeff's father packed his suitcase and left the house. That's why Jeff knows the divorce is all his father's fault. How is Jeff feeling? What advice would you give Jeff?

CHILD: Maybe like his mother was yelling at him and that's why he left. It could be both of their faults.

COUNSELOR: That's right. Even if his mother were yelling at him there were probably other times when he was yelling at her. Anyway, divorces don't happen just because of one incident, but build up over a long period of time. Usually neither parent is at fault.

Maternal Blame

Card

The way Sue figures it, when a person breaks their marriage vows like her mother did, that makes them a bad person. How is Sue feeling? What advice would you give her.

CHILD: That sometimes you can't stick by the rules. Sometimes you just have to [divorce] because your parents, well, they don't love each other anymore and they fight too much.

COUNSELOR: I think that's right. *Both* parents stopped loving each other so it's really neither one's fault.

Self Blame

Card

Tommy took for granted living with his parents. Now since they've divorced he wonders what he could have done to keep them together. How is Tommy feeling? What advice would you give Tommy?

CHILD: You can't keep them together. They were probably fighting over things and all that.

COUNSELOR: Parents get divorced because of adult things and it has nothing to do with the kids.

Fear of Abandonment

Card

Doug's mother told his father, "I never want to see you again!" What if she says that to him? What would he do? That worries Doug a lot. How is Doug feeling? What advice would you give Doug?

CHILD: She'll probably never say that.

COUNSELOR: Why not?

CHILD: It's different. Because your parents fight a lot about different things. Like many problems and all that. They wouldn't fight over him.

COUNSELOR: How is it different?

CHILD: 'Cause he's their son.

COUNSELOR: And the kind of love that parents have for their children is very different. They may get mad at their kids sometimes, but their love for them is always there. But sometimes its difficult to see that.

Hopes of Reunification

Card

Ted just knows that his parents will get back together again. He remembers they were separated before and got together again. Why should that not happen again? How is Ted feeling?

TED: "Mom, I think you and Dad will get back together again. Just like you did the last time you separated."

CHILD: Down in the dumps. He's feeling aggravated.

COUNSELOR: Why?

CHILD: He's trying to get his parents back together again. He probably thinks he can do it.

COUNSELOR (playing role of child):   Mom, I think you and Dad will get back together again. Just like you did the last time you separated.

CHILD   (playing role of parent):   No.

COUNSELOR: But you got together before.

CHILD: We had two chances together. We just couldn't stay together.

COUNSELOR: So this is for real?

CHILD: Yeah.

Single Parenting

Card

It's one thing for his mother to date, Andy thinks. But when her date stays overnight, it really makes Andy angry. How else is Andy feeling? What advice would you give Andy?

CHILD 1:   Down in the dumps.

CHILD 2:   Naughty, naughty, naughty!!

COUNSELOR: What does that mean?

CHILD 2:   It's wrong.

CHILD 1:   Well, I think he's feeling very mad because maybe he wants his privacy. And maybe the date has to sleep around him and snores and keeps him awake and the kid can't do anything.

CHILD 2:   Really, Mom does have the decision because it's her house and it's really not his. And you can't really tell her who to go out with and who not to. It's really her decision. You can try to like him. You can get together and meet each other and maybe you'll like him. I didn't like my sister's boyfriend when he was putting up a tree with us at my sister's house before they got married. And now I like him.

Visitation

Card

Rita likes to visit her father, but she feels bad because her mother looks hurt when Rita wants to spend time with him. How is Rita feeling? What advice would you give Rita?

CHILD 1:   My mom's glad I go visit my father so she can go out.

CHILD 2:   Tell her you have to be with your dad too.

CHILD 1:   Yeah, you miss him.

COUNSELOR: What could she tell her mother?

CHILD 1:   That she misses her dad and still wants to visit him.

COUNSELOR: Yeah. A lot of parents may look kind of hurt, which is real natural but deep down inside they really want their kids to have a good relationship with *both* parents. So most parents would understand if this is said in a nice way.

SUMMARY AND CONCLUSIONS

In clinical practice the *Changing Family Game* has been found to be engaging and effective in improving children's divorce related problem solving and communication. Based on a cognitive-behavioral orientation, the game utilizes cognitive restructuring and behavioral rehearsal; self-disclosure is, however, also stimulated by play of the game.

Two important features of the game are (1) the integration of assessment of divorce related problems with the intervention for those problems, thereby facilitating the optimum individualization of a therapeutic program, and (2) the safe yet therapeutic environment the game provides by not demanding personal self-disclosure unless the player wishes.

Several research studies assessing the utility of the game are under way. One very encouraging finding is that the adequacy of solutions that children offer to problems improves over game-playing sessions (Berg, Hickey, and Snyder, 1985). Through coaching and selective reinforcement of adaptive elements of children's responses, it was hypothesized that the adequacy of children's advice would improve across four game playing sessions. Responses were rated on a five-point scale by two raters blind to the session from which the response was drawn. Interrater reliability was high ($r = .81$), and adequacy of advice was found to improve across sessions ($F = 3.95, p < .01$). Another study (Snyder, 1984) found that the posttest scores on the *Children's Separation Inventory* (after three game playing sessions) correlated highly ($r = .51$) and significantly ($p < .01$) with the adequacy of their responses to the game cards; that is, children evidencing fewer problem attitudes on the *Children's Separation Inventory* gave the most adequate responses. Both these findings are important since they suggest, respectively, (1) that there is measurable improvement with play of the game and (2) that assessment of problem attitudes is important in that it is predictive of children's responses to the game cards.

   A number of research questions have yet to be addressed. (1) What is
the optimum number of game playing sessions? (2) What problem attitudes are most and least resistant to change? (3) Is improvement in divorce related problem-solving related to sex and age? and (4) To what degree and in what areas do skills acquired in playing the game generalize
to the child's own environment? This is only a partial list of questions;
readers will doubtlessly pose many more of their own.

REFERENCES

Bard, J.A. and Fisher, H.R. (1983). The rational-emotive approach to underachievement. In A. Ellis and M.E. Bernard (Eds.), *Rational-emotive ap-
   proaches to the problems of childhood* (pp. 189–210). New York: Plenum.
Berg, B. (1979). *Children's attitudes toward parent separation inventory.*
   Dayton, OH: University of Dayton Press.
Berg, B. (1980, May). *Children's attitudes toward parental separation inven-
   tory: Reliability and validity.* Paper presented at the meeting of the Mid-
   western Psychological Association, St. Louis, MO.
Berg, B. (1982). *The changing family game.* Dayton, OH: Cognitive-Behavioral
   Resources.
Berg, B., Hickey, N., and Snyder, L. (1985, May). *The changing family game:
   Efficacy of cognitive-behavioral intervention for children of divorce.* Paper
   presented at the meeting of the Midwestern Psychological Association
   meeting, Chicago, IL.
DiGiuseppe, R. (1983). Rational-Emotive therapy and conduct disorders. In A.
   Ellis and M.E. Bernard (Eds.), *Rational-emotive approaches to the prob-
   lems of childhood* (pp. 111–138). New York: Plenum.
Grieger, R.M. and Boyd, J.D. (1983). Childhood anxieties, fears and phobias.
   A cognitive-behavioral-psychosituational approach. In A. Ellis and M.E.
   Bernard (Eds.), *Rational-emotive approaches to the problems of childhood*
   (pp. 211–240). New York: Plenum.
Kelly, R. and Berg, B. (1978). Measuring children's reactions to divorce. *Jour-
   nal of Clinical Psychology, 34*, 215–221.
Kendall, P.C. and Fishler, G.L. (1983). Teaching rational self-talk to impulsive
   children. In A. Ellis and M.E. Bernard (Eds.), *Rational-emotive ap-
   proaches to the problems of childhood* (pp. 159–188). New York: Plenum.
Knaus, W.J. (1983). Children and low frustration tolerance. In A. Ellis and

M.E. Bernard (Eds.), *Rational-emotive approaches to the problems of childhood* (pp. 139–158). New York: Plenum.

Kurdek, L. and Berg, B. (1983). Correlates of children's adjustment to their parents' divorce. In L.A. Kurdek (Ed.), *Children of divorce: New directions in child development* (pp. 47–60). San Francisco: Jossey-Bass.

Snyder, L. (1984). *The changing family game: Efficacy of a treatment program for children of divorce*. Unpublished master's thesis, University of Dayton, Dayton, OH.

CHAPTER 6

Family Communication and Problem Solving with Boardgames and Computer Games

ELAINE A. BLECHMAN, CLAIRE RABIN, and MICHAEL J. McENROE

Communication and problem-solving training, major components in behavioral family therapy, use standardized, well delineated sets of instructions to teach family members how to discuss and solve behavioral problems. Much like the instructions embedded in the popular boardgames played by families since the late nineteenth century, the core instructions in communication and problem-solving training act as controlling stimuli for family interaction behavior, for what family members say and do with one another while they are playing the game, or while they are involved in a training session. In fact, design of a boardgame useful in family communication and problem-solving training requires only a thorough description of a desirable sequence of family interaction behavior, and an equally thorough description of the obstructive behavior in which troubled families engage when therapists attempt to shape desirable family interaction. This chapter covers the theoretical and practical aspects of communication and problem-solving training, and describes boardgames and computer games designed to enhance the skills of families.

FAMILY COMMUNICATION AND PROBLEM SOLVING

Communication and Problem-Solving Deficits and Behavior Problems

A family's influence on its members is communicated through antecedents (spoken rules, unspoken expectations, and examples) and conse-

129

quences (rewards and punishments) (Cook and Dreyer, 1984; Mealiea, 1976). Dysfunctional families use their influence to obstruct communication and problem-solving attempts (Alexander and Parsons, 1973), often through coordinated attacks on one another's personality (Aldous, 1971; Turner, 1970). In these families, unsolved problems and dissatisfactions accumulate, and deviant behaviors become habitual, promoting further deterioration in communication. Enduring remediation of problem behaviors requires that family members learn to talk to each other about mutual problems and to develop effective solutions together.

Problem-solving skills determine how a family identifies and defines problems and generates and implements solutions (D'Zurilla and Goldfried, 1971). Communication skills determine how family members send messages to one another about problems and solutions (Baldwin, Cole, and Baldwin, 1982; Christensen, Phillips, Glasgow, and Johnson, 1983; DeLorenzo and Foster, 1984; Robin and Canter, 1984). These two broad categories of skills easily translate into observable, quantifiable units of behavior, permitting a determination of whether family members: (1) pay attention to what each other says, (2) talk about one problem at a time, (3) generate specific problem definitions, (4) send clear, brief, assertive messages with congruence between verbal and nonverbal channels, (5) send few hostile messages, (6) reward each other's communication and problem-solving attempts with interest, attention, and praise, (7) suggest problem solutions, (8) ask for and offer concessions, help, and compromises, (9) negotiate conclusive, timely, mutually acceptable agreements, and (10) cooperate in implementing, evaluating, and refining agreements (Blechman and McEnroe, 1985; Gottman, Markman, and Notarius, 1977; Liberman, Wheeler, de Visser, and Kuehnel, 1980).

Effective and Ineffective Families

In families that communicate effectively, the group as a whole attends to all members' reactions to a given problem. In families that solve problems effectively, the group only adopts solutions that respond to each one's individual needs and which are acceptable to all family members.

Parents influence their families' problem-solving and communication styles by the type of leadership they provide (Baumrind, 1968, 1978), and by the type of social power they exercise (Blechman, 1980; French and Raven, 1959).

Couples who have achieved a healthy balance of power, in which each partner can openly, comfortably, and successfully express needs and work toward fulfillment of those needs, are likely to feel satisfied with marriage and to share child-rearing responsibilities in a manner that benefits parents as well as children. These couples are prepared to act in an authoritative manner when their children are old enough to take part in discussions of family problems and plans. Authoritative parents, whether coupled or single, promote verbal exchanges among family members, and give children a voice in decision making proportionate to their ability to implement solutions and deal with consequences. They exercise social power by providing expert information. Because useful information becomes increasingly important as children mature, affiliations with authoritative parents grow stronger and more positive as children move through adolescence and adulthood. In sum, effective families are likely to have one or two authoritative parents as leaders.

Couples who have failed to arrive at distributions of power and responsibility which satisfy the needs of both husbands and wives, and who are consequently dissatisfied with their marriages, are likely to inject the battle of the sexes into the child-rearing arena. Couples in which one partner's needs are the primary focus of the relationship often become authoritarian parents. Couples in which both partners fail to express their needs and to take responsibility for satisfying those needs often become permissive parents. Ineffective families can be headed by one or two authoritarian or permissive parents. A combination of an authoritarian and a permissive parent is not unusual.

Authoritarian parents discourage a free flow of ideas in the family and preempt most decision-making power. They exercise social power through coercion, threats, and punishments. Because children are increasingly able to avoid parental coercion as they mature, affiliations with authoritarian parents remain negative and grow weaker as children move through adolescence and adulthood.

Permissive parents encourage children to air their reactions to problems, but fail to influence the family to adopt solutions with good short- and long-term benefits for all concerned. They exercise social influence by means of reward power, in the form of noncontingent positive reinforcement, and by means of referent power, as they establish friendly relationships with their children. Since the combination of reward and referent power blurs age and power differences between the generations, promotes rivalry between parents and children, and overdependence of children on parents, affiliations with permissive parents grow stronger and more negative as children mature.

Families ineffective at problem solving and communication rapidly accumulate unresolved conflicts and problems. Some of these families eventually request clinical treatment of marital conflict, parent-child conflict, or of specific child and adolescent behavior problems.

GAME-GUIDED FAMILY PROBLEM SOLVING

Family Problem-Solving Training

Family problem-solving training is designed to improve communication and problem solving, while remedying the specific behavioral complaints of family members in accord with detailed procedural modules. To accomplish this dual objective, family problem-solving training draws on principles of operant conditioning and observational learning, and emphasizes the interdependence of maladaptive individual and group behavior.

Researchers and clinicians have long recognized the need to develop treatment programs that promote generalization and maintenance of therapeutic gains (Patterson, 1971). Family problem-solving training consists of a series of instructional modules, each designed to train clinicians in the resolution of specific problems (Patterson, 1971) and, at the same time, to promote generalization and maintenance of communication and problem-solving skills.

Interactive Family Problem-Solving Games

The first family problem-solving training module to be developed used a boardgame to guide contingency contracting. A contingency contract is a written contingency management plan negotiated and consented to by all family members. Distressed couples (Jacobson, 1978), children with behavior problems (Gordon and Davidson, 1981), and delinquent adolescents (Alexander and Parsons, 1973) have benefited from contingency contracting.

Early excitement about contingency contracting led to indiscriminate use and poor results. At this point, it is clear that the background, needs, and problems of a family must be considered before involving the group in contingency contracting (Blechman, 1980), that the family, not the therapist, must determine the content of the contingency contract, and that the therapist must, after exposing the family to contingency contracting, use social reinforcers to shape successful problem-solving and contract compliance (Blechman, 1977).

Family problem-solving-training boardgames were designed to lead families through the contingency contracting process while minimizing dependence on a therapist and hastening the generalization of new skills to the family's natural environment. The basic steps in group problem solving and contingency contracting are embedded in several of these games: identification of a target problem for resolution, generation of potential solutions, selection of a trial solution, specification of details of the solution, and agreement to implement and evaluate the outcome of the solution.

The Family Contract Game (*FCG*) was designed to help parents and children resolve conflicts about things that happen at home (Blechman, 1974). The *FCG* board is partitioned into 14 squares which instruct players to make a statement, ask a question, or give a reply. Game pieces include four card decks (problems, rewards, risk, and bonus), contract forms, charts for recording the occurrence of target behaviors, and the contingent provision of rewards, play money, red and blue markers, pencils, and a timer. Family members create their own problems and reward deck—drawing from and elaborating on standard problem inventories. Bonus and risk card decks provide humorous instructions to receive, or pay, play money.

After a few practice games with a therapist, families play the game on their own. Two family members can play, or the family can divide up into two teams (red or blue). The player with the red marker begins the game by stating the problem, and suggesting a new pleasing behavior that the target of the complaint could substitute for the displeasing behavior. Once blue agrees to engage in the pleasing behavior, players agree on a contingent reward for blue, and decide on the details of the contract, such as when and how the reward will be given and who will keep track of the pleasing behavior. Players then select a bonus card and earn play money after reaching an agreement.

Throughout the game, players select a risk card and lose play money after a disagreement. Whenever a disagreement occurs, the player who disagrees is instructed to make a counterproposal. Counterproposals are traded back and forth, until an agreement is achieved. A time limit of 15 minutes encourages participants to follow rules and focus on problems at hand, rather than engaging in irrelevant and fruitless arguments (Blechman and McEnroe, 1985).

Players who move around the game board within the time limit write a contract based on a bilateral exchange of desirable behavior. Repeated game play provides practice in charting contract compliance, and in negotiating and renegotiating viable contracts.

The *FCG* was evaluated in several single-case experimental design studies involving a mother and her 14-year-old symptomatic son (Blechman, Olson, Schornagel, Halsdorf, and Turner, 1976), four single-parent families with problem children (Blechman and Olson, 1976), and six families with children exhibiting behavior or interactional problems (Blechman, Olson, and Hellman, 1976). These families were videotaped during game play and during unstructured problem-solving sessions; results indicated that the *FCG* exercised stimulus control, significantly increasing the frequency of on-task and problem-solving behaviors. In an additional study, Bizer (1978) demonstrated generalization of improved problem solving from clinic use of the *FCG* to the home.

Solutions, a game whose format resembles the *FCG*, was designed to improve family problem solving and children's school performance (Blechman, Kotanchik, and Taylor, 1981; Blechman, Taylor, and Schrader, 1981). When a family plays *Solutions*, they formulate a contract which specifies a back-up reinforcer for a "good news note." The note is sent home by the teacher when children perform above their baseline average in a particular academic subject. No note is sent on a day when children perform below their baseline average, and parents are instructed to say nothing when no note comes home. Thus, families who move around the *Solutions* game board within the time limit write a contract arranging for positive reinforcement of school work of good quantity and quality relative to the child's own prior performance.

Two early-intervention studies tested the impact of *Solutions* on children's academic performance. In both studies, children whose academic performance was extremely variable during baseline were identified, and their families were recruited. In the first study, recruits were randomly assigned either to a *Solutions*-generated, home-note system or to an untreated control. The academic performance of the *Solutions* group improved significantly more than that of the control group (Blechman, Kotanchik, and Taylor, 1981). In the second study, recruits were randomly assigned either to a *Solutions*-generated, home-note system, to a home-note system that involved no family problem solving, or to an untreated control. The academic performance of the *Solutions* group improved significantly more than that of the other two groups, and generalization to nonreinforced probe days was greater in the *Solutions* than in the home-note comparison group (Blechman, Taylor, and Schrader, 1981).

The Marriage Contract Game (*MCG*) (Blechman and Rabin, 1982) was designed both to provide guidance in problem solving and contingency contracting, and to encourage open and warm communication. The *MCG* does this by directing partners to make precise statements, provide each other with contingent positive feedback, make honest statements of trust and confidence in one another, and talk openly about feelings.

The *MCG* guides couples in contingency contracting so that they: (1) select one problem to negotiate, (2) convert a specific complaint into a target behavior, (3) select a cooperative behavior, to be enacted by the complainant, that will help the target behavior occur, and (4) sign a contract describing details of the agreement and of charting responsibilities.

Single-case study evaluations of the *MCG* found significant improvements in couples' interactions as measured by self-report, by direct observation of problem solving and affective behavior, and by conflicted couples' readiness to resolve child-behavior problems (Rabin, Blechman, Kahn, and Carel, 1985; Rabin, Blechman, and Milton, 1984).

Stimulus Control Over Effective Family Interaction

A stimulus with a high probability of eliciting a specific response (Keller and Schoenfeld, 1950) exerts stimulus control. Boardgame instructions both elicit desirable interactional behavior and reinforce its occurrence. Games designed to capitalize on the principle of stimulus control can rapidly elicit complex, unfamiliar interactional patterns. In less than an hour, a literate family motivated to resolve an intragroup conflict, with no prior experience in contingency contracting, can use a boardgame to come up with a technically correct agreement. Families with literacy problems or families with a vested interest in the maintenance of intragroup conflict can use a boardgame to come up with a technically correct agreement with the support of a skilled therapist. These same families might be resistant to change directed solely by the therapist.

A potential disadvantage of stimulus control is the possibility that new responses governed by tight stimulus control might not generalize. Thus, a family that has learned to communicate effectively in the presence of a specific game instruction might not transfer their new communication patterns to situations from which the instruction is absent. Fortunately, when a boardgame is the medium of stimulus control, generalization is readily promoted by encouraging the family to carry the game along with them and use it in as many situations as possible. Thus, a family might use the game to solve problems at home and when traveling away from home.

Once family members have overlearned effective communication and problem solving in response to game instructions and have practiced these skills, guided by the game, in a multitude of real-life situations, a loosening of stimulus control will augment the generalization of new skills (Becker, Engelmann, and Thomas, 1975). The family can achieve this result by frequently discussing problems without the game, while trying to follow game instructions from memory.

Motivation for Effective Family Interaction

During a successful group game, players work toward clearly defined and desirable goals by making decisions and carrying them out, and experiencing the good and bad consequences of their decisions (Van Sickle, 1978). By offering immediate intrinsic rewards, such as a sense of mastery over the game, power over other players' fates, and opportunities to laugh at (rather than be upset by) one's own and other's mistakes, successful games motivate players to attend to every aspect of game play and to make careful decisions (Coleman, 1968; Rabin, 1983).

The successful group game creates an unusual atmosphere that encourages goal-directed behavior, risk-taking, cooperation, and playfulness. Although very little is known about the atmosphere created in a family by a successful group game, or by a successful therapist, such an atmosphere appears to be a necessary condition for acquisition of new communication and problem-solving skills and for resolution of serious behavior problems.

Types of Therapeutic Games

Consistent with the work of Varenhorst (1973) who categorized simulation games, Rabin (1983) has categorized therapeutic games in respect to their rules (structured or unstructured) and procedures (cognitive or behavioral) and has recommended that clinicians should keep this typology in mind when selecting a game for therapeutic use.

The more rules a game has about procedures, behavioral constraints, environmental responses, and goals the more structured it is (Varenhorst, 1973).

The procedures of cognitive games emphasize new knowledge, insight, and understanding of problems. Cognitive games often use postgame discussion sessions to achieve the game's goal (Caracappa, Nasy-McMenamin, and Yuschak, 1977; Chaisson, 1977; Zweben and Miller, 1968).

The procedures of behavioral games promote rehearsal of new skills, or skill elements, starting with simple, easily mastered responses, and gradually targeting more complex behaviors. Behavioral games use contingent positive reinforcement, material and social, to achieve their goals. Behavioral games have been used successfully to increase safety skills in latchkey children (Peterson, 1984), honesty in schoolchildren (Flowers, 1972), and communication skills among teenagers (Corder, Whiteside, and Vogel, 1977), married couples (Blechman and Rabin, 1982), parents and school-aged children, and parents and adolescent children (Blechman and Olson, 1976).

COMPUTERIZATION OF BEHAVIORAL GAMES

Computers, Games, and Behavior Therapy

The goals and procedures of contemporary behavioral interventions are particularly well-suited to computer applications. In these interventions, the role of the therapist is usually delineated by a very specific protocol or treatment manual. Choice points in intervention are, at least in theory, guided by objective data about client behavior (Blechman, 1981). Although the relationship between the client and the therapist is a medium for communication whose importance cannot be discounted, development of the relationship between client and behavior therapist is a secondary goal of treatment. The primary goal is the transmission of new knowledge and skills in a way that insures their survival after treatment is over. It is for this reason that behavior therapists welcome procedures which rapidly reduce client defensiveness, discourage client dependency on the therapist, and enhance maintenance of new skills in the client's natural environs. Since behavior therapists aim for generalization of new skills to the natural environment, they welcome treatment procedures that reduce the need for the therapist to act as a controlling stimulus for new behavior.

In many as yet unrecognized ways, computers can hasten accomplishment of the goals of behavioral interventions. Computer-assisted treatment is more easily standardized and disseminated than any treatment wholly guided by a human therapist. While human therapists can only gather, analyze, and integrate into treatment limited amounts of data about client behavior, microcomputers have the capacity to gather large amounts of information about client behavior either through keyboard entry or on-line acquisition, to process this information quickly, and to rapidly recommend the next step in treatment. A positive aspect of computerized therapy appears to be reduced client defensiveness, and dependence on the therapist (Slack and Van Cura, 1968).

Computerization of Structured Behavioral Games

The *FCG*, *Solutions*, and *MCG*, highly structured behavioral games, are easily translated into computer programs because of their well-defined procedures and predefined response options. Some of the demands of structured behavioral games are more efficiently executed by a computer program than by a boardgame. And, a computerized game is capable of functions that could never be performed by a boardgame, even in combination with a skilled therapist and research technician. For example, during a boardgame, players must keep track of timing, money, and markers, which may distract them from the goals of the game. In contrast, a computer game can manage all these control procedures and free the players to concentrate on the game's objectives. Data about player interaction during a boardgame must be coded by trained raters at great expense and with the risk of low reliability. Yet, a computer game can collect critical interaction data on-line at a very low cost and with high reliability. Despite the advantages of computerization of structured behavioral games, initial development of these games does require a substantial investment of time and money, and entails some problems that are worth considering.

Obstacles to Computer-Assisted Mental-Health Services

Cost is no longer a major impediment to computer-assisted mental-health services, now that the price of microcomputers has dropped. Uneasiness with computers is no longer a major impediment, now that the computer has become a familiar educational and recreational device in classrooms and private homes. Progress in interactive programming is, however, impeded by difficulties in writing software acceptable to mental-health practitioners, researchers, programmers, and users as well as by difficulties envisioning the flow of prompts and responses appropriate to various therapeutic contexts (Myers, 1978; Selmi, Klein, Greist, Johnson, and Harris, 1982). Even if all these problems are resolved, an important question remains to be answered. Will the computer merely replace unskilled technicians and mimic skilled clinicians? Or, will the computer provide services beyond the capabilities of the most skilled clinician?

Psychologists have just begun to design complex computer-assisted therapies. Selmi, Klein, Greist, Johnson, and Harris (1982) designed a computer-assisted cognitive behavioral treatment for depression that permits continuous on-line interaction between the computer and the patient during each therapy session. Although outcome research on this computerized cognitive therapy treatment is still in progress, the procedure is a good example of the use of computers to structure the treatment process. Clark and Schoech (1984) programmed an adventure game (in the popular *Dungeons and Dragons* format) on a DEC-20 to teach impulse control to adolescents; the game improved client interest and attention to therapy.

The Computer Marriage Contract Game

We (Blechman and McEnroe) designed a computer version of the *MCG*, believing that the time was ripe for development of software to facilitate dyadic and group problem-solving efforts, that such software could be used as a central component of marital or family therapy, and that it could stand alone as a counseling procedure for relatively well-adjusted people. Most important, we were convinced that such software would, for the first time, permit on-line continuous recording of the flow of interaction between therapeutic software and family group, and among family-group members, and that data collected in this manner would contribute to basic knowledge about mechanisms of family communication and problem solving. Our experience computerizing the *MCG* has more than confirmed these expectations.

Despite all of the advantages of boardgames as therapeutic tools, they had some shortcomings which we hoped to remedy by converting the *MCG* into an interactive computer game: the *Computer Marriage Contract Game* (*CMCG*) (Blechman, McEnroe, and Carella, 1985). First, it is extremely difficult to use boardgames to assess patterns of family interaction, but on-line data acquisition during a computerized game is quick and reliable. A second disadvantage of the original boardgames is that there is no way to insure that the group that plays the game always learns from past mistakes and adjusts future game play accordingly. In contrast, we found during development of the *CMCG* that computerized games can be designed to recall past mistakes and select appropriate pathways in future games. A third disadvantage of the original boardgames was the difficulty in tailoring game play to each family's problem-solving expertise. During development of the *CMCG*, we found that game play could be tailored to suit families who were novices and those who were experts at problem solving and communication.

The rules, format, and goals of the *CMCG* are identical to those of the *MCG*. The computer version, designed for an IBM PC, provides a different method of presenting the game to players, collecting objective data, recording responses, and insuring consistent play from game to game. The *CMCG* has not yet been tested, as has the *MCG*, for therapeutic value. However, a recent study (Blechman, McEnroe, and Carella, 1985) investigated how seriously couples would approach problem solving, during the *CMCG*. An A-B-A single case design (Hersen and Barlow, 1976) was used with seven couples, two of whom reported clinically significant marital distress (on the Marital Adjustment Test, Locke and Wallace, 1959). Each couple played the game three times, with a 20 minute time limit for each game. During their first and third games each couple confronted a problem area they had previously identified as "most difficult" to solve; during their second game they confronted an "easy to solve" problem. If couples approached problem-solving seriously during game play, they should have spent much more time on the first and third games than on the second. The results confirmed this expectation; the couples did spend more time discussing difficult problems, and they disagreed more often when trying to resolve difficult problems.

Distressed and nondistressed couples had no trouble playing the game, although none had prior familiarity with the software, and few were computer literate. Of the two distressed couples, one expressed considerable pleasure with the game, and the other refused to complete the third game (the husband believed the game was biased against him). These results indicate a need to determine which distressed couples are most likely to be receptive to the game and which will fare better with a human therapist.

CONCLUSION

This chapter has described the development and effects of structured-behavioral boardgames and the development of a computerized game. The transition from therapy wholly guided by humans to therapies which rely for assistance on boardgames and on computer games deserves thoughtful inquiry. The widespread social impact of these technological innovations should be studied now, during the process of transition (Lepper, 1985).

REFERENCES

Aldous, J. (1971). A framework for the analysis of family problem solving. In J. Aldous, T. Condon, R. Hill, M. Straus, and I. Tallman (Eds.), *Family problem solving: A symposium on theoretical, methodological, and substantive concerns* (pp. 265–281). Hinsdale, IL: Dryden.

Alexander, J.F. and Parsons, B. (1973). Short-term behavioral intervention with delinquent families: Impact on family process and recidivism. *Journal of Abnormal Psychology, 81*, 219–225.

Baldwin, A.L., Cole, R.E., and Baldwin, C.P. (1982). Parental pathology, family interaction, and the competence of the child in school. *Monographs of the Society for Research in Child Development, 47* (5, Serial No. 197).

Baumrind, D. (1968). Authoritarian vs. authoritative parental control. *Adolescence, 3*, 255–272.

Baumrind, D. (1978). Parental disciplinary patterns and social competence in children. *Youth and Society, 9*, 239–276.

Becker, W.C., Engelmann, S., and Thomas, D.R. (1975). *Teaching 2: Cognitive learning and instruction*. Chicago: SRA.

Bizer, L. (1978). *Generality of treatment effects in single parent-child problem solving*. Unpublished doctoral dissertation. University of Massachusetts, Amherst.

Blechman, E.A. (1974). The family contract game: A tool to teach interpersonal problem solving. *Family Coordinator, July*, 269–281.

Blechman, E.A. (1977). Objectives and procedures believed necessary for the success of a contractual approach to family intervention. *Behavior Therapy, 8*, 275–277.

Blechman, E.A. (1980). Family problem-solving training. *The American Journal of Family Therapy, 8*, 3–21.

Blechman, E.A. (1981). Toward comprehensive behavioral family intervention: An algorithm for matching families and interventions. *Behavior Modification, 5*, 221–236.

Blechman, E.A., Kotanchik, N.L., and Taylor, C.J. (1981). Families and schools together: Early behavioral intervention with high-risk children. *Behavior Therapy, 12*, 308–319.

Blechman, E.A. and McEnroe, M.J. (1985). Effective family problem solving. *Child Development, 56*, 429–437.

Blechman, E.A., McEnroe, M.J., and Carella, E.T. (1985). *Computer-assisted marital problem solving*. Manuscript submitted for publication.

Blechman, E.A. and Olson, D.H.L. (1976). The family contract game: Description and effectiveness. In D.H.L. Olson (Ed.), *Treating relationships* (pp. 133–150). Lake Mills, IA: Graphic.

Blechman, E.A., Olson, D.H.L., and Hellman, I.D. (1976). Stimulus control over family problem solving behavior. *Behavior Therapy, 7*, 689–692.

Blechman, E.A., Olson, D.H.L., Schornagel, C.Y., Halsdorf, M., and Turner, A.J. (1976). The family contract game: Technique and case study. *Journal of Consulting and Clinical Psychology, 44*, 449–455.

Blechman, E.A. and Rabin, C. (1982). Concepts and methods of explicit marital negotiation training with the Marriage Contract Game. *American Journal of Family Therapy, 10*, 47–55.

Blechman, E.A., Taylor, C.J., and Schrader, S.M. (1981). Family problem solving vs. home notes as early intervention with high-risk children. *Journal of Consulting and Clinical Psychology, 49*, 919–926.

Caracappa, M., Nasy-McMenamin, D., and Yuschak, M. (1977). *Assylumation*. Unpublished manuscript, Rutgers State University, New Brunswick, NJ.

Chaisson, G. (1977). Life cycle: simulating the problem of aging and the aged. *Health Education Monographs, 5* (1, Pt. 1).

Christensen, A., Phillips, S., Glasgow, R.E., and Johnson, S.M. (1983). Parental characteristics and interactional dysfunction in families with child behavior problems: A preliminary investigation. *Journal of Abnormal Child Psychology, 11*, 153–166.

Clark, B. and Schoech, D. (1984). A computer-assisted therapeutic game for adolescents: Initial development and comments. In M.D. Schwartz (Ed.), *Using computers in clinical practice: Psychotherapy and mental health applications* (pp. 345–353). New York: Haworth.

Coleman, J. (1968). Social processes and simulation games. In S. Boocock and E. Schild (Eds.), *Simulation games in learning* (pp. 29–53). Beverly Hills, CA: Sage.

Cook, W. and Dreyer, A. (1984). The social relations model: A new approach to the analysis of family-dyadic interaction. *Journal of Marriage and the Family, 16*, 679–687.

Corder, B., Whiteside, M., and Vogel, M. (1977). A therapeutic game for structuring and facilitating group psychotherapy with adolescents. *Adolescence, 12*, 261–268.

DeLorenzo, T.M. and Foster, S.L. (1984). A functional assessment of children's ratings of interaction patterns. *Behavioral Assessment, 6*, 291–302.

D'Zurilla, T.J. and Goldfried, M.R. (1971). Problem solving and behavior modification. *Journal of Abnormal Psychology, 78*, 107–126.

Flowers, J. (1972). Behavior modification of cheating in an elementary school student: A brief note. *Behavior Therapy, 3*, 311–312.

French, Jr., J.R.P. and Raven, B.H. (1959). The bases of social power. In D. Cartwright (Ed.), *Studies in social power* (pp. 150–167). Ann Arbor: University of Michigan Press.

Gordon, S.B. and Davidson, N. (1981). Behavioral parent training. In A.S. Gurman and D.P. Kniskern (Eds.), *Handbook of family therapy*. New York: Brunner/Mazel.

Gottman, J., Markman, H., and Notarius, C. (1977). The topography of marital conflict: A sequential analysis of verbal and nonverbal behavior. *Journal of Marriage and the Family, 9*, 461–477.

Hersen, M. and Barlow, D.H. (1976). *Single case experimental designs: Strategies for studying behavior change*. New York: Pergamon.

Jacobson, N.S. (1978). Specific and nonspecific factors in the effectiveness of a behavioral approach to the treatment of marital discord. *Journal of Consulting and Clinical Psychology, 46*, 442–452.

Keller, F.S. and Schoenfeld, W.N. (1950). *Principles of psychology*. New York: Appleton.

Lepper, M.R. (1985). Microcomputers in education: Motivational and social issues. *American Psychologist, 40*, 1–18.

Liberman, R., Wheeler, E., de Visser, L., Kulhnel, T., and Kulhnel, J. (1980). *Handbook of marital therapy. An Educational approach to treating troubled relationships*. New York: Plenum.

Locke, H.J. and Wallace, K.M. (1959). Short marital-adjustment and prediction tests: Their reliability and validity. *Marriage and Family Living, 21*, 251–255.

Mealiea, Jr., W.L. (1976). Conjoint behavior therapy: The modification of family constellations. In E.J. Mash, L.C. Handy, and L.A. Hamerlynck (Eds.), *Behavior modification approaches to parenting* (pp. 152–166). New York: Brunner/Mazel.

Myers, R.A. (1978). Exploration with the computer. *The Counseling Psychologist, 7*, 51–55.

Patterson, G.R. (1971). *Families: Applications of social learning to family life*. Champaign, IL: Research Press.

Peterson, L. (1984). The "Safe at Home" game: Training comprehensive prevention skills in latchkey children. *Behavior Modification, 8*, 474–494.

Rabin, C. (1983). *Towards the use and development of games for social work practice*. Unpublished manuscript.

Rabin, C., Blechman, E.A., Kahn, D., and Carel, C. (1985). Refocusing from child to marital problems. *Journal of Marital and Family Therapy, 11*, 75–86.

Rabin, C., Blechman, E.A., and Milton, M.C. (1984). A multiple baseline study of the Marriage Contract Game's effects on problem solving and affective behavior. *Child & Family Behavior Therapy, 6*, 45–60.

Robin, A.L. and Canter, W. (1984). A comparison of the marital interaction coding system and community ratings for assessing mother-adolescent problem-solving. *Behavioral Assessment, 6*, 303–314.

Selmi, P.M., Klein, M.H., Greist, J.H., Johnson, J.H., and Harris, W.G. (1982). An investigation of computer-assisted cognitive-behavior therapy in the treatment of depression. *Behavior Research Methods & Instrumentation, 14*, 181–185.

Slack, W.V. and Van Cura, L.J. (1968). Patient reaction to computer-based medical interviewing. *Computers and Biomedical Research, 1*, 527–531.

Turner, R.H. (1970). *Family interaction*. New York: Wiley.

Varenhorst, B.B. (1973). Game theory, simulations, and group counseling. *Educational Technology, 13*, 40–43.

Van Sickle, R. (1978). Designing simulation games to teach decision-making skills. *Simulation Games, 9*, 413–428.

Zweban, J. and Miller, R. (1968). The systems game: Teaching, training, psychotherapy. *Psychotherapy: Theory, Research, and Practice, 5*, 73–76.

CHAPTER 7

The "Instant Replay" Game to
Improve Rational Problem Solving

STEWART BEDFORD

Instant Replay is a game to help children learn problem-solving methods. It can be used with some children as young as 2½ years old, and with variations in language style, the philosophic framework of the game can be used with any age. The theoretical foundation for the game is based on cognitive restructuring in general and on Rational-Emotive Therapy (RET) in particular. The game was first published by The Institute for Rational-Emotive Therapy in 1974 in the form of an illustrated booklet for children and an accompanying pamphlet for parents, therapists, and child-care people. (The institute has given permission for the game to be described in this chapter.)

Albert Ellis originated RET in 1955. One of the first cognitive therapies was RET and Ellis dates it back to the stoic philosopher Epictetus, who was at one time a Greek slave more than two thousand years ago. Epictetus said, "People are not upset by things, but by their ideas about things." This idea is fundamental to RET and also to the *Instant Replay* game.

An idea that Ellis described in his book *Reason and Emotion in Psychotherapy* became an important beginning for *Instant Replay*. Ellis said:

> It is my contention that all effective psychotherapists, whether or not they realize what they are doing, teach or induce their patients to re-perceive or rethink their life events and philosophies and thereby to change their unrealistic and illogical thoughts, emotions, and behavior. (Ellis, 1962, p. 36)

In the beginning stages of RET, Ellis described the "ABCs" of rational and irrational thinking that he developed to help people understand how their thinking often resulted in unpleasant emotions and problem behavior. After further research, Ellis added D and E to the alphabet of RET. In RET, A stands for "activating event," and C stands for "consequence." Ellis showed how many people believed that their activating events (As) caused their consequences (Cs) they encountered. Ellis did not think this was true. He postulated that it was not activating events that caused consequences, it was the "belief systems" (Bs) of the people. He showed people how to understand their irrational belief systems and then learn to "dispute" (D) them. He taught people that when they learned to dispute their irrational beliefs with rational ones, they could have new and more pleasant "effects" (Es). This, in a nutshell, is the ABCDEs of Rational-Emotive Therapy, and it works.

I started playing *Instant Replay* with my own children and I have taught a good many other parents how to play the game with their children in my practice of psychotherapy. It is a game that can be played by a parent and child and it can also be played by an entire family. It can also be played in a schoolroom setting or in other types of groups. One of the primary goals of the game is to teach people how to play the game by themselves as they face the inevitable problems of their day-to-day living. In brief, it is a game to help people learn to use rational problem solving in their daily lives. *Instant Replay* can be used in conjunction with other therapy methods with children and families and it can be taught to parents and other child-care people for use in working with children.

HOW TO PLAY INSTANT REPLAY

I usually introduce the RET technique during an intake interview with a family. I ask each person to tell me about fun and "unfun" things in their lives. After they have all done this, I ask one of them (usually a child) to tell me more about an unfun event, which I label as a "rough spot." After the child has described the rough spot, I have him or her tell me what happened next or as the result of the rough spot. This part I label as a "consequence" (or consequences). We now have the A (activating event) and the C (consequence) of Ellis' ABCs. During this discussion, I explain to the parents that I don't want them interrupting their children and I tell the parents that they will have a turn in a little while.

After a child has talked about the rough spot and the consequences of the rough spot, I say something, such as "Please tell me what you were thinking to yourself during the rough spot." If the child has taken some action, I might say, "Please tell me what you were thinking when you decided to _____" (here I would fill in what they had done). This can lead into some detail on the B (beliefs) of RET's ABCs.

I have found that this part of the game can be very helpful as a diagnostic tool in understanding the underlying dynamics of family systems. After each family member has done something like this, some family members have also begun to see more about their systems.

After everyone has had a chance to go through the ABC part, I pick one—usually a child—and suggest that they think of other things they could have thought (or done) when they were in their rough spot. This part I label as "other options" and I suggest that they think of as many as they can. Other family members can be drawn in here and some interesting "brainstorming" can result. This phase corresponds to Ellis' D (disputing), in that it has people dispute the idea that there is only one thing they can do when something happens in their lives.

After other options have been explored, I have the children speculate about what the consequences might be to each of the new options they have thought of. This corresponds to the E (effects) part of RET theory. This part can also be diagnostic, but it is also into the phase of actively teaching new problem-solving methods.

Homework is an integral part of the practice of RET. Homework also fits in with the use of *Instant Replay*. Parents are taught how to play the game and they are urged to play it at home. I also suggest that they keep some notes on the homework and bring them in for the next session. I caution parents to wait until their children have settled down some after rough spots as it is harder to learn the method when upset than it is when emotions have subsided.

A form of *Instant Replay* bibliotherapy can be used with parents and with children. For this, the little illustrated booklet can be used. The booklet is published by The Institute for Rational-Emotive Therapy (Bedford, 1974) and it comes with a manual for parents. Here is the text of the booklet to illustrate the technique. (Permission to use this was granted by The Institute for Rational-Emotive Therapy.)

One day Sandy was playing hopscotch with her little brother. Father was snoozing in his hammock, and mother was reading a book. All of a sudden there was a loud "Ow!" and little brother ran screaming down the street.

Mother dropped her book and ran after little brother. Father fell out of his hammock. Sandy just stood there by the hopscotch place and smiled a funny little smile.

Father picked himself up and asked, "What happened, Sandy?"

Sandy told father that little brother had gone "Nyahh, nyahh, nyahh" to her, and then had run down the street.

Father asked Sandy why little brother was yelling "Ow!"

Sandy said, "I guess it's because I hit him when he went 'nyahh, nyahh, nyahh' to me."

Father thought for a moment and then said, "I have an idea. Let's play a game called *Instant Replay*. First, you tell me everything you can remember about what just happened."

And Sandy said, "I just did."

Father explained that he wanted Sandy to pretend that it was a television replay and to "run it through" again and to tell everything she could think of that had just happened.

Sandy said, "Well, little brother and I were playing hopscotch and he cheated and said he won and he went 'nyahh, nyahh, nyahh' and I whopped him and he ran down the street. You have to whop them when they cheat and say they won and go 'nyahh, nyahh, nyahh.' "

Then father asked, "How did you feel when you decided to hit little brother?"

Sandy said, "I didn't decide to hit him, I just hit him."

Father asked again about how she felt, and Sandy said, "Mad."

Father asked, "What were you telling yourself when you got angry?"

Sandy thought a little and said, "I told myself he cheated so he really didn't win, so he can't go 'nyahh, nyahh, nyahh' to me."

Father asked, "Can you think of anything else you said to yourself before you decided to hit little brother?"

Sandy said, "He always thinks he's better than me."

"Yes, go on," said father.

Sandy thought and thought and thought and then said, "That's all."

Father said, "Okay, let's pretend you could do it all over again, what else could you have done instead of hitting little brother?"

"I could have kicked him, or I could have bit him," Sandy said.

Father asked Sandy to think of other things she could have done, and Sandy said, "I could have gone 'nyahh, nyahh, nyahh, *nyahh*' back to him!"

Father said, "Yes, go on."

And Sandy answered, "I could have tattled and I could have told him I wouldn't play hopscotch with him if he cheated and . . . I can't think of any more."

Father listened carefully and then asked, "What do you think would have happened if you had done those other things?"

Sandy thought and thought and thought, then she said, "Well, if I'd kicked him or bit him, I'd be in worse trouble than I am now."

Then Sandy said, "If I'd gone 'nyahh, nyahh, nyahh, *nyahh*' to him, he'd have gone 'nyahh, nyahh, nyahh, *nyahh, nyahh*' back to me."

Father asked Sandy to go on, and she said, "If I'd tattled, you'd have been mad and said, 'Settle your own fights.' "

"You're probably right," father said, "go on."

Sandy said, "If I had told him I wouldn't play hopscotch if he cheated, maybe he'd have stopped cheating. He likes to play hopscotch."

As little brother and mother were coming back down the walk, Sandy whispered to father, "If we could have instant replay, I'd tell him not to cheat any more."

Father just smiled and gave Sandy a big hug and kiss and said, "I love you, Sandy."

Then Sandy went over to little brother and gave him a big hug and said, "I'm sorry I whopped you. I love you, little brother."

And little brother began to smile again and they were both very, very happy.

CASE ILLUSTRATIONS

The first example of *Instant Replay* comes from some family therapy. The case involved a nine-year-old boy, Tim, who was referred by the school because he was having difficulties learning to read which they felt were related to emotional problems. Tim was in special classes for reading and spelling and his teacher had told his parents that he had a "mental block" in relation to reading. Tim's family consisted of his mother, father, and a younger sister who was (naturally!) a good reader and speller.

In the first session, I saw Tim and his family together. I started out by asking each of them to tell me about some fun things they liked to do. Tim could not think of anything. His sister said that she liked to read and spell. Tim's father was amazed that Tim had not told me about Little League. Father said to Tim, "Little League has to be the most fun thing you have ever done!" Tim sat in a dejected manner and looked at the floor. Father became noticeably upset. At that point, I described "rough spots" as "unfun" things and asked each of them to tell me about a recent one. Tim said, in a weak voice, "Little League."

Father really came unglued and said he was "speechless." He then proceeded to make a speech about the joys of Little League and the fact that he had wanted to be a professional baseball player when he was younger. I identified the "rough spot" that father was having and said that I wanted him to tell me about his. I told father he would have a turn, but that right now I wanted him to listen to Tim.

I asked Tim to tell us about a recent rough spot with Little League. Tim said, "I'm standing there at bat. There are two men on and two outs. I can hear Dad up in the stands yelling at me, the pitcher, and the umpire. Then I start to shake and I can't see the ball anymore and I strike out."

That was a very graphic description of a rough spot—an A (activating) event if I ever heard one. I then asked Tim to tell us what happened next and how he felt.

Tim said, "I felt funny inside. Like sick. Like shaky. Like down." His Cs (consequences) were not pleasant.

I then asked Tim to tell us what he was thinking to himself while his rough spot was going on. He said, "I thought 'I hate this but I better not let dad know. He's going to give me a bad time 'cause I'm going to strike out. Then he'll say I didn't try.' "

I asked Tim what he was thinking to himself when he heard his father yelling. He said, "I think he's mad at me and I think he don't like me 'cause I'm not good enough."

I then asked father to describe Tim's rough spot. I explained that it was very important for him to let Tim know that he had heard all that was said. I said that this was a form of "active listening" (Gordon, 1964) and it was a way of showing people that you have heard what they have said even if you didn't understand all about what they said.

Father repeated most of what Tim had said. I then asked father to tell us the feelings he had in relation to the rough spot he seemed to experience while Tim was talking. Father said, "I had a pain in my stomach. It was like I got hit in the guts with a line drive."

I then asked father what he was thinking to himself as Tim talked about "father's yelling." Father said, "I was thinking, 'I can't believe what I'm hearing. Then I thought about how I wished I'd had Little League when I was little. Maybe I would have been better. I wasn't all that good and I want Tim to be the best.' Then I thought, 'Where did I go wrong.' "

In considering "other options," Tim wasn't able to come up with anything. Fortunately, father was. He thought of ways he could dispute (D) some of his irrational thinking and help Tim (and himself) have some new effects (Es).

The second example also comes from some family therapy and it is an example of how *Instant Replay* can be used in crisis intervention. This case involved Sue, a seven-year-old girl. Her parents brought her in late one Saturday afternoon on an emergency basis. The visit was the first time I had seen any of the family. In addition to Sue, there was a five-year-old brother, a mother, and a father. They all came in.

The stated problem was that the family home had caught fire that morning and Sue was home alone and she refused to talk to her parents or the fire department about the fire. No one was injured and the main damage was from smoke and water. A set of drapes in the living room was the main thing that had burned. Sue herself had put the fire out by dragging a garden hose in from the patio.

At the beginning of the session mother described the fire and the family's concern that Sue refused to talk to them. Sue listened to this but didn't say anything. I said that I would like to know all of them better and I asked each of them to tell me about some fun things in their lives. Father thought it was fun to fish, mother thought it was fun to work in her home office, little brother liked to go to the playground in the park, and Sue liked to go to the library for books. I then asked each of them to tell me about anything they could think of that was unfun. Both mother and father thought it was very unfun to have the house catch fire. Brother thought it was unfun to go to the library, and Sue thought it was unfun to have her mother break promises.

I explained *Instant Replay* and asked Sue to tell us about the rough spot she was talking about—the most recent time she believed her mother had broken a promise. Sue said that it had happened that morning. She said that her mother had promised to take her to the library for books but that she ended up taking little brother to the playground. Mother started to interrupt, but I asked her to wait and listen. I asked Sue to tell me more about what had happened. Sue told us that her mother had been promising all week to take her to the library. She said that her mother had then told her that she (Sue) could either go to the playground and get some exercise or stay home by herself.

I repeated what Sue had said about the rough spot that morning and asked her to tell how she felt. She said she felt sad and lonesome. I then asked her what she thought to herself when her mother took her brother to the playground. Sue said that she thought, "Mom likes little brother better than she likes me."

I asked Sue to go on and tell me what else she thought. She said, "Mom's always busy at her desk or she's doing something for brother." Then she added, "I'm as good as him and it's not fair when she doesn't keep her promises."

After this, I asked Sue what happened next that morning. Sue said that the telephone had rung and she had gone to her mother's desk in the corner of the living room to answer it. She said it was for her mother and that she had taken the message. With a little probing and support to keep talking, Sue said that she had crumpled the message up and put it in her mother's ashtray and lit it on fire with her mother's lighter. This fire had then gone to the drapes and Sue had dragged in the hose and put the fire out.

In talking about other options, Sue decided that she could have gone to the playground with her mother and her brother and she thought the different effect might have been that she could have talked her mother into stopping by the library on the way home. When the whole family considered other options, the parents decided they wanted to learn some new ways of talking and listening so that they could solve problems in a better way than they had in the past.

In both of these examples, the families were able to get some important information with *Instant Replay*. They did not solve all of their problems. In both situations the families continued in consultation. They also continued playing the game at home. (Both of these examples were also cited in the book, *Look Mom, Paper Tigers: How To Teach Children About Stress*, Bedford, 1985.)

A third case illustration of *Instand Replay* comes from some consultation I was doing in an elementary school. The boy involved, we'll call him Ted, was in the fourth grade. He was sent to the principal's office from the playground for allegedly starting a fight. Since I happened to be in the school at the time, I got the referral hot off the field of battle. I talked to Ted awhile and got him calmed down with some relaxation and deep breathing methods. I then explained the game and related it to television replays of sports events. The "fight" had started during a game of work-up baseball at recess. Ted liked to watch sports events on television so he was very familiar with instant replays.

This is Ted's instant replay of the activating event. "We was playing baseball and I was running from first to second when the second base guy tripped me." I asked Ted what happened next and he said, "I got up and shoved him, then he hit me, then we stopped playing baseball and started to fight."

I asked Ted what feelings he had and he replied, "Mad!" I then asked him what he was thinking to himself when he decided to shove the other boy. Ted thought for awhile and said, "It isn't fair to trip people in baseball." I agreed that that was the rule and asked Ted what he thought next. He said, "He shouldn't do it and when he does I've got to get even." We then talked some about his beliefs in relation to "shoulds" and "getting even." He got into his beliefs about what other people thought of him when he did not get even, and he recognized that several of the other players thought that he had deliberately run into the other boy and that he (Ted) had started it. We then talked about the consequence of the incident and the fact that this sort of thing frequently happens to him. We considered other options and other effects and Ted decided that if he had gotten up and gone on to the second base, the other players might have thought that he was a good baseball player. This did not solve all of Ted's problems, but it got his attention and his interest.

SUMMARY AND CONCLUSIONS

Instant Replay is a simple game that can be played with children to teach them a method of rational problem solving. The theoretical background for the game comes from Rational-Emotive Therapy (RET), a form of cognitive restructuring psychotherapy. The game can be played in the course of therapy with children and families. It can also be used in group or classroom situations. It can even be used in some crisis intervention circumstances. In my practice of psychotherapy, I have used it directly with children and families and I have taught the game to parents and families to use between sessions in homework exercises.

In the game, parents and children recall events that have occurred in their lives and describe the events to each other. They also discuss what they were thinking to themselves prior to the events and while the events were occurring. They then go over the consequences that followed the event (usually behavioral or unpleasant emotional reactions). Following this, they speculate about other options they may have had and the consequences that might have come about if they had chosen the other methods of acting or reacting. In the course of this procedure, it is very often possible to help them see that their thinking plays a very important part in their behavior and emotional reactions. When they can see this, is is usually much easier for them to restructure their cognitions and thus gain a new dimension of control over their lives.

In the ABCDE framework of RET, people learn about their activating events (As), see the consequences (Cs), discover their belief systems (Bs), consider other options and dispute their beliefs (Ds), and formulate new effects (Es) they might like to have in their lives. The game can be combined with Gordon's (1964) active listening and it fits in with the systems approach to family therapy.

The research that I have done with *Instant Replay* has all been empirical. More formal and systematic research could easily be done in conjunction with either diagnostic or therapeutic techniques. Research could also be done in various settings, such as child guidance clinics, family therapy units, stress management programs, and schools and preschools.

BIBLIOGRAPHY

Ard, Jr., B.N. (1966). *Counseling and psychotherapy*. Palo Alto, CA: Science and Behavior.

Bedford, S. (1974). *Instant replay*. New York: Institute for Rational Living.

Bedford, S. (1985). *Look mom, paper tigers: How to teach children about stress*. Chico, CA: A & S.

Ellis, A. (1962). *Reason and emotion in psychotherapy*. New York: Lyle Stuart.

Ellis, A. (1974). *Humanistic psychotherapy: The rational-emotive approach*. New York: Julian.

Ellis, A. and Harper, R. (1961a). *A new guide to rational living*. Englewood Cliffs, NJ: Prentice-Hall. (Revised in 1975.)

Ellis, A. and Harper, R. (1961b). *Creative marriage*. New York: Lyle Stuart. (Revised in 1973.)

Ellis, A. and Wolf, J. (1972). *How to raise an emotionally happy child*. Hollywood, CA: Wilshire.

Gordon, T. (1964). *Parent effectiveness training*. Pasadena, CA: Gordon.

Hauck, P. (1967). *The rational management of children*. New York: Libra.

CHAPTER 8

Feedback and Could This Happen: Two Therapeutic Games for Children of Divorce

YAKOV M. EPSTEIN

In this chapter, I describe *The Children Helping Children Game* and *The Could This Happen Game* and present case illustrations of each.* The games are an important aspect of the Children Helping Children Program, a group-based program for children of divorce, but could easily be adapted for other purposes and other populations. At the conclusion of this chapter, some of these possible modifications are discussed. To begin, I will share my reasons for using games as a therapeutic tool.

WHY USE GAMES?

Children are frequently reluctant to attend therapy sessions. The meetings conflict with other activities that interest them. Typically, meetings occur in the evening after an exhausting and trying day at school. Candidates for child psychotherapy are also likely to suffer peer ridicule or the reproach of teachers and parents. By the start of the therapy hour, they have accumulated considerable frustration and anger which they frequently vent on fellow group members. They are likely to tease, taunt, fight, bully, or "put down" others. Not only are these actions a response to accumulated frustrations, they are also an accepted and enjoyable aspect of

*Fictitious names are used when describing case material.

159

children's social interaction patterns. Teasing another child is fun—
though being teased is anything but fun. Prevailing in a contest of opinions is so universally a cause for celebration that a voluminous lexicon of
victory slogans (I owe a debt of gratitude to my daughter, who, over the
course of many years, has given me numerous opportunities to observe
these patterns), including "moted" as in "ooh—you're moted" (a California expression intoned in a singsong voice), "you're beat" (the current
New Jersey counterpart), or a covey of less polite epithets could easily be
compiled. Even when children are too tired to concentrate on learning,
they have more than enough energy to engage in these contests.

Adults working with children can find these patterns disruptive and an-
noying. In a therapy session it is difficult to discuss children's feelings or
focus on their fears when some children are bickering, or teasing others.
My own approach is to engage in "psychological jujitsu." Rather than trying to curtail these behaviors, I try to harness them. If children are motivated to tease, then I will give them the opportunity to do so in a manner
that promotes learning. Teasing, after all, involves pointing out another
person's shortcomings. This is equally true in giving feedback to someone. The difference, however, lies in the destructive intent. I utilize the
motivation of teasing as an aspect of *The Children's Feedback Game*
which teaches feedback skills while avoiding the destructive aspects of
teasing.

Games are also exciting: they license competition. At the same time,
they promote collaboration between teammates who might otherwise be
antagonists in an effort to beat the other side. With, what sometimes
seems like, acrobatic skill group leaders balance the competitive spirit
against an incentive system which favors collaboration between opposing
teams. Just how this is done will be explained shortly.

The desire to win is also a powerful incentive to discuss topics and engage in actions that would otherwise be shunned. In the guise of a game,
children can deny the reality of their words. By invoking the belief that
"it's only a game" children allow themselves the luxury of feeling emotions and expressing beliefs that would otherwise be verboten. The *Could
This Happen Game* is based on this premise.

I believe that a frequent consequence of divorce is a precipitous dimi-
nution of the power of the child. The youngster's oft unheeded plea to the
parents to stay together is perhaps emblematic of his or her inability to influence the course of these trying events. Clinicians have targeted the

rapid decline in power and influence as an important contributor to mental illness (Ackerman, 1958). Hence, I take every opportunity available to demonstrate to the children in our program that they are not powerless— they will be heard. The structure of the game provides an opportunity to drive this point home. When games are employed in the context of children's therapy groups, the adult therapist recedes into the background, becoming an observer or referee, while the children assume a focal role. This shift in influence diminishes restraints on disclosure and spontaneity that may otherwise occur when children interact directly with an adult therapist. It also increases their commitment to the group and may even enhance their self-esteem.

There are additional reasons for elevating the child's influence in the program. Researchers have recently begun investigating the efficacy of using peer-mediated approaches to promote children's positive social interaction. In a review of this literature Odom and Strain (1984) conclude:

> Numerous studies have demonstrated that socially competent peers who, at times receive training from teachers or clinicians, can effect positive changes in the social behavior of children exhibiting social interactional deficits. (p. 555)

While the basis for the studies cited in this review is largely atheoretical, there is nonetheless literature in social psychology to support the value of using peers as change agents.

In a classic paper dealing with opinion change processes, Kelman (1958) distinguished between *compliance, identification,* and *internalization. Compliance* is changed behavior in response to external reinforcement contingencies. The compliant individual changes his or her opinions to obtain available rewards or to avoid the punishment or censure of others. Compliant change is comparatively easy to engineer with the proper schedule of reinforcement. However, researchers have found that compliant change is superficial, limited only to circumstances in which the change agent can monitor the actions of the subject. The individual does not value the new behavior more than the old habit. Given the opportunity to revert to the old pattern, he or she is likely to do so.

Identification produces changes which are more enduring than those rooted in compliance. The individual adopts behaviors and opinions which are valued by someone he or she esteems and seeks to emulate.

Like compliant change, however, the new behavior is not valued in and of itself. Should the esteemed other fall from grace or the relationship deteriorate, the subject is likely to revert to the old behavior pattern.

The deepest and most enduring change is based on newly acquired values which are *internalized*. The person whose values have changed considers the new behavior better and more worthwhile than the old way of acting. Even in the absence of surveillance and despite disillusionment with a former idol, internalized values are likely to maintain changed behaviors.

Adults typically employ compliance- or identification-based strategies to change a child's behavior. Rarely do they succeed in creating internalized change. In what was perhaps the most extensive research program dealing with persuasive communication, Hovland, Janis, and Kelley (1953) demonstrated the importance of the communicator's *credibility*. The failure of adults to promote internalized change may stem from their lack of credibility. When adults criticize children, these youngsters attribute the censure to a fundamental characteristic of the adult role. Grownups are expected to criticize the behavior of children: peers, however, are not supposed to do so. Therefore, for children, peers may be more credible evaluators.

Festinger (1954) postulated that the desire for social comparison with peers drives social behavior. Children wish to know how they are evaluated by their friends and classmates. Often, they are given the summary comments without being privy to the full review, as it were. Children know when their peers dislike them. They recoil from the taunts of other children which are often freely offered. But these same peers rarely share information about their reasons for disliking these children. Even when they do, the feedback is usually not offered constructively. Adults must find a way to transform these hurtful communications into productive messages which can stimulate internalized change. *The Children's Feedback Game* was designed to fill this need.

Yalom (1970) postulated a number of "curative" factors in group psychotherapy. Games are an effective vehicle for introducing these factors discussed by Yalom:

1. Sharing, expressivity, and catharsis.

2. Legitimizing the expression of negative affect.

3. Experiencing the universality of a problem (in this case the problems created by divorce).

4.   Receiving help from peers considered similar to oneself. Help includes: advice, skill, training, experimentation with new behaviors, and direct emotional support.

5.   Giving help to others in a similar situation. By learning to help others, the child learns to help himself or herself.

6.   Instilling hope. This often follows from learning new ways to cope with problems and thus feel less helpless.

7.   Receiving feedback from similar peers and learning to take more responsibility for oneself.

8.   Using similar peers as models.

In describing the features of the two games, we will show how they incorporate many of these curative factors.

THE CONTEXT IN WHICH THE GAMES ARE USED

The *Children Helping Children* program is a two to three month program consisting of a children's group and a concurrent parents group each meeting weekly for 1½ hours. The activities of the children's group are based on a number of assumptions about families of divorce. One such assumption is that these families frequently organize themselves either as competitive systems or as individualistically oriented groups in which each person attempts to satisfy his or her own needs without regard for the needs of others. Children's aggressive or competitive behavior may model the parental conflicts they witnessed. Further, children may also emulate their parents' attempts to satisfy their own social and emotional needs, thereby reducing their commitment to the common goals of the family unit. This individualistically oriented stance results in a sense of aloneness for family members: mutual social support, one of Yalom's (1970) curative factors so necessary for coping with the stress of divorce, is reduced. In an effort to promote a supportive family climate, the *Children Helping Children* program attempts to teach cooperation. By creating a cooperatively oriented children's group, the members are able to benefit from the support of other children. Hopefully, the cooperative behaviors they learn in the program can be transferred to behavior at home. However, if children are to behave cooperatively, they must acquire several essential skills. They must learn to (1) take the role of the other per-

son, (2) give and receive feedback, and (3) share and take turns. The
Children's Feedback Game teaches these skills.

Another assumption is that children are often confused about numerous
aspects of the divorce experience and are reluctant to discuss their fantasies and anxieties. Frequently, they experience shame and guilt, thinking
that they are unique in their feelings and beliefs. Our program encourages
children to air these secret thoughts. We believe that such public expression can foster social comparison and enable children to feel "in the same
boat" with other group members. The "we-feeling" is likely to be experienced as social support and contribute to a cooperative atmosphere in the
group. The _Could This Happen Game_ is used to reduce children's secre-
tiveness and foster an open discussion of beliefs and concerns, thereby
incorporating several of Yalom's (1970) curative factors.

Taken together, the two games build on one another. The skills of giving and receiving feedback acquired in the _Children's Feedback Game_ increase the effectiveness of communication in the _Could This Happen
Game_. Likewise, the discovery of common experience resulting from the
Could This Happen Game promotes the cooperative group structure
which the _Children's Feedback Game_ seeks to develop. As the group becomes increasingly cohesive and supportive, children's initial defensiveness begins to dissipate and the likelihood of sharing anxiety-arousing
material in the absence of a specific game format increases.

DESCRIPTION OF THE GAMES

The Children's Feedback Game

This game was developed by Epstein and Borduin (in press) as a means of
reducing the disruptive, silly, and aggressive behavior which occurred
frequently in the initial meetings of the _Children Helping Children_ program. Such disruptiveness seems to be common to group programs for latency age children. In conjunction with a group program which she conducted, Rhodes (1973) observed that:

> Authorities in the use of groups with preadolescent children agree that a re-
> curring problem is the handling of aggressive behavior (Barcai and Robin-
> son, 1969). Certainly, with these groups, _the most difficult aspect was the_

*management of the chaos and disorganization which tended to be present at times. . . . * The leaders found that from the very beginning the children tested the limits of the situation by a wide range of disruptive activity. This included breaking into small groups, whispering, getting up and engaging in individual or joint activity apart from the group and occasionally chasing one another. (p. 212)

Ginott (1961) devoted an entire chapter to discussing the need for the adult therapist to set limits in order to circumvent children's disruptiveness. However, I believe that peers can be more effective than adults in changing disruptive behavior and that such change is more likely to be internalized. Rhodes (1973) notes, in reference to the group described previously, that "When the group could be engaged to confront the group member with his impulse ridden behavior, it was far more effective than when the leader did so . . . " (p. 212). The *Children's Feedback Game* facilitates this process while also teaching the children observational skills, training them to give constructive feedback, and increasing their motivation to attend to their own behavior.

The *Children's Feedback Game* is "data based." The data consists of salient events pertaining to the group members. The use of the game motivates children to attend to their own behavior and the behavior of others. Group leaders provide summary information to the children to help them recall these events. They videotape and audiotape group sessions and prepare summaries based on this recorded material. A typewritten summary of the previous session is distributed to the children at the start of each session. The summary contains a separate paragraph for each member as well as a paragraph summarizing what happened to the total group. Each member's paragraph begins with the following heading:

WHAT HAPPENED TO . . . . . (name of child)

Reviewing the recorded information is time consuming (though extremely valuable) and alternative procedures could be substituted. Rather than listening to a recording of the session, leaders could compose a brief paragraph about the salient events which occurred for each child during the session. These paragraphs could be typed and distributed to group members.

The use of summary information is consistent with the program's underlying goal of maximizing the children's likelihood of success. Children may initially be unable to provide feedback to others for lack of information. We therefore supply them with data on which to base the feedback. Alternatively, children may have sufficient information but be ignorant of which items are worth sharing and how to communicate them constructively. The summary models the feedback process while the game motivates the children to read the transcript and learn how to provide the feedback appropriately. In all, providing information and a means of absorbing it increases the likelihood that a child will succeed at giving feedback to members of the group.

The *Children Helping Children* program uses an incentive system to promote group member interdependence by increasing the children's involvement in the games. Toward the beginning of the program a point system is introduced. Points accumulated through participation in several different activities are used to acquire items for a group party held during the last meeting of the group. A party chart prominently displayed in the room allows children to determine their current point accumulation. The chart, which looks like a ladder, includes a number of subgoals. Each subgoal corresponds to an item to be acquired for the party (e.g., ice cream, balloons, etc.). The group is divided into two teams who compete for points in the various games. The competition is exciting and motivates participation. However, despite the competition, the games promote cohesiveness since points earned by each of the teams are totaled and applied to the common goal of a group party.

The game begins by dividing the group into two teams. Next, the leader reads a description of an incident which occurred in a previous meeting. The description does not identify the child involved in the incident. The wording of the description omits gender cues. For example, a description might read: "This child made fun of other children in the group and didn't participate in the game we played." The children's task is to guess which child is being described. Typically, the children are eager to demonstrate their ability to identify the *target* child. The leader encourages them to huddle with their teammates so as to arrive at a team consensus. In so doing, each child has to check his or her impulsive tendencies and learn to consider the ideas of other children.

Several rounds are played. On each round, the teams alternate being the guessing team. After the spokesperson announces the team's guess, the leader gives the other team an opportunity to "challenge." The challengers disagree with the guess and offer an alternate name. If the guessing team is correct, they earn one point. However, if the challengers are correct, they earn two points while the guessing team loses one point.

The competition between teams heightens interest in the game. But the competition is embedded in a larger cooperative context. Points earned by each team are cumulated and applied toward the common goal of a group party. Thus, each team is pleased at the success of its opponent. This overarching cooperative goal is consistent with the program's values.

The children also have an opportunity to earn a variety of *"bonus points."* A child can earn a *feeling* bonus point by describing how he or she felt when the target child behaved as he or she did. *Owning* bonus points can be earned by the target child for acknowledging the feedback and guessing how other group members reacted to this behavior. The target child can also earn a *change* bonus point by suggesting changes in his or her behavior in future situations. Finally, children can earn *advice* bonus points by advising the target child about alternative ways of acting. Thus, the use of bonus points motivates the children to engage in behaviors which promote several of Yalom's (1970) curative factors.

Points are recorded on a blackboard. During the game, each child is given a turn to be "scorekeeper," a highly desirable role. An equally sought after job is "party chart recorder." The child performing this task fills in "rungs" on the party chart "ladder" with a magic marker to indicate progress toward the group goals. The "scorekeeper" and "recorder" roles are used as reinforcers as well as teaching tools. Children learn to cooperate in taking turns at these roles. Appointing children to these roles also affords an opportunity to address children's feelings of deprivation resulting from not being chosen for the task. Other roles can also be created. For example, teams can have "captains." The decision to add roles is but one of many choices which should be made after assessing the strengths and weaknesses of each child, their distinct familial problems, and the characteristic interaction patterns of group members. The game is an adaptable means to attain therapeutic goals. It can be used most effectively when modified to best meet the particular needs of each unique group.

We capitalize on the ability of games to stimulate discussion and extend the discussion as far as possible. All children are encouraged to participate in the discussion. Indeed, the leader often asks children to share anecdotes in which they acted like the target child. This procedure seeks to help children see themselves through the eyes of others and learn how others react to their behavior. Taking the "role of the other" toward one-self is a critical ingredient in the socialization process (Mead, 1934) and an important element in developing a cooperative group.

Case Illustrations

The *Children's Feedback Game* has been used successfully with several different groups. Some background information about the children described in the case illustrations will provide a basis for assessing the impact of the game.

David, a very bright nine-year-old boy, was caught in the midst of his parents' turbulent and mercurial relationship. The vicissitudes of their relationship are exemplified by the changes which occurred within the space of one two-week period. During this brief time span, they fought so violently that the father called for police intervention lest he literally murder his wife. This incident, witnessed by David, was followed not one week later with a reconciliation. David's father moved back into the home. Shortly thereafter, the fighting resumed and he once again left. Against this backdrop of "Sturm und Drang," David, who was by nature shy and had difficulty expressing feelings, became confused, antagonistic, and acted out his frustration and anger. In this time of loneliness, when he was most in need of support, his actions in the group only served to alienate him from his peers.

During the third meeting of the group, David frequently left the room, curled up in a bookcase, and played with the microphone. At first, the other children paid attention to David's actions and some even imitated his behavior. The resulting chaos made it difficult for the leaders to involve the children in discussions of divorce related material. Some of the children complained that David was interfering with the group's activities yet they did not tell him how they felt about his actions. By the end of the fourth group meeting, David had earned the reputation of group "deviant" and was treated as a scapegoat. In response, he distanced himself even more from group activities wrapping himself in a mantle of exaggerated indifference to their reaction to him. Less than 30 days after meeting a new group of children, David was mired in an uncomfortable role from which he could not extricate himself.

Joseph's parents separated when he was less than one year old. He had limited contact with his father and never witnessed the conflicts which were so much a part of David's world. However, Joseph's mother felt continuously angry with Joseph, primarily because she viewed him as an impediment to fulfilling her career and social needs. In response to her anger, she distanced herself emotionally from Joseph who, in turn, escalated his demands for attention. Unable to satisfy these needs at home, Joseph's appetite for attention from other adults became insatiable. In the group, he was attentive and delightful when he had the leader's ear. But he refused to relinquish the floor to any other group member. Like David, he too sought a great deal of attention. When he was not in the limelight, he disrupted conversations, attempted to dominate the discussion or, failing that, acted silly.

During the fifth meeting of the group, the leaders introduced the *Children's Feedback Game*. Whenever we introduce a new procedure, we give the children some practice trials to familiarize them with it. The practice question said:

> This child interrupted group discussions several times. Often, when other children wanted to talk this child didn't give them a chance. Instead, this child insisted on talking. When the leaders stopped this child and let other kids talk, this child acted silly. Guess which child we are describing.

The description referred to Joseph. On an index card, each child wrote the name of the child he or she thought was being described. Enthusiastic shouts of "Ooh—I know who it is" had to be contained and the children were instructed to consult their teammates to reach consensus. The guessing team was unanimous in its belief that the incident referred to David. David's team, the challengers, were likewise inclined to agree with this guess, but David prevailed on them to challenge. Reluctantly, they acceded to his demands and offered Joseph's name instead. To their surprise, the other team's chagrin, and David's utter delight, the group was informed that the incident indeed referred to Joseph. David's dogged determination to resist group pressure and the subsequent vindication of his stance enhanced his self-esteem and contributed to his stature among his teammates. In a productive discussion which ensued, the children examined the reasons for attributing Joseph's behavior to David. The discussion focused on the issue of obtaining a "bad reputation" and being blamed for the misdeeds of someone else. The children realized that their conclusion did not fit the data. They had indicated a child who had steadfastly refused to participate in group discussions as the group member who dominated conversations. They had overlooked this discrepancy because they deemed David the candidate most likely to engage in any undesirable behavior.

The discussion provided important feedback to David about the reputation he had earned. It also provided a forum in which he was able to hear not only the negative reactions children had to his disruptive behavior, but also the positive feelings—the caring they felt for him and their wish to be his friend. In order to earn *advice* bonus points, they suggested ways in which he could change. Dawn advised David to sit down and refrain from wandering around the room in the future. In order to earn a *feeling* point, she also told him that she thought he was much more attentive now than he had been in previous sessions and she liked him as she saw him now. David seemed to enjoy the positive feedback. It provided a face-saving means by which to change his behavior. By following the advice of group members, he indicated that he valued their opinions and they, in turn, appreciated him more.

David's behavior changed dramatically in subsequent sessions. He rarely left the room, never again climbed into the bookcase, and stopped playing with the microphone. Although he did not share very many of his feelings during this or other games, he was extremely attentive and actively participated on a cognitive level. Given the inner turmoil which we suspect he was experiencing, it is our opinion that he was incapable of discussing the turbulent emotions he harbored within him. Whereas this agitation had heretofore driven him to literally run from discussions of emotionally charged topics, he was now able to sit quietly and have the opportunity to vicariously absorb therapeutic benefit from the discussions he witnessed. I attribute the change in David to a desire to be regarded favorably by his peers. The game broke the cycle of reciprocal antagonism and afforded an opportunity to bring an otherwise alienated youngster back into the supportive fold of the group.

Silent members are often ignored by other children. Because they do not disrupt ongoing activity they rarely evoke feedback. The leaders wanted to help Carl, a silent member, break out of his shell. They hoped that the game would provide a forum to discuss Carl's silence and facilitate his entry into the group. Accordingly, they constructed the following item:

> This child is very quiet during group meetings. This child almost never says anything when the rest of the group is having a discussion.

The children correctly identified Carl as the subject of this description. Carl acknowledged his silence and discussed his view of the situation. He found it difficult to break into existing conversations. According to his recollection, he had attempted to speak several times but was ignored by others who were unwilling to relinquish the floor.

This interchange was the beginning of a productive dialogue between Carl and the other group members. It provided a nonthreatening arena to discuss Carl's silence and an opportunity to consider some ways to change this situation. In an effort to earn *change* bonus points, Allison, Joseph, and Dawn told Carl that they would like to see him talk and participate more. Carl welcomed the opportunity and promised that he would try to change. The leaders praised Carl for making this public commitment and exhorted the other children to increase Carl's chance of succeeding. They taught the children the importance of listening when Carl talked so that he would feel successful. This discussion appears to have been fruitful. For the duration of the program, Carl was the most actively involved group member.

Joseph continued to act the clown and competed for attention paid to other children. During the sixth session the leaders described a child who tried to focus the conversation on his concerns and, failing to do so, acted silly. The children easily identified Joseph as the culprit. Allison said to him: "When you act silly I get so mad at you I want to beat you up." Carl told him: "When you act silly I think it's because you want to get all of the attention. You just act like a big shot. I don't like that." Joseph agreed that he behaved this way and promised to try to change.

It would be gratifying to report that following this interchange Joseph stopped acting silly and seeking the limelight. Unfortunately, this was not so. However, now the children would say "Joseph, you're acting silly again" or "cut it out Joseph" and he would acknowledge his action and halt. The game seems to have created a mechanism for rapidly bringing Joseph's behavior under control without eliminating its cause. The leaders attributed much of the cause of Joseph's actions to intractible family patterns and were therefore gratified by their "limited success."

In addition to modifying disruptive behavior, the game can also be used to help a child appreciate some of his or her positive qualities. This is how the leaders used it to help Dawn.

Dawn coped daily with a most confusing family environment. Her parents disliked one another intensely and agreed to separate six months before the start of the program. Dawn's mother was employed in a fairly prestigious professional position. However, the downturn in our nation's economy had cost her father his job. Financially destitute, he continued to live in the marital home maintaining separate quarters and waiting for a time when he would be able to rent his own apartment. Each of Dawn's parents was romantically involved with another person and each introduced Dawn to this individual. Dawn's mother had a negative opinion of her daughter. Her description of Dawn as "my little monster" had a critical rather than a playful edge to it. She was quick to dismiss Dawn's good qualities. When the leader complimented Dawn for sharing candy with the other children her mother quickly dismissed it explaining that Dawn gave her candy away because she wasn't allowed to eat it at home. This constant belittlement contributed to Dawn's inability to appreciate her good qualities.

The leaders read a description of a child who acted kind in the group and cared about other children. Group members guessed that the description referred to Dawn. She, on the other hand, dismissed the praise thinking she didn't deserve it. However, the discussion gave the children an opportunity to share with Dawn their positive feelings for her. She seemed to relish this feedback and became centrally involved in the group.

Concluding Comments about The Children's Feedback Game

As the program progressed toward its later phases, the children were encouraged to give feedback to one another in the "here and now." Indeed, having learned to give feedback in response to the incidents described in the game, the children rapidly developed the ability to point out each other's negative behavior in the present. They described these behaviors and shared their emotional reactions to them. They attended more closely to one another's behavior. Rather than acting out their negative reactions or complaining to the leader about a child's misbehavior they talked directly with this person. Moreover, children confronted with feedback developed the habit of acknowledging rather than instinctively defending against and denying the information.

Experience using the game demonstrated that it is easier to train children to spontaneously criticize constructively than to praise freely. However, by modeling praise, and reinforcing the children's imitation of these behaviors, the leaders succeeded in heightening awareness of positive behavior as well as increasing positive feedback.

Use of the game was beneficial in a number of related ways. Because the children had learned to give and receive feedback they were often able to rapidly curtail undesirable behavior. By gaining this control over disruptive behavior the group was able to work more productively and reduce the level of friction in the group. This reduction in tension promoted the development of a cohesive and cooperative group. Finally, the frequency with which feelings were expressed and the depth with which they were explored showed a noticeable increase after the introduction of this game. In all, the Children's Feedback Game has been a valuable therapeutic tool in the *Children Helping Children* program. I shall now describe a second useful game, the *Could This Happen Game*.

The Could This Happen Game

The *Could This Happen Game* is introduced after the children have had an opportunity to play the *Children's Feedback Game*. The *Feedback Game* teaches children how to express their feelings. This skill is further honed in the *Could This Happen Game*.

Children of divorce are often reluctant to discuss their feelings concerning divorce related family problems. Likewise, many of these children have never aired their fears and worries. Some of these concerns (such as a parent's inability to pay bills) may be realistic. Others, however, may be based on misinformation, overheard snatches of conversation, or information which they misunderstood and never felt free to check out with an adult. Thus, they may be needlessly burdened with guilt which could be alleviated through discussion with their parents. The *Could This Happen Game*, developed by Epstein and Borduin (in press) was designed to facilitate a discussion of these problems and fears.

The game begins with a division of the group into two teams. Each team selects a name. Pencils and index cards are distributed to each child. The leader posts a newsprint chart containing the following four alternatives:

1.   I'm sure this could happen
2.   I think this could happen but I'm not sure
3.   I don't think this could happen but I'm not sure
4.   I'm sure this could not happen

The leader informs the children that they will be told about a hypothetical situation and asked to guess whether or not it could really happen. The newsprint chart is displayed and each of the four alternatives explained. The leader invites the children to practice playing the game by answering a sample question. Each child writes his or her name on the index card and one of the four numbers listed on the chart. The cards are collected and the leader reads each child's choice. The child is questioned to ensure that he or she understood the meaning of the chosen alternative and that it indeed represented his or her belief. The leader counts how many children voted for each of the four alternatives and announces which of the four was the most popular alternative.

Team representatives ("reps") are selected. They stand in front of the room and, in contrast to their teammates, do not answer the questions. Instead, their task is to guess which of the four alternatives received the most votes (from both teams combined). Their team receives *one* point for *each* person who voted for the alternative the "rep" thought was most popular. Suppose, for example, that the question said: "Two brothers share a room and never fight with each other. Could this happen?"

If three children select alternative 3 (I don't think this could happen but I'm not sure) and one child selects alternative 4 (I'm sure this could not happen), and Team A's rep guesses that the most popular answer is alternative 3, his or her team gets three points because three children voted for that alternative. However, if Team B's rep guessed that the most popular answer is alternative 4, he or she earns one point because only one child voted for that alternative. It is possible for both "reps" to select the same alternative.

In addition to points earned by the rep, the other team members can earn *bonus* points. One type of bonus point is the *evidence* point. A child earns an *evidence* point by presenting "evidence" in support of his or her chosen alternative. In the previous example, a child might tell how he and his brother fight constantly over when to turn off the lights at night, as evidence that brothers could not possibly share a room harmoniously. His desire to earn the bonus point and prove to others that he is correct uncovers information which can be used to discuss the sibling relationship.

Building on the skills acquired in *The Children's Feedback Game*, the children are also given an opportunity to earn *feeling* bonus points. Disclosing "evidence" related to divorce often stirs up powerful feelings. The availability of *feeling* bonus points removes many of the restraints against discussing these feelings. As the children begin to express their feelings, the leader praises them, thus encouraging them to be even more forthcoming. Hearing other children express their feelings reassures the listener by validating his or her own experience, and contributes to a sense of group solidarity.

The *Could This Happen Game* can be used to explore almost any topic. The initial catalog of questions was drawn from the concerns voiced by some of the children in the group, from worries which researchers have attributed to children of divorce, and from our concern about children's feelings of powerlessness and disappointment with their parents. Records of childrens' responses can provide valuable sources of research data.

At the start of the game, a number of "warm-up" items are used. Typically, the content of these items is not divorce related. Here is one of the warm-up items we have used:

> An eight-year-old child runs in a race with members of the Rutgers University track team. The eight-year-old child wins the race. Could this happen?

This warm-up item was selected for several reasons. Its content is nonthreatening so it is readily answered. Its unlikely outcome encourages the children to consider the plausibility of the question. It also challenges the children to dredge up evidence supporting their answer. I have found that one or two items of this sort are all that is needed to provide a sufficient introduction to the game. However, I attend to the level of anxiety in the group and increase the warm-up time if it seems high.

A second warm-up item is designed to provide a transition between nondivorce and divorce related items. "A woman is elected President of the United States. Could this happen?" This is a valuable transition item because it can lead to an important divorce relevant discussion of the relative power and status of women, and of male-female relationships. As children express their opinions about the plausibility of the item's premise, the leaders guide the discussion to a consideration of what parents have said about opportunities for women. The discussion can then be shifted to a consideration of men's views of women and, more specifically, of fathers' views of mothers.

Case Illustrations

The cases selected to illustrate the use of this game will be drawn from the same group of children described in the material illustrating the use of the *Children's Feedback Game*. Using this same group eliminates the need for additional background material and provides a view of additional facets of the psychological world of these children.

As noted previously, I consider the child's feelings of powerlessness an important consequence of the divorce experience. The following question facilitates a discussion of power:

> A child wants hamburgers for dinner. His parents hate hamburgers. The parents want spinach pie for dinner. The child hates spinach pie. The family discusses what to have for dinner and the parents decide to make hamburgers. Could this happen?

The underlying issue posed by this item is a parent's weighting of a child's expressed preferences against their own. The item raises the question of whether parents place their own needs ahead of their child's. Several children believed that the parent would make hamburgers because that's what the child wanted. However, some children disagreed and spontaneously connected this item with their parents' divorce related choices. Carl noted that parents don't always do what their child wants. He said that parents are often too busy to listen to the important things a child wishes to say. He said "I asked my mom to help me with homework and she said 'I'm too busy.' When my father was living with us, I asked him to help me and he said 'I'm too tired. I need a rest badly.' They don't have time for me." Then Carl gave a more poignant example to support his contention. He said:

Once, my dad went to Florida without even telling me. I didn't know where he was. He never called me. I asked my mom 'why doesn't my daddy call?' and she said 'I don't know.'

On his return, his father's lack of contrition precipitated an argument between father and son. Carl discussed how hurt he felt by the way his father treated him during this incident. Were it not for the game, Carl would have been unlikely to describe this incident. Moreover, this initial description led to more painful revelations of other ways his dad had discounted him.

The "hamburger" item is a nondivorce item which stimulates valuable discussion. Careful thought must be given to the transition from the nondivorce to the divorce content items. The children's responses are often helpful in determining the proper pace for the transition. In my opinion, it would be a mistake to suggest a hierarchy of the sequence of items or guidelines about the timing of specific items. Such an overly uniform approach might inhibit the children's spontaneity and impede the group's progress.

When the leader thinks the time is ripe, he or she could approach the content of the "hamburger" item more directly with the following question:

A child's father tells his family that he plans to get divorced. The child asks her father to stay married. The father agrees to remain married. Could this happen?

This item could stimulate children to discuss instances in which they asked their parents to stay together and how their parents responded. It is a useful item for generating cameraderie since so many children have tried to reconcile their parents and failed. Hearing other children discuss these feelings can help the child feel he or she is not alone.

The experience of discussing items whose content does not specifically pertain to divorce, eases the transition to a discussion of emotionally charged divorce-related items. The content of these items is drawn from background questionnaire material provided by the parents, from the contents of problems which parents are discussing in the parent group, and from problems reported in the divorce literature. The following question

deals with one such topic—a noncustodial parent who withholds financial support.

> A child's parents are divorced. The child needs braces for her teeth. The
> mother does not have enough money to pay for the braces. The father has
> enough money but refuses to pay for the braces. Could this happen?

Arlene eagerly volunteered to answer this question. She was a very
bright youngster with low self-esteem. Both of Arlene's parents were angry with one another and attempted to recruit Arlene as an ally in their
marital conflict. During my first meeting with her prior to the start of the
program she repeatedly informed me that she was incapable of drawing,
that she was "no good at anything," that she had no opinions on any
topic, and that she had no feelings about any of the tactics her parents
were using to involve her in their conflict. However, the game provided a
forum in which she was free to express opinions and strong feelings about
these actions. Arlene stated that she was sure that it was possible for the
father to refuse to pay for the braces. As "evidence" she stated, "My father is supposed to give my mother some money and he refuses to give it.
My mom has been working the night shift and she hasn't been seeing me
that much. Every time I want to see her, there's always a babysitter
around instead." In attempting to earn a *feeling* bonus point, Arlene
openly discussed her sadness at not seeing more of her mother and her anger at her father's behavior.

The ability to express feelings which was stimulated by this game generalized to other areas of Arlene's day-to-day activities. Indeed, her
mother noticed these changes and, several weeks after the conclusion of
the program, wrote me to share her observations and reactions. In her letter, she stated that "many people have noted the growth in Arlene in the
past few months." To illustrate this growth, she sent me a photocopy of a
composition which Arlene had written in school. In this essay entitled
"Divorce," Arlene wrote:

> People are busy all the time. I never get to see my mom and dad. My mom
> and father are getting divorced. I feel that they are trying to pull me apart.
> It's not fair to me. I hate it so much. . . . They both love me. They want me
> to live with them. . . . It's hard to have to choose my mother or my father. I
> hate divorces.

Arlene, a girl who six months previously had been unable to express any feelings concerning the divorce, was now able to talk openly and spontaneously about her feelings. The lure of the game induced her to drop her guard and set into motion a self-perpetuating process of change. For other children, however, the challenge of the game itself may not be sufficient to induce therapeutic movement. However, other curative factors related to the game may provide the needed spark. Lieberman, Yalom, and Miles (1973) report that a group member who is initially reluctant to participate in group activities can assume the role of "spectator." By watching others and vicariously sharing in their experiences, the spectator's motivation to participate is increased and an opportunity for therapeutic benefits derived from participation becomes available. This, indeed, is what happened to Craig.

Craig was a butterball whose disposition belied the "fat men are jolly" adage. In his mother's opinion, he was more "seriously disturbed" than the other children in the group. She doubted that the program could benefit a child as unbalanced as he. Combative at home, especially with his younger brother, he was shy and uncommunicative during the first four sessions of the group. But sitting quietly as he was, he must have been an avid spectator for Arlene's disclosure unleashed in him an outpouring of emotion that was to change his participation in the group and his behavior at home. He followed Arlene's disclosure with these words:

> When I was at my old house, Friday night, my dad said he was going to a meeting. I said "Daddy, why do you have to go to a meeting" and he said "I have to." He didn't go to a meeting. He was moving to another place without me. He was lying to me, my sister, and my brother. My mother had to call the police and say I'm missing a husband.

Perhaps Arlene's expression of anger at her father demonstrated to Craig that other children also experience this emotion and that it's okay to express this feeling. Perhaps Craig connected Arlene's anger at her father's "betrayal" with his own anger about this issue. While it is impossible to determine what caused what, it is clear that Craig's behavior following this incident was noticeably different. He became much more communicative, affectionate, and helpful in the group. His mother reported similar dramatic changes at home.

A second recurring problem, ineffective communication between family members, was the impetus for another game item. In many two-parent families, children are taught that giving feedback to parents is disrespectful and should be avoided. Likewise, voicing one's concerns may be equated with complaining, another negatively sanctioned activity. Although these prohibitions may not cause great problems for children living in a salutory environment, they are likely to severely hamper children of divorce who may refrain from discussing the stresses they are experiencing. In order to open a discussion of beliefs about communication, a necessary prelude to training in communication skills, the following question was devised:

> A parent says something that hurts a child's feelings. The child tells her parent that the parent hurt her feelings. The parent gets angry at the child and punishes her. Could this happen?

Discussion of this question is usually accompanied by role plays in which the child is encouraged to communicate with his or her parent. The leader provides feedback about the strengths and problem areas exhibited by the communicator. The viewing children are encouraged to use the skills they acquired in *The Children's Feedback Game* to share their reactions about what they observed. Often they are able to effectively point out that a child is whining, or acting silly when he or she is communicating a serious concern. Children are asked to take the role of the parent and imagine how a parent would react to this entreaty. Following the role plays, the leader asks each child to identify a concern about which he or she suspects his or her parent is unaware. The children are then given a "homework" assignment. They are asked to communicate the concern they identified as effectively as possible. To maximize the likelihood of success, the leader of the concurrent parent group is informed prior to the meeting that the children will be practicing new approaches to communication in the upcoming week. The leader communicates this information to the parents and discusses effective ways in which they can respond to the new initiatives.

When the children meet the following week, they discuss the outcome of their assignment. The ensuing discussion is often the source of new items for the game. For example, one child mentioned that he talked about how upset he became when his mother constantly described his father as a bad person. A number of children noted that they had similar experiences. Knowing that this problem was widespread, the leaders of a subsequent program constructed the following item to stimulate discussion of this topic:

> A father tells a child that the child's mother is a bad person. Could this happen?

As anticipated this item stimulated a productive discussion. Betty stated that her parents were involved in a custody dispute and shared her feelings about this matter. She stated that her father had urged her to live with him because "my girlfriend and I are better than your mother . . . who never does things or gets things for you." Betty never told her father how his words affected her. She revealed to the other children, however, that her father's statements frightened her so much that she would hide in her bedroom after talking to him. In the ensuing group discussion, she revealed that what most frightened her was the possibility of going to court and being asked to publicly choose between her mother and father. The children offered her considerable support and provided several helpful suggestions related to her difficulties.

As children can sometimes be supportive, they too can be cruel—their cruelty often far outstripping their kindness. Teachers have reported that children from intact families often tease children of divorce. To open discussion of this issue, I posed the following question:

> Children in school tease a child because her parents are divorced. Could this happen?

Carl thought this could definitely happen and said "I don't think it's very nice of the kids to make fun of her because its not her fault that her parents are divorced. They make fun of me. They say 'Oh Carl, your father doesn't live with you. And he doesn't take you anywhere.' " Arlene chimed in "Same with me. They tease me—'your father's got a girlfriend. Your father's going to marry her. And then your mother's going to be by herself with you. . . . 'I don't do anything when they say that but I feel mad." The ensuing discussion revealed that many of the children had shared this same distressing experience. Since knowing the trials of others can provide limited consolation, the children seemed to draw strength from the recognition that they were not unique in their harsh treatment.

I have also constructed questions which help the children to recognize the anguish their parents experience. By so doing, I help them take the role of their parent and see their mothers and fathers in a less stereotypic fashion. In this regard, one question I have found useful is:

A father was talking about something sad with his children. Suddenly he started to cry. Could this happen?

All of the children said that it could definitely happen. Joseph mentioned a time when his mother cried and he and his brother tried to console her. The leaders mentioned that it was good for parents as well as children to share their feelings with one another and encouraged the children to support their parents and in turn draw support from them.

The parents often provide us with material for questions. In one parents group meeting, the mothers complained how they were frequently the recipients of their child's anger while the noncustodial fathers were treated as the "good guys." Based on this information I constructed the following question:

A child is angry at his father. But instead of acting angry at his father, he acts nice with his father and acts angry with his mother. Could this happen?

I used this question in a special joint session of parents and children together. Discussion of this question helped to strengthen the parent-child bond. The children all felt that the hypothetical situation could definitely happen. Carl stated that he got angry at his father and took it out on his mother. Carl's mom suggested that Carl is worried that if he expresses anger at his father the father will stop seeing him. Carl said "I feel sorry for my mom because she's the one getting dumped on." His mom expressed how good she felt hearing Carl share this sentiment and grant psychological weight and validity to her concerns.

The items described give a flavor of the types of questions that can be developed and the impact they have on group discussion. It should be clear to the reader that any issue can be phrased as a game item and used productively. I urge others to unleash their imagination and create questions which can be discussed in the *Could This Happen Game*.

Using the Game as a Teaching Tool

The game provides the leader with an opportunity to provoke discussions about cooperation, to raise issues about male-female relationships, and to delve into feelings about belonging and rejection. The method of choosing teams is one such opportunity. The leader can choose from among several alternative methods of team composition. If a discussion of male-female issues is desirable, the leader might divide the group into one team of boys and one of girls. Alternatively, if the leader would like to discuss the sociometric patterns in the group as a prelude to discussing feelings of rejection, he or she might allow the children to choose their own teams.

Another excellent teaching opportunity arises when team reps offer their guesses concerning the most common answer. A rep choosing an unpopular answer may be ridiculed by his or her teammates. Should this occur, the leader can encourage the child to discuss his or her feelings and provide feedback to the tormenters using skills acquired in the *Children's Feedback Game*. The discussion can then be focused on experiences of being ridiculed at school and in neighborhood play situations. The group can then explore positive alternatives to ridicule and blame.

SUMMARY AND CONCLUSIONS

The *Children's Feedback Game*, though specifically developed for use with children of divorce, is equally suitable for use in other situations. Training classmates to give feedback to one another could eliminate much of the time consuming and emotionally draining disciplinary activities of teachers. Parents too could use this game to reduce sibling rivalry manifested in taunting, teasing, and tattling.

The *Could This Happen Game* could also be used with populations other than children of divorce. The game capitalizes on children's desire to demonstrate to others that they are "correct" and their willingness to offer evidence to prove it. Though I have constructed items which highlight beliefs and anxiety about divorce, different items could be constructed to open discussion about other areas of concern. For example, guidance counsellors could use this game to discuss test anxiety. They might offer the following item:

A child got a failing grade on a test. When he told his mother about his grade she stopped loving him. Could this happen?

Here the guidance counsellor could explore some of the pressures children may feel to perform well lest their parents reject them. Teachers could also use the game to discuss sex-role stereotypes. Here is a possible question:

A girl liked playing baseball and didn't like playing with dolls. None of the girls in her class wanted to be her friend. They all made fun of her. Could this happen?

The game could also be used to open discussions about prejudice, stereotypes, career aspirations—the list of possibilities is limited only by the imagination of the user. By judiciously choosing items, productive discussions are likely to ensue. Even children who are silent spectators can gain from these discussions as they listen to the concerns voiced by other children and realize that they are not alone in their worries. Further, the use of this game legitimizes the assignment of plausibility to *any* concern. Thus, it may encourage children who might otherwise think their worry is "ridiculous" and thus keep it to themselves, to share it with an adult and have the opportunity to discuss their fears and possibly have them allayed.

Throughout this Chapter, I have suggested tht the *Children's Feedback Game* and the *Could This Happen Game* can be creatively used to positively influence child psychosocial development. I have pointed out only a few of the therapeutic and teaching possibilities the games afford. Before using the game, the leader is encouraged to carefully consider the needs of the children in the group and to exercise much flexibility in adapting the game to meet these needs. Above all, the leader is exhorted to give great weight to the playful attitude with which most children approach games. Although the games were designed as therapeutic and teaching tools, I feel strongly that children learn most when they are given the freedom to laugh and to behave with a large measure of spontaneity. And what could be better than joyful learning?

REFERENCES

Ackerman, N. (1958). *The psychodynamics of family life*. New York: Basic.

Epstein, Y. and Borduin, C. (in press). Could this happen: A game for children of divorce. *Psychotherapy: Theory, Research, and Practice*.

Festinger, L. (1954). A theory of social comparison processes. *Human Relations, 7*, 117–140.

Ginott, H. (1961). *Group psychotherapy with children*. New York: McGraw-Hill.

Hovland, C., Janis, I., and Kelly, H. *Communication and persuasion*. New Haven, CN: Yale.

Kelman, H. (1958). Compliance, identification, and internalization: Three processes of attitude change. *Journal of Conflict Resolution, 2*, 51–60.

Lieberman, M., Yalom, I., and Miles, M. (1973). *Encounter groups: First facts*. New York: Basic.

Mead, G.H. (1934). *Mind, self and society*. Chicago: University of Chicago Press.

Odom, S. and Strain, P. (1984). Peer mediated approaches to promoting children's social interaction: A review. *American Journal of Orthopsychiatry. 54*, 544–557.

Rhodes, S. (1973). Short term groups of latency age children in a school setting. *International Journal of Group Psychotherapy, 23*, 204–216.

Yalom, I. (1970). *The theory and practice of group psychotherapy*. New York: Basic.

CHAPTER 9

Therapeutic Games for Children

CONNIE BEHRENS

A moment of truth: verbal children, who are acutely aware of their emotional pain and want relief, are frequently the most successful in therapy and, in the process, the therapist experiences enormous gratification in the helping role. My experience since 1967, in treating troubled children, reveals that such motivated youngsters are the exception rather than the rule. Most troubled children have a history of poor self esteem and few gratifying experiences with peers and adults. They assume excessive blame for problems and experience a diminished sense of power in controlling their lives. The eventual outcome is children who lack confidence in the value of their own thoughts, opinions, and feelings. They have seldom felt understood and respected, so they treat others with a lack of sensitivity. They are used to being blamed for problems, frequently told how to behave, and rarely asked about their feelings. With this type of adult involvement, such youngsters have few alternatives for handling stress and conflict, and they show a definite lack in successfully negotiating their situation with others.

The parents of these youngsters suffer their own pain, frustration and anger. They do not deal with feelings very effectively and, often out of a sense of helplessness, take on too much power to remedy the situation without involving their children in the process. A slow, growing distancing takes place during which parents blame children, children blame parents, no one talks to each other and, if they talk, they do not listen. The outcome is predictable: resistive children feeling powerless, worthless, and not very trusting of adults to be supportive, understanding, or helpful.

Both *The Problem-Solving Game* and *Picture That* are available for purchase from Connie Behrens, 1130 Aylesford Road, Charlotte, North Carolina 28211

A surprising phenomenon, which takes place in the therapeutic setting, is that many such children do like to talk about themselves. With 100 percent of an adult's attention for an hour, they will have little problem sharing information about themselves; however, they are very often resistive to sharing problems, concerns, fears, and worries. Their solutions to interaction conflicts frequently reflect the hurt and anger they have experienced so often "to resolve is to retaliate" and are devoid of creativity and sensitivity. The therapy process is often another arena in which to perfect their withholding, resistive tactics, or it is a situation too threatening to their lack of experience in sharing feelings that a therapist feels overwhelmed at his or her inability to get the children to open up. The children also seem to sense the pressure of the situation and little is accomplished or, if so, very slowly.

All of the dynamics discussed thus far reflect a very widespread condition of many latency age children: a tremendous void in their interpersonal problem-solving skills. To me, problem-solving consists of four steps: (1) helping the child explore the conflict situation (what happened? how did it start? how did the child react? how did the other person react? what was the final outcome?); (2) helping the child share his or her feelings about each part of the situation, as well as helping him or her put himself or herself into the other person's shoes with regard to how that person probably felt based on his or her reaction; (3) exploring together what alternative ways the child could have handled himself or herself in that same situation and relate to how the outcome could have been different with each alternative; and (4) giving the child the autonomy to make a decision for the future handling of similar conflict situations, reinforcing the fact that this is one area in which he or she can control his or her life, his or her reactions to others.

The task of improving problem-solving skills is not an easy one. However, it is an essential educational component to successful relationships. Any adult can help a child with this, and it has been my experience that adults learn additional skills in the process of helping the child. A key to the process is to remember that there are no right or wrong alternatives, but rather more effective and less effective ones. The greatest difficulty encountered is the one of being creative with a variety of solutions. If you can help a youngster choose a style that is both more adaptive than his or her original choice and more in line with his or her own style or relating, the opportunity for success will be greater. In other words, it would be very difficult for an aggressive, assertive child to ignore a conflict situation. Helping that child to be verbally assertive and to learn this adaptive skill would be more compatible with his or her basic style of handling relationships. Likewise, to expect a shy child to join a group of peers would likely be impossible; however, a reasonable alternative may be to encourage him or her to seek one child to start a friendship.

In an effort to relate more constructively to such situations, therapeutic games provide a vehicle for helping children to be more relaxed and productive in looking at their behavior. Games offer a level of competition, power, and control to which children can relate. A game attracts interest, encourages motivation, and the desire to win, all of which may mean greater involvement. When these qualities are present in a game which helps children deal with problem behavior, inappropriate responses, and sharing of feelings, the results are positive and often lasting.

The inspiration for *The Problem-Solving Game* came from a nine-year-old boy I will call Trent. He had been in therapy since preschool and remained a rigid, inflexible withholding child. He lacked self-esteem and he displayed hostile and insensitive relating skills with adults and peers. Trent was manipulative and resistive to talking about his problems, fears, and worries, so that "talking therapy" was ineffective. He skillfully managed to avoid involvement in important issues when "play therapy" was introduced so, out of sheer frustration on my part and strong pressure and concern from his parents and teacher, I confronted Trent with "the problem." The session went as follows:

THERAPIST: Trent, I've got a big problem and I need someone to help me with it. You are a bright boy, you know a lot about a lot of things, and I think perhaps you can help me. (With this introduction, Trent pulled up a chair in front of me and said: "Tell me about your problem.")

THERAPIST: You came to Children's House a while ago and we have been friends for a long time. You have had problems getting along with adults and children and have not made much progress. In our sessions together, you try every way imaginable to get out of talking about these important things, and now your parents and teacher are on my back to make things better. My problem is that I cannot make things better for you without your help so, in that way, it's your problem too. What are we going to do with our problem?

Trent got up, proceeded to stack two cube seats on top of each other and perched himself on a "throne." He instructed me to bring him pairs of rubber animals and dinosaurs and to put them in front of his "throne." He told me to make up a problem for each one and he would provide a solution. For the remainder of this session, I brought the animals to Trent with various problems identical to the ones he was having, and he provided creative, reasonable solutions for them to try. For the next six weeks, during at least half of each session, Trend chose to play this game and, as a result, he was able to generalize the problems and solutions directly to his own situation. Trent and I finally began to experience some success; talking about himself became easier; he felt less threatened by his problem behavior and the reactions of others and, above all, his behavior at home and at school began to improve.

Giving this youngster a "seat of power" to draw on his own creativity and intellect to deal with the problems of others gave him a less threatening way to discuss issues of high anxiety about himself. I decided to transpose this activity into a game utilizing the same philosophy which worked to help Trent open up. Similar success has been noted with other resistive and scared children; ones who lacked the experience in talking about issues of importance, who have never been given a chance to express their ideas, and who lacked problem-solving skills have benefitted from the use of this game.

DESCRIPTION OF THE GAME

The format of *The Problem-Solving Game* is simple; it includes a stack of "problem cards" (each worth one or two points based on color) and a bag of wooden chips (distributed by the "banker"). The game can be played with groups of children or in a one-on-one setting. Players receive chips for responding to their chosen problem card, and they can receive extra chips for helping a fellow player, if help is requested. The written material on the cards is reflective of the most common problems I have encountered in working with children in the age range of 6 to 12 years. Situations deal with shy, aggressive, fearful, confused, angry, and handicapped children. Cards include adults (parents and teachers) in need of help and issues, such as divorce, separation, death, fears, firesetting, stealing, bedwetting, parental conflict, adoption, stepparents, siblings, anger, grades, child-parent relationships—the list is extensive. The player is asked to help by coming up with a solution to the problem on the card. To elaborate on the response, as an avenue for additional discussion, is useful. To personalize the situation with questions such as "Has that ever happened to you?" "Has anyone ever treated you that way?" or "Have you ever handled a problem like that?" helps bring the discussion into a more individualized focus. I have found that, before children realize it, they are sharing information about themselves, sometimes for the first time, and find that it is not as scary and threatening as they had always thought. Chips are given regardless of the type of response. With instances of maladaptive or inappropriate solutions suggested by a child, the adult can offer an alternative resolution of more effective coping without challenging the child's idea as wrong. By pursuing the child's ineffective solution with further discussion and enlarging on the contents of the "problem card," you can deal with how others may respond to this solution and decide if this would magnify the problem or resolve it.

In view of the nonthreatening setting of this game, interaction can be dealt with on a more intellectual level. The problems on the cards ask the child to help *someone else* in difficulty. This is an important element because many troubled children cannot look at all angles of their own problems due to their anger and hostility, which so often mask hurt, sad feelings. The opportunity for objectivity, in dealing with a problem situation, enables even the most troubled child to deal with the situation more productively.

The game ends either after all the cards have been used or after a designated period of time has elapsed. The player with the most chips is the winner.

A fellow social worker, and partner in practice at Children's House, developed a unique therapeutic game, *Picture That*, which relates to affective responses and body language recognition as a means of expressing feelings. A group of cards, with pen sketches of children displaying various facial expressions and body postures, are selected by the players to depict how one may feel in response to a "situation card," which states an example of interaction between two people. The cards have point values to keep score and determine a winner.

The therapeutic value of this game is obvious: it is another vehicle to help children talk about feelings. However, it is more specifically designed to heighten a youngster's awareness of the messages inherent in body language and facial expressions. It helps children go beyond the often obvious feelings of anger and happiness to consider the sad, scary, hurt, and embarrassed feelings which are often masked by anger. *Picture That* has value by itself, and I have found the picture cards useful to use in conjunction with *The Problem-Solving Game* as a creative second step to dealing with another facet of understanding and considering solutions to problems. My experience with using *Picture That* is that children begin to realize that any one interaction (positive or negative) can actually create a variety of feelings in another person. For example, a strict father scolding his child, for unacceptable report card grades, may leave the child feeling angry and sad. If the child's poor performance were an attempt to rebel against his father's control, there may be present also feelings of pleasure and satisfaction. Through this game, all these feelings can be related to and awareness can be heightened.

CASE ILLUSTRATIONS

Professionals have reported success using *The Problem-Solving Game*. With defensive children, not only does it provide a vehicle for conversation, but it also affords a way to look at the maladaptive defenses children use in coping with peers and authority figures. A particularly hostile, defensive 11-year-old girl, who was highly resistive to talking about herself, agreed to play the game. After reading her first problem card, she got angry, pushed the cards and chips on the floor and accused the therapist of trying to trick her into talking about her problems. The therapist calmly collected the game parts and explained that she was not trying to trick her, but merely thought it would be easier for her to talk about others' problems than it had been to talk about her own. In the next session, the girl reluctantly asked to try "that game" again and played for 30 minutes. In that time, the youngster revealed more about herself than she ever had in the past and chose to play often in subsequent sessions. As a vehicle to "opening up," the game also became a productive method of allowing this resistive child to look at her own behavior and begin to consider change. A final note to the case is that, by the time therapy terminated, this girl had written 30 additional "problem cards." Her reason was that she felt the person who "made up" this game had left out some important things that happen to children. This is control and power to the very end, but more adaptive nevertheless.

A seven-year-old girl, who was shy, anxious, and lacked creativity in problem-solving skills, entered the therapy situation with much hesitancy. She had a great need to "do the right thing" and please adults, so that attempts to talk about her problems appeared to cause her embarrassment. Efforts to discuss difficulties with her were unsuccessful and resulted in a variety of manipulative behaviors. For this child, therapeutic games provided the only way for conversing and sharing. What she revealed was an attitude that all of her problems were the result of others' behavior and that she did not view herself as responsible in any way. While playing *The Problem-Solving Game*, this youngster had many creative resolutions to the situations presented; however, she had no creative resolutions to some of her own peer problems. This was pointed out to her and she had no explanation, but did recognize the discrepancy. In the course of therapy, she began to "loosen up" and frequently presented her therapist with the day's dilemma. Unable to draw on the creativity the girl possessed and in sheer frustration, the therapist decided to present back to her, in the form of a "problem card," each situation she brought to the session. To the amazement of both, this child came up with some very original and creative solutions to her own concerns and problems, but could only do so when they were addressed as someone else's problem. Therapy continues with this youngster and *The Problem-Solving Game* is rarely used; however, her version is used frequently and with success. This child is less anxious, more independent in relation to her own social problems and is more verbal regarding her feelings.

A final illustration is that of a bright, verbal 10-year-old boy who was experiencing intense feelings of helplessness and pressure from the expectations of adults in his life. The burden of a learning disability increased feelings of inadequacy and vulnerability. His typical response to any stress was an angry aggressive outburst, frequently resulting in loss of control and hitting. This occurred with conflict interaction toward adults and peers. By use of *The Problem-Solving Game*, this youngster began to realize that a variety of responses were available to him and often caused fewer negative reactions from others. Discussions of alternative solutions gave him an increased sense of power and control over a portion of his life, and the feelings of helplessness began to diminish. Being an assertive child, he had a need to be actively involved in interaction and would use his therapy hour to discuss the best way to handle a problem, then implement the plan on his own. Changes in his behavior were dramatic once he realized that being verbally assertive, in a positive way, carried more weight and respect from others than his previous explosive behavior.

SUMMARY AND CONCLUSIONS

The Problem-Solving Game, as a therapy tool to facilitate conversation, discuss feelings, and develop self-awareness in resolving interpersonal conflicts, has been established in this chapter. An additional use for the game is gathering diagnostic information about children. Based on their responses, one can determine basic styles of handling conflict situations and assess adaptive or maladaptive defenses used for coping. Children will reveal basic attitudes regarding authority and responsibility, as well as demonstrating qualities such as flexibility, sensitivity, and self-esteem. Since this is a game, the element of competition is present, and children can be seen in a win-lose situation with adults and other children. Although *The Problem-Solving Game* is not designed to be a specific diagnostic tool, the information to be gathered about children and their functioning is limitless.

The focus of this chapter has been related to using the game in the therapy setting. It is significant to use in any social group and with families as a way to enhance and improve verbal skills, communication, and sharing. Since the family setting is the primary social learning situation for children, any improvement in the functioning of the unit, particularly in problem-solving skills, will enhance the quality of everyone's relating.

THREE

Ego-Enhancing Games

The chapters in this section describe the use of games to enhance the ego functioning of children. This particular use of games emphasizes the competitive, challenging aspects of game playing. Competitive games involve more than just an enjoyable form of play; they challenge children to apply their skills to win the game. Under these conditions, the opportunities to observe the child's ego processing are many. Feelings of competence or self-doubt, impulse control and frustration tolerance, reality testing, intellectual skills, locus of control, self-image, and concentration are among the ego functions that are revealed during competitive game play. In therapy, the child often faces the prospect of playing against an adult who is superior in intellect and experience. As a result, feelings of competition, aggressiveness, trust, and helplessness in relation to adults are often revealed in the child's manner of play. The diagnostic information gathered during game play can then be used to formulate dynamics of the child's psychological functioning and to plan treatment strategies. Therapeutic interventions in the form of ego-level interpretations, modeling of appropriate responses, and teaching of adaptive behaviors can be made during competitive game play.

Contemporary uses of games for ego enhancement represent a continuation of the psychoanalytic tradition of bringing play and games into therapy to engage children in the therapy process and provide a vehicle for expression of emotions and conflict. Today, ego enhancing game play remains identified, but not exclusively so, with the psychoanalytic theoretical orientation. Ego enhancing game play typically takes place in a one-to-one, rather than group, therapy situation. Relatively simple, well-known games, such as checkers, target games, card games, *Sorry*, *Connect-Four*, and so on are preferred, on the assumption that children feel more comfortable with and derive more enjoyment from familiar games rather than unfamiliar "therapeutic" games, and therefore are more likely to project their own personality into their game play. More recent developments in game therapy have seen games applied within other theoretical frameworks, such as cognitive-behavioral therapy. The trend is toward greater specialization; that is, to use games to help children improve specific ego skills, such as self-control, visuospatial ability, reflective thinking, and basic cognitive skills relevant to academic learning.

CHAPTER 10

The Use of Competitive Games
in Play Therapy

IRVING N. BERLIN

BRIEF HISTORY OF THE USE OF GAMES IN PLAY THERAPY

Play therapy was developed as a way of understanding the nonverbal communications of disturbed children whose feelings, thoughts, and conflicts are often more easily discerned through play than through "talking" therapy. Hug-Helmuth in 1911 (1921) first used play as a therapeutic tool. In different periods in the 1920s Klein (1932) and Anna Freud (1928) expanded on the meanings and uses of play in a therapeutic setting. Later, a number of psychoanalysts contributed to the understanding of the symbolic meaning of play in a psychoanalytic context, followed by Levy (1938) and others who developed a play technique called "structured play," in which traumatic events encountered by a child were replicated with toys, much like a stage set, to provide an opportunity for catharsis and working through the specific trauma encountered by the child. Axline (1947) and Taft (1933) developed specific play techniques which reflect their particular theoretical framework for understanding the psychopathology of children.

Today, the use of games as active play to bring about communication has become a frequent part of play therapy. The increased use of games to some extent reflects a change in the kinds of children and adolescents we work with in treatment. We rarely see the neurotic child who, at six or so, can play and talk out his or her conflicts and benefit from interpretations. More often, we see children with more serious psychopathology resulting from severe neglect or abuse, and these children seldom communicate in words. Among older children, preadolescents and adolescents, it has become commonplace to find they come from homes where talking with

197

parents and among other adults is unusual. The behavioral problems that bring these young people to us point strongly to an orientation which emphasizes action, rather than talk. Thus, play therapy, and the use of games in that context, has become an increasingly important method of establishing therapeutic communication.

Over the past decade, a number of child therapists have employed various game strategies to break through the communication barrier, with various results. It has become apparent that certain attitudes about the self are readily displayed in game playing. Bettelheim (1972) described his use of poker and chess for specific purposes in play therapy. Others have used the games of *Monopoly* and *Risk* to focus on specific aspects of feeling helpless and the need to feel powerful and aggressive. Winnicott (1971) introduced the squiggle game as a means of quickly reaching the child's fantasies, which otherwise could not be talked about or were slow in emerging. Gardner (1971) and other child therapists devised storytelling games in which the therapist collaborated with the child to tell a story which usually helped reveal hidden feelings and conflicts; these same child therapists developed structured games—like Gardner's *Talking, Feeling, Doing Game*—in which each participant draws a card which tells him or her what to do or talk about. The impersonal nature of being instructed by a card to describe a feeling, thought, or engage in an action, combined with the equal participation of the therapist, seems to make expression of ideas and feelings easier. Gardner has commented that the structure of this game helps bypass the superego and permits the ego greater freedom of expression.

Most of us in our training in play therapy have been warned specifically against playing competitive games, such as checkers, because they inhibit the free associative aspects of free play and its accompanying fantasy. While these anticipated drawbacks may be in some degree true, I have found competitive games very useful in certain therapeutic situations. Further, I think with few exceptions we often find in practice that children who need to use competitive games easily find ways to introduce them into the playroom, often in the rudimentary forms of tic-tac-toe and hangman.

WHY AND WHEN COMPETITIVE GAMES ARE USEFUL

It has been my repeated observation over a number of years that competitive games permit many silent children and preadolescents easier access to unacceptable feelings of hostility, hate, and vengeful feelings toward parent figures and siblings, as well as broader competitive feelings with adults. They also provide an opportunity for dealing with the need to win and feel powerful and competent, in contrast to the actual feelings of helplessness. The therapist as competitor becomes not only a person to defeat, but also one to identify with, especially in the therapist's expression of attitudes about losing and winning. The child may identify as well with many other feelings expressed by the therapist in the play of a game.

An important aspect of game playing is how both therapist and patient deal with the universal need to cheat. An equally important aspect is the patient's opportunity to experience the therapist's regard and respect, which are clearly demonstrated by his or her various attitudes towards the patient in his or her efforts to learn the game, need to cheat, and so on. Also, the therapist's empathy with the patient's feelings when the patient wins or loses are important to the therapeutic alliance. The game provides repeated opportunities for the therapist to model how a variety of feelings can be openly expressed.

I prefer to play those games in which each move permits the therapist and later the patient to express feelings. Thus, I prefer to play the card game *War* with very young children, dominos with somewhat older children, and checkers with the most mature children. I avoid chess because it is difficult for children to learn and requires too much concentration on the therapist's part to play a good game and attend at the same time to the variety of details in the therapeutic interaction.

It is critical that the game be played in such a way that each player has a good chance to win. In doing this, the therapist shows his or her respect for the competitor and enhances the patient's self-esteem. The methods of promoting such attitudes in competitive play will be described.

SOME CONCERNS ABOUT THE DIFFERENCE BETWEEN PLAYING AND PLAY THERAPY

One of the major obstacles to the therapeutic use of competitive games is the need of many therapists, who are themselves very competitive, to win. This may reflect a strong need to assert and be reassured about their own competence and power. Such therapists very easily slip into playing the game only to win. If being defeated by a child arouses in the therapist anger, hurt, or a sense of loss of status, he or she can be sure that what is occurring in the session is not therapeutic. Play therapy of all kinds requires an ability and effort to understand the child's behaviors as they are expressed by posture, gestures, speech, and affect. Such attentiveness to the patient is not possible if the therapist is playing the game largely for his or her own satisfaction.

On the other hand, therapy falls just as far short when the mutual enjoyment of the competitive game precludes the kind of attentiveness just described. Naturally, mutual pleasure in playing often occurs in therapy; however, in the nontherapeutic instance the enjoyment of the game and often the relief at having the child engaged with the therapist, rather than sullenly silent, may lead the therapist into seeing the competitive game as being sufficient if it provides mutual fun. This greatly reduces therapeutic effectiveness.

Young therapists who have not resolved their own competitiveness with siblings and parents and are not yet sure about the process of play therapy are most vulnerable to using the competitive game as an end in itself, rather than a means to an end. They still need to learn and experience that the essence of play therapy is the facilitation of communication. Their efforts must be to follow the child's activities closely in order to comprehend the expression of conflict, no matter how disguised. They must also attempt to communicate a personal receptiveness and a desire to understand the child's troubles and to help the child reduce his or her distress and troublesome behavior.

A DEVELOPMENTAL APPROACH TO COMPETITIVE GAMES

By age four many children are aware of the existence of rules; certainly the six-year-old knows that rules exist for behavior at home, school, and in other organized settings. Problems with observing rules often stem from laxity at home about the necessary rules for living, especially noted in a very permissive home setting with what amounts to no rules. Conversely, an overly strict, harsh, unreasonable, and punitive family attitude tempts the child to overtly comply and covertly defy the rules. In the case of the abused and neglected child, the difficulty is often compounded in that the rules may be terribly harsh and punitive, but enforced at one time and not at another, so that the child learns to do as he or she pleases, since punishment may occur under any circumstances and at any time.

Competitive games, in common with other games, have rules. At their simplest, the rules require taking turns. The working through of the use of a set of rules may be the first area of conflictful interaction the therapist must face. This must be done in accordance with the child's cognitive development. How does one begin to deal with taking turns? One way is to inquire whether the youngster understands the idea of taking turns so that a game can be played. If this is hard, and there is no taking of turns, then the child is playing the game alone and that is fine if the child wants to play that way for a while. Most children find that playing alone is no fun, since there is no interaction. If the therapist initiates the turn taking and compliments the child on being able to await his or her turn, the child experiences some real pleasure at the interaction. I have found that the problem about taking turns occurs most often in games, such as *War* and some boardgames, in which the child must amass cards or must reach "home" to win. When one emphasizes that the youngster didn't really beat the therapist and, therefore, didn't really have the fun of winning, most children quickly become eager to win by actually beating someone.

CHEATING IN COMPETITIVE GAMES

Many children and adolescents need to win at all cost in any competitive game. These are youngsters who are very unsure of themselves and have a very poor self-image. They frequently are very angry at the adults in their life. Often the anger stems from intense sibling rivalry and a feeling that the sibling is preferred and gets the parents' attention, love, and also material things as signs of preference. Their need to win, by forcing others to give in to them, often represents being successful or triumphant over siblings and parents. At times, the need to win may represent being the victor in an oedipal struggle. The parent of the same sex is frequently hostile and threatening. More often than not, the strong need to win results from a developmental arrest, usually during the separation/individuation stage as described by Mahler, Pine, and Bergman (1975). The most needy of these children appear to be those who were neglected and/or abused around age two. Most of these young people have not enjoyed the experience of being cherished and valued as an individual: Their efforts at exploration were not stimulated; their charming ways and engaging comments were neither applauded nor encouraged. Thus, the practicing subphase and subsequent phases are not lived through in a benign and caring environment. The child who must win appears to be convinced that he or she is superior and deserves to be admired and cared about.

In time, the therapist's emphasis on making the game fair and competitive, as well as his or her efforts to teach the child to win fairly will reduce the need to cheat. With some youngsters in whom the need to cheat is overpowering, it may be important to extend one's self to provide a means for winning. For instance, if the therapist is ahead, he or she can exchange the piles of cards, reverse the board in checkers, or change places in dominos so that the child or adolescent can experience the therapist's desire to help him or her win.

Often the youngster will want to play the game by his or her rules. Such alterations in rules may profitably be permitted, but there must be a clear understanding that any change in rules will apply to both players. The therapist's understanding comments about the child's need to win, while permitting and encouraging winning, is perhaps more effective than sticking to the game rules at the outset. Helping the patient stick to whatever set of rules are established at the beginning of the game with candid comments about how the therapist feels, that is, angry and frustrated that a real game cannot be played helps the child play by the rules.

At some point in the therapy, the child will be receptive to being helped to learn to play effectively and to win legitimately. The therapist must be alert to use this moment of the patient's willingness to play correctly. The therapist needs to acknowledge his or her pleasure in helping the child or adolescent to learn, and to compliment the young person on his or her courage in wanting to learn.

Since I use each game to dramatically express my feelings, I take care to show the child a different affective partner when he or she cheats: Mild protests with no major affective displays are a sharp contrast to the free expression of affect which is pleasurable to the child or adolescent and which results in his or her responsive behavior of either smiling or mild derision. In such situations, the playfulness is a powerful aid to playing fairly.

THE PRESCHOOL CHILD IN THE PLAYROOM

Very frequently we begin by playing *War*. For the uninitiated, in this game the players divide the deck in half, each taking a stack of cards. The individual piles are placed face down. Simultaneously, the players turn over the top card in their stack, and the highest card takes the trick. When each player exposes the same-numbered card, they both shout "war!" and the next turned card determines who takes in both piles of cards. The therapist helps the child recognize the number printed on the card by calling out his or her number and encouraging the child to call out his or her card. This game permits the therapist a great deal of emotional expression: "Oh, darn it, your queen is taking my best jack; you're skunking me!" or "Oh boy, my king is taking your queen; I'm really going to beat you!" The therapist's loud declaration or shout of "war!" when the same numbers surface is soon imitated by the child, as are other exclamations. A good deal of affective interaction can occur with each turn of a card. When the therapist finds himself or herself with a much larger pile and a young child who *needs* to win, he or she can offer to exchange piles with the child to help him or her win. However, the therapist needs to be clear that on each turn of the card, the player with the highest number on his or her card does in fact take both cards. Sticking with that rule shows respect for the child's ability to play and win by the rules.

With some young children I use dominos as a competitive game. Though a game of chance, learning how to block an opponent is important in winning the game. When the therapist assists the young child in learning how to block, the child's self-confidence is bolstered. The child sees, or I demonstrate that when he or she blocks, that is, figures out that I do not have any dominos with certain numbers of dots and plays those numbers, then I must hunt for more pieces because I can't match any of the dominos in play. If the child can continue to block, I will have to keep hunting, which increases his or her chances of winning. I always mention aloud what numbers are open to be played on. The triumph of a four- or five-year-old who understands how to block is a delight to observe. The expressive possibilities are rich: Gleeful when matching the dominos in play or dejected and fearful of losing when hunting for more dominos and increasing his or her pile. The winner is the one who is out of dominos first, and the loser must add up the total number of dots on his or her remaining dominos. Each player keeps a total until the end of the contest, and often the therapist must help the child count the number of dots and add it to the total for him or her. In preparation for this game, I may play several games with both players' piles turned face up so that the manner of playing the game becomes clear to the child.

CASE ILLUSTRATION

Alice, a bright four-year-old, came to treatment because she had been hitting other children at preschool and attacking her infant brother at home, as well as refusing to obey her mother. Her father, a trucker, was rarely home. When he was, she obeyed him. Alice had nightmares about creatures from outer space taking her away to another planet.

In the playroom, I explained the rules about being able to play with any toys as long as she didn't break anything or hurt herself or me. She soon tried to smash a toy truck with a long block. When I prevented this and held her so she could not hurt me or break anything, she screamed and kicked the floor, but then relaxed. In preschool and at home, Alice was a nonverbal child, and it soon became clear that there was little talking at home by either parent.

In the second session, I prevented her abortive attempt to stamp on a doll and I held her again. She was relaxed in my arms. I reached for the dominos and tumbled them out of the box. I picked one up with a six and four on it and asked if she could find a domino that matched either end of the one I had. She counted the dots on each end silently and finally found a six/three and laid it next to my six. We continued to match dominos and created a nice pattern on the floor. Towards the end of the hour, she whispered the numbers on my domino she had to match, imitating my calling the numbers of each domino aloud. The next hour she came in, sat down, picked up the dominos and began the matching play, enjoying the taking of turns and my comments of "Oh my, where will I find a seven to match yours?"

Then I explained the game to her, how we each started out with seven dominos, and so forth. Because I knew how to play, I handicapped myself by taking ten instead of seven dominos. We played one "open" game and then a regular game; she won both. She chortled triumphantly whenever I would lament, "You've really got me stuck!" as I hunted for a matching domino. When I would find a matcher and loudly exclaim that I was going to beat her, she'd say very softly, "Oh no, you're not." In a few weeks, she was screaming she'd squash me when she matched my domino and crying out, "You stinker, you!" when I managed to block her. These were words I'd used at various times, and the affects were good imitations of feelings I had voiced.

As Alice's verbalizations became louder and more fervent, her hostile behavior lessened considerably at preschool and at home. When she learned to block me, she very proudly told her mother when she went into the waiting room.

After about four months, Alice began to use some of the Flagg family dolls to enact a number of themes. But when she began to feel threatened by what she was playing out with toys, she'd return to the game of dominos. Her joyous triumphant cries or mock cries of horror if I had a good run, which were appropriately responded to by me, seemed to ease her tension and she could return to play with the dolls and dollhouse. This repetitive play dealt with sibling rivalry and oedipal themes. After two years of therapy, Alice was a much changed girl, doing well in school, home, and with peers.

At age eight, Alice came back to see me for a short time when her father was hospitalized after an automobile accident. Alice had been immobilized and very depressed. In the playroom she picked out the dominos for us to play, but she also began to talk about her fears of her father's death and how her mother was so scared and helpless that Alice felt she had to take care of everyone. While we played a perfunctory game of dominos during each session, the game was primarily a means Alice used to talk out her anxieties. When her father came home, and I was able to convince both parents that couple's therapy was in order, Alice stopped seeing me.

The dominos were useful as a way of getting angry, hostile, fearful, gleeful, and victorious feelings out in the open, as well as the sad feelings that accompanied losing. As Alice learned to play well, and especially to block, her self-attitudes became positive and her self-image changed from a frightened, insecure child to a self-confident, effective one.. Playing dominos led to her ability to express feelings in symbolic play.

THE SCHOOL-AGED CHILD

The school-aged youngster is well aware of rules and his or her need to win is not clouded by lack of understanding how games are played. In my experience, children of this age who are unable to talk easily and tend to be silent and withdrawn have often suffered serious abuse and neglect. To trust an adult will take time. For school-aged children, playing checkers is usually of interest, although playing with an adult may be anxiety producing. Sometimes an evident need to cheat reflects the parents' or other adults' lack of concern about the child, particularly in terms of helping him or her to become a competent, effective person. This may lead, and often does, to the child's conviction that beating someone else and winning at any cost is the important goal, not being an effective person.

Children are keenly aware of adult superiority in games, and they are sensitive to the lack of respect for them shown by an adult who gives them permission to play unfairly or to win illegitimately. The therapist who communicates a lack of respect or concern for the dignity of the child or adolescent is repeating their previous experiences with adults and damaging the therapeutic relationship. The therapist must also be aware that there are some children whose need to win—even knowing they are being allowed to win—is symptomatic of serious neurotic oedipal conflicts. Their omnipotence may need to be deliberately bolstered early in treatment as a therapeutic phase.

It is important with school-aged children to play a trial game to find out how good each player is and to determine how much of a handicap is necessary to have a good hard-fought game. By doing this through one or more trial games, the therapist lets the child know that he or she really wants him or her to have a good chance to win the game and to learn to enjoy the playing. The therapist must also convey that he or she does not want to win through the opponent's lack of skill or by thoughtless errors by either player. When a child makes a silly or haphazard move, the therapist should ask him or her to reconsider the move. In checkers, the youngster sometimes needs to be shown repeatedly how a particular move will lead to being jumped and perhaps beaten, and alternative moves should be suggested. Occasionally, a child will insist stubbornly on his or her original move, no matter what the consequences, and the therapist must decide whether to go along with the move or to demonstrate once more how this move will probably end in the youngster's loss. After asking the youngster several times to reconsider the move, the therapist may need to say he or she cannot play this way, and that perhaps they can play another game of checkers at the next session.

The therapist's choice in this situation may well depend on the child's developmental stage, as well as on the degree of characterologic impulsiveness. For the child who is beginning to want to learn to play by the rules—at age seven or so—it may be better to stop the game. The therapist should make it clear that it is no fun for him or her and the child seems not to be ready to learn to play a good game or to enjoy playing.

With the very impulsive child, the therapist's willingness to stop this game and begin another may demonstrate to the child that his or her mistake has not lost him or her the game, although impulsive, angry behavior has prevented him or her from winning. Readiness to try again expresses the therapist's hope that he or she will want to learn how to play better next time. In either case, the child gets the message that the therapist wants him or her to play well. This is a message he or she may have seldom or never received from an adult. His or her desire to be the equal of the adult, even in a few areas, rarely has been acknowledged or encouraged. Once the child recognizes the therapist's concern in helping him or her achieve mastery in a game, the child will begin repeated testing of the sincerity and extent of that concern.

Most competitive games permit the therapist to demonstrate how one can fully express feelings of anger and hurt on losing, and triumph, glee, or pleasure on winning. Checkers, however, permits such demonstration of feelings with almost every move. When I am jumped, I scream with anguish and anger about possibly being beaten or almost losing, and I playfully accuse my opponent: "You skunk, you're trying to smash me!" When I jump my opponent, I chortle with glee about how I will demolish him or her. I crow when I win a game, usually bragging about how good I am. If I lose, I'm equally dramatic in my dejection. Since I exaggerate the affect, with obvious enjoyment of my own histrionics, the youngsters seem to enjoy it. It does not take long for even a very silent, withdrawn child to begin to imitate my behavior, at first tentatively, and to begin to express his or her hurt and anger on losing a game after a bad move and his or her pleasure on winning or at a good move.

In the following clinical material, the youngsters I describe are developmentally delayed in some cognitive, social, sensory-motor, or psychologic-interpersonal areas as a result of psychopathology and the resulting problems arising at various periods of their development. Exacerbation of difficulties with major maladaptation occurs when conflicts in the current developmental stage reinforce the original trauma and maladaptation of previous stages of development.

CASE ILLUSTRATIONS

Herb, a six-year-old boy who was very hyperactive, hostile, aggressive, and had a poor attention span, was referred by the school. At the time of treatment, he was in a foster home, but had been severely abused until age four. He came sullenly and worriedly into the playroom, sat down at the low table, and would not accompany me to look at the toys available for him to play with. When I asked him what he'd like to do, he shrugged his shoulders and looked both scared and hostile. I took down the checkerboard and checkers and asked him if he knew how to play; he barely nodded yes. I explained our playing a trial game to find out how many checkers I needed to take off for it to be a good and fair game. He withdrew and looked uncomfortable. It was clear he knew the moves of the game.

When I stopped his moving his checker because I'd get a double jump, he seemed surprised. When I complimented him on a good move, he stared suspiciously at me. After handicapping myself three checkers, we played a close game. Herb reacted with a slight smile when I moaned, "Oh no, you're not going to jump me again." Thus, while we played for four weeks in near silence, Herb seemed to be less apprehensive each time and also appeared to appreciate my instructions which helped him make better moves and my warning him of potentially bad moves. After about a month, Herb would whisper after me comments like "Darn it you're going to trap my man" or "Oh boy, have I got you!" Each time he whispered, he looked fearfully at me. In another few weeks, he moved from echoing my words to exclaiming with muted glee when he was about to jump me or expressing annoyance. In time, he became very boisterous as he imitated my remarks. He'd greet me joyously when he came in. He learned to play well for his age. His foster father once inquired with a mixture of annoyance and pleasure how I had taught Herb to play so well that he could often beat him. Through our playing checkers, Herb worked out a great deal of his anger, hostility, fear, and hate and his behavior at school improved markedly. He was clearly more trusting of adults. He also learned to express feelings of closeness, saying "this is fun," and to enjoy those moments. Herb's learning improved, attention span increased, and there was no evidence of hyperactivity.

Nine-year-old Sammy was brought to treatment because of hyperactive, destructive behavior in school. He was frequently ejected from his classroom and sent home, and had fallen two years behind in basic subjects. He displayed aggressive, overactive behavior with his mother and two younger siblings, but was less aggressive and overactive around his father. However, he inadvertently broke things when he and his father worked in the yard, on the car, or made appliance repairs. These were activities which Sammy usually enjoyed. At the time I saw him, repeated expulsions from class, along with the anger of teachers, administrators, and parents, had resulted in Sammy's becoming a sullen, defensive child.

He was brought in to be evaluated for minimal cerebral dysfunction. There were no developmental data to confirm the diagnosis and no abnormalities revealed by neurologic and neuropsychologic examinations.

Sammy was very large for his age and demonstrated some of the clumsiness of large nine-year-olds, as well as an inability to sit still; but his coordination in physical games and gross motor skills were excellent. Developmentally, Sammy was not yet ready to spend much time sitting still. His fine motor skills, while good, were not refined, so that he could not write easily. While he could read and concentrate, he needed to be up and about frequently. Given a model to build, however, he spent an hour without interruption.

After several introductory sessions, Sammy was still uncommunicative, wandering from toy to toy, silently discarding tinker toys, trucks, and the like, just moments after he picked them up. I asked if he would like to play checkers. He nodded glumly. I explained our trial games, and after I had beaten him handily in several, he agreed to my being handicapped by playing with two less checkers. In our first game, after a few opening moves which showed he knew how to play, he made an impulsive move that would give me a triple-jump. I refused to move and asked him to reconsider, explaining it would be no fun to beat him simply because of a careless mistake. He refused to reconsider or change his move. I removed the checkers from the board and said we would play another time. For the remainder of that play session, Sammy wandered around the playroom disconsolately kicking at toys. I said several times that I was sorry we could not continue the game, but it was no fun unless we played well enough to make it tough for me to win.

At the next session, Sammy heeded my warnings and even asked my advice about a move. We both tried to figure out which move would be better. On one occasion he tried to cheat by moving a checker straight across squares so that he could make a double jump. When I mildly remonstrated, muttering, "I sure do know how much you want to win," he shamefacedly replaced the checker. He narrowly lost this game, and at the end I praised him for the great fight he had put up. In the 10 minutes left in the session, he began to arrange furniture in the doll house quietly and systematically, without comment.

In a session sometime later, he stopped me when I had made an unthinking, stupid move, saying he could not move until I had reconsidered. When I soberly thanked him, he grinned and approved my next move. Sammy learned to play well and became less concerned with winning than with playing a good game.

His subsequent play with other toys became more serious, and he began to talk about the behavior and feelings of the dolls in the dollhouse. He seemed to take it for granted that I would listen attentively, try to understand him, and treat him with dignity. At this juncture, he had made the transition from essentially nonverbal, concrete, competitive play to verbal fantasy, and we entered the next phase in therapy.

Chester, at the age of 13, used checkers to communicate in various ways. He was a brilliant boy from a brilliant family, but emotionally he was very constricted and depressed. He was brought to treatment because he had begun to stay in his room, refusing to go to school or to see his friends. He complained of assorted aches and pains and was eating little. His symptoms had begun shortly after the onset of puberty and his promotion to high school.

I suspected developmental problems, especially the recrudescence of previous conflicts about self-worth which had previously led to depression, combined with adolescent anxieties as he was being flooded with sexual impulses. There was also evidence of rebellion at unrelenting parental demands for scholarly excellence which in no way reflected his parents' pride in his talents and achievements, only in fulfilling their expectations.

Chester was passive and silent in the interviews. After failing to get him talking by commenting several times about the kinds of feelings adolescents might experience, I suggested a game of checkers. He snorted, saying it was a child's game and he had been the state junior chess champion in junior high school. I said that I did not play chess well enough to make it interesting. With unexpected graciousness, he sighed grudgingly but humored me. In our trial game of checkers, he won easily so I suggested a handicap of one checker for him.

In the ensuing game, he reacted with subdued glee to my agonized cries when he jumped me. When I beat him occasionally, my triumphant cries were met with his half angry, half derisive comment, "You were just lucky."

When I made it clear that we could not allow stupid moves, he began to stop me when I was making an error with the expletive, "Stupid!" Then he would show me some alternate moves. Gradually, when he began to realize that I wanted to learn and did not resent his teaching me, he stopped me more gently. When he won, he began to crow with increasing expressions of pleasure. Once my playing clearly showed I had benefited from his ever more patient teaching, we began to play without handicapping him. Our games were fairly even, though "Chet," as he now asked me to call him, won most of them.

Chet could predict who would win after two or three moves, just as he had learned to do in chess. Since I did not have this capacity to visualize the end of the game, I would insist we play the game out, with all the attendant drama I initiated. After a time, Chet enjoyed the opportunities for expressing feelings himself, and he stopped making predictions. As he himself more freely expressed feelings of dismay, hurt, anger, pleasure, and victory, it became easier for him to laugh and enjoy my histrionic displays in victory and defeat, which he had earlier labeled as childish.

At this point, Chet began to use our game of checkers in a new way. When it was time for him to move, he would pick up a checker, hold it or toss it thoughtfully in the air, and talk, as if to himself, about something that concerned him. I was careful to hear him out and follow his lead, making my comments or questions of clarification or interpretations while I also thoughtfully considered a move. Most of our therapeutic work was done while ostensibly playing checkers.

It was evident that the game permitted communication at several levels, as well as permission to identify with me. My communication of respect for his brilliance was not coupled with any demands, except for my request that he help me play a game which would be mutually challenging and interesting. Thus I, a feared and despised adult, wanted and needed to learn from him. He felt superior to me in this role and, as I've noted, early imitated my displays of feelings in a limited way, which generally meant deriding me or expressing anger that someone as "stupid" as I should win. When I did not retaliate, he recognized the metacommunication: I was not disturbed by his derision, was not tempted to retaliate, and enjoyed both his instruction and excellence of his playing.

As he began to imitate my more open and exaggerated expression of feelings, which seemed to him a safe make-believe way of expressing deep, disturbing, and dangerous feelings of anger, he watched guardedly for my reactions. To express open anger toward me when I won a game seemed frightening; he cut his comments short and suggested starting another game. But when he saw his anger did not alter our relationship, he seemed to accept my laconic comment, "It feels pretty good to me when I get angry." As he became more open about his feelings, he began to tease me when I made a poor move or was trapped. The difference was that it was a healthy, gentle teasing that led to his trying to be helpful. By the time he initiated talking over checkers, expression of affect seemed less difficult for him.

During the seven months of therapy, Chet's behavior at home changed markedly. He went to school, worked, took gym, studied, and again began to associate with friends. Attitudes towards both parents became more relaxed as some of his early anxieties and fears of his father's irrational, unexpected, explosive anger and of his mother's seductiveness emerged and were discussed, and he was also able to repeatedly open up the conflicts about whom he had to please with his schoolwork. He finally decided if he worked effectively for himself that his parents would also be satisfied. These discussions occurred while we played at checkers. Chet was also able to work out some of his anxiety about the enormous anger he had to suppress, and at the same time to express his concurrent anxiety about retaliation and loss of support and nurturance from important people, as if he were a small and vulnerable child. The safer it became for Chet to experience and express many of his feelings, the more gentle and nurturant his teaching of me became in the game situation.

SUMMARY AND CONCLUSIONS

Competitive games, especially checkers, can provide a developmentally appropriate means of communication between a therapist and a non-verbal child or adolescent patient. With school-age children who are cognitively beginning to learn the use of rules, the rules in checkers provide a basic framework for the relationship. A number of therapeutic issues can be approached and explored in the context of the games. The child's need to win at all costs, often by cheating, can be worked through. Moreover, cheating can be made unnecessary by handicapping the more expert player. Refusal to permit impulsive or obviously thoughtless moves helps the youngster to think about strategies and to accept help in planning his or her moves. Also, such efforts to enhance the competence of the child and to build his or her self-esteem reflect the adult's respect for the child. When the child is able to play well enough so that the therapist can learn from him or her, there is a major opportunity to experience and later express mutual respect and pleasure.

One of the problems in playing competitive games is the therapist's need to win. Feelings of competitiveness from the past, usually sibling rivalries or rivalry with a parent, may interfere with playing the game therapeutically. Such interferences need to be worked out by the therapist, usually in supervision. Another interference may be that enjoying a competitive game with a previously sullen, uncommunicative child may become an end in itself. In both instances, the therapist is not able to carefully observe the patient's interactions and respond therapeutically to the youngster's need.

Checkers and some other competitive games provide a medium by which the therapist can model feelings of hurt, anger, and hopelessness after a very poor move or defeat. Similarly, feelings of pleasure and triumph can be demonstrated in relation to excellent moves and winning. Both victory and defeat present opportunities to model ways in which attendant feelings can be expressed fully. Each game is a separate opportunity for modeling, and it encourages the child to behave similarly when he experiences the same kinds of feelings during the game. What the youngster sees is that he or she can display feelings that can be accepted by his or her therapist without being labeled "silly" or "bad." Since the experience is a repetitive one, the child begins to feel safer about the fuller expression of feelings.

Feelings generated and expressed in the context of playing checkers often are generalized later to other aspects of play therapy. With an older child, they can be generalized in the way he or she talks about difficulties and problems, perhaps during the actual game.

Nonverbal children are difficult to work with in psychotherapy. They may not speak easily because of the severity and type of their psychopathology or because of their sociocultural background. Under the conditions of play described previously, there is no pressure or demand from the therapist for the child to participate in exposing or talking about his or her feelings and thoughts before he or she is actually ready to do so. Thus, the negativism resulting from expectations and demands, which these children have experienced with other adults, may be reduced.

In summary, then, competitive games like checkers, dominos, or *war* can be utilized so that in the rivalry between adult and child, as players, they are on relatively equal terms. Full expression of feelings can be demonstrated by the adult and later imitated by the child. Such capacity to experience and communicate on a feeling level in the therapeutic situation is critical to therapeutic effectiveness and often extremely difficult to achieve with nonverbal children and adolescents. Competitive games provide a reliable means for therapeutic engagement of youngsters who, by virtue of their developmental problems, their particular psychopathology, or their sociocultural antecedents, are difficult to engage in ordinary play or "talking" therapy.

REFERENCES

Axline, V. (1947). *Play therapy*. Boston: Houghton-Mifflin.

Bettelheim, B. (1972). Play and education. *School Review, 81*, 1–13.

Freud, A. (1928). *Introduction to the technique of child analysis*. New York: Nervous and Mental Disease Publishing.

Gardner, R. (1971). *Therapeutic communication with children: The mutual storytelling technique*. New York: Science House.

Hug-Helmuth, H. (1921). On the technique of child analysis. *International Journal of Psychoanalysis, 2*, 287–305.

Klein, M. (1932). *The psychoanalysis of children*. London: Hogarth.

Levy, D. (1938). Release therapy in young children. *Psychiatry, 1*, 387–389.

Mahler, M., Pine, F., and Bergman, A. (1975). *The psychological birth of the human infant: Symbiosis and individuation*. New York: Basic.

Taft, J. (1933). *The dynamics of therapy in a controlled relationship*. New York: Macmillan.

Winnicott, D. (1971). *Playing and reality*. London: Tavistock.

CHAPTER 11

The Game of Checkers in Child Therapy

RICHARD A. GARDNER

It is important to state at the outset that I consider the game of checkers to be relatively low in therapeutic efficiency when one compares it to the wide variety of other therapeutic games generally utilized in child psychotherapy. My main reason for taking this position is that the game's potential for eliciting fantasy is low and, therefore, it is not likely that the therapist will learn as much about unconscious processes as he or she would from games that more directly elicit projective material. The more structure and rules a game has, the less the likelihood that such material will emerge. Conversely, the closer the game resembles a "blank screen" the more likely the therapist will obtain material derived from unconscious processes. This drawback notwithstanding, the game has a definite place in the child psychotherapist's armamentarium. The game of chess, however, is of far lower psychotherapeutic value. Whereas a game of checkers can generally be completed within 10 to 15 minutes, the game of chess rarely can and usually goes beyond the standard 45 to 50 minute session. Continuing in the next session is impractical because the likelihood of all the pieces being in the same place at the time of the next session is extremely small. Furthermore, playing a 10 to 15 minute game of low therapeutic efficiency still leaves a significant portion of the session available for more highly efficient therapeutic modalities. Playing chess does not provide this opportunity.

The author's search of the literature has revealed very little on this subject. Other than articles by Loomis (1964, 1976), Levinson (1976), and the author (Gardner, 1969), only occasional references to it were found—and then in the context of discussions of other aspects of play

215

therapy. This is not surprising in that its low therapeutic efficacy does not lend the game to extensive discussions of its psychotherapeutic value.

DESCRIPTION OF THE GAME

Because the vast majority of readers are probably familiar with the game of checkers, a detailed description is not warranted. The game is well known throughout the western world and has been popular for thousands of years. It was played in the days of the Pharaohs and is mentioned in the works of Homer and Plato. Basically, the game consists of a board of 64 squares, 32 black interspaced with 32 red. One player is supplied with 12 red checkers and the other with 12 black checkers. The players place their checkers on the black squares only, in the first three rows. Accordingly, because there are eight rows, the two center rows remain unoccupied at the onset of play. The checkers may only be moved diagonally along the black squares. The initial aim is to progressively advance one's checkers to the row closest to the opponent in order to obtain a king (a double checker). Regular checkers can only proceed in the forward direction one space at a time, in the direction toward the opponent. Kings, however, may move in any direction. The primary aim of the game is to jump an opponents piece and remove it from the board. Jumping can only be accomplished when an opponent's piece is on the contiguous black diagonal square and the square beyond the opponent's piece is unoccupied. The player then jumps over the opponent's piece and removes it from the board. If the player is in a position to jump, then the rules require that the jump be made even if such jump then exposes the player to significant retaliation by the opponent, for example, a responding double or triple jump. The game ends when one player has been completely depleted of playing pieces.

CASE ILLUSTRATIONS

The game can be of both diagnostic and therapeutic value. The manner in which the player plays the game and the comments made during the course of the game can provide the therapist with material of diagnostic value. In addition, the therapist's responses and the interchanges that evolve from the players' behavior and statements can be therapeutic. However, it is important for the reader to appreciate that much of the time may be spent in interchanges and activities that are of little, if any, therapeutic value. I will focus here on the potentially diagnostic and therapeutic material that may emerge.

Self-Esteem Problems

Insecure children will sometimes hesitate to begin playing the game because of the fear that they may lose. Instead, they may suggest a game of pure chance in which there is less likelihood of humiliation. Such a child may ask, "Are you good?" in the hope that the therapist will be a poor player and thereby increase the child's chances of winning. They may insist on going first each time, again in the hope of reducing the likelihood of losing. In the course of play such children may frequently interrupt the game in order to count the checkers in order to determine who is winning. Children with feelings of low self-worth are typically "sore-losers." Sore-losers are usually children with profound feelings of inadequacy whose need for winning to compensate for their feelings of low self-worth is exaggerated. They will often play a hard game, put all their energies into it, and moan at every loss or disadvantage. It is as if their whole worth as human beings depends on the outcome of the game. The therapist, however, should not fall into the trap of invariably allowing these children to win. The world will not be so benevolent and the child is not being provided with a reality experience. Allowing such children to win tends to perpetuate the use of the sore-loser reaction as a way of manipulating others into letting them win. (Many children appreciate at some level that the adult is doing this.) Parents and therapists may so indulge the child, but peers are rarely going to do so.

Such a child, when playing with great tension and fear of losing, might be told, "You think that my whole opinion of you is based on the outcome of this game. That's just not so. My opinion of someone is based on many things and most of these things are much more important than whether or not the person wins or loses at checkers. What do you think about that?" My hope here is that the child will then engage in a discussion of my comments. But even if this overture is not successful (commonly the case with most children) the child's actually having the experience that the therapist does not laugh at or humiliate him or her for losing can be a corrective emotional experience. Alexander and colleagues (1946) empha- sized this important aspect of the therapeutic process.

Self-esteem must, at least in part, be based on *actual* competence, not delusional or fantasized competence (Gardner, 1973b). It is common practice on the part of parents and teachers to attempt to enhance chil- dren's feelings of self-worth by praising them in an abstract way, for ex- ample, "What a nice (kind, good) boy you are" and "What a lovely girl." Such comments are often meaningless. Because they do not direct their attention to some specific quality or area of competence they are not likely to be successful in enhancing feelings of self-worth. And, if the child senses that he or she is being "buttered-up" this may lower self- worth—especially in the sensitive child who appreciates that the adult is utilizing these gratuitous compliments because of the fact that the praiser cannot think of anything genuine to praise. Far more effective compli- ments are: "What a beautiful model boat you built," "Good catch!" and so on. These focus on the actual qualities and accomplishments that are proof of the child's capabilities. In the game of checkers one can accom- plish this with such comments as, "That was a very clever move," "Gee, I fell right into your trap," "Boy, you really had me sweating there for a while."

Related to the issue of competence is that of competition. In fact, it is very difficult to separate entirely the two issues. One cannot truly assess one's competence without measuring it against the competence of others. And this comparison process inevitably introduces an element of compe- tition. There are those who believe that all competition is psychologically detrimental and ultimately ego-debasing, both for the winner and the loser. I am not in agreement. I believe that one must differentiate between healthy and unhealthy competition. In healthy competition there is re- spect for one's opponent and the aim is to win but not to degrade and hu- miliate one's adversary. In unhealthy competition these undesirable fac- tors may become predominant. If not for healthy competition, we might all still be living in caves. Unhealthy competition, however, has resulted in much grief in the world and has resulted in many people suffering sig- nificant pain, torture, and even murder. Winning a hard-fought game of checkers—in a benevolently competitive way—can provide the child with an increased sense of self-worth.

Holmes (1964) emphasizes this point. He describes the fiasco that re- sulted in the physical education program of his adolescent residential treatment center when rivalry and scorekeeping were eliminated when games were played. The boys refused to attend. However, when a vigorous program of training and competition was instituted, Holmes reports, "The boys left the gymnasium perspiring, panting, and bone-weary. They complained lavishly and in chorus. They were bright-eyed, square-shouldered, and flushed with pride in the aftermath of battle. The boys follow a year-round schedule of coaching in tackle football with full equipment, basketball, boxing, baseball, and track. Each of these endeavors requires many consecutive weeks of monotonous drill, all without a prospect of immediate reward. When they have acquired sufficient skill and strength to qualify for competition, the boys are forthwith subjected to the "threat" of winning and losing. The approach has provided them with an earned and well-deserved sense of masculine accomplishment."

A number of years ago, the author had an experience while playing checkers with a child that demonstrates some important points related to competition, winning, and ego-enhancement. While playing checkers with a five-year-old boy, he exhibited what I thought was an exaggerated investment in whether or not he was winning. In order to help alter what I considered to be an inappropriate attitude, I said to him, "Andy, the important thing is how much fun you have while playing, not whether you win the game." To this he replied, "No, you're wrong, the *important* thing is whether you win the game!" The boy was for the most part right. We pay lip service to comments such as mine, but who of us would enjoy tennis, bridge, or chess were there no winner. My revised advice to him would be, "There are two important things: how much you enjoy playing the game and whether you win; both can be fun."

The issue of competition and the therapeutic benefit of winning leads necessarily to the question of whether the therapist should let the child win. This may be a dilemma. If the therapist plays honestly and wins most games, this can be antitherapeutic in that the child may be humiliated and deprived of the feeling of accomplishment associated with winning. If the therapist purposely loses, the child may benefit from the gratifications of winning, but the therapist is being dishonest with the patient, and the child may sense this and lose trust in him or her. Although the author is a strong proponent of being honest with children (generally it is a *sine qua non* of therapy), this is one of the situations in which the author considers falsification of the truth to be justified. He allows the child to win or lose depending on what is therapeutically indicated at that time for that particular patient. He has not found his patients to have basically lost trust in him over this "duplicity," probably because there is so much openness and honesty in compensation, and possibly because winning and losing is usually so balanced that the child does not become suspicious. Such duplicity, used sparingly and with discretion, serves to enhance the children's self-esteem and makes them feel worthwhile and competent.

The child with feelings of low self-worth may try to change the rules in the middle of the game in order to improve his or her chances of winning. For example, the rules of the game are that one *must* jump if one is in the position to do so. Insecure children may recognize that complying with this rule will place them in a particularly disadvantageous position and may then refuse to jump. To such a child, I will generally say, "Look, this game is no fun if we don't play by the rules. If you want to continue playing with me you're going to have to follow the rules. I'm sure that if you tried to change the rules in the middle of the game with your friends, they probably wouldn't want to play with you again." My response here is based on the assumption that if the child were to be allowed to change the rules, the sense of ego-enhancement that might then come from winning would be compromised by the knowledge that the success was not honestly attained. Furthermore, some useful information is provided the child regarding peer relationships. My hope here is that if I am heard, my advice will improve the child's relationships and thereby enhance feelings of self-worth. However, after making this comment I might add, "If you want to make up special rules for the next game, rules that apply to both of us, I'll be glad to try them. But remember, once we agree to the rules at the beginning of the game, they can't be changed in the middle of the game."

One should observe whether the child is having fun while playing the game. Pleasure enhances self-esteem and serves as a universal antidote to many psychogenic problems. It has been said that "pleasure is the food of the ego." I am in full agreement with this statement. While one is having fun, one is less likely to be dwelling on one's psychogenic problems. With joking and laughing even further therapeutic benefit may be derived from the game. If, however, the child is not deriving pleasure from the game, it behooves the therapist to attempt to ascertain why. And such failure to enjoy it may be the result of a variety of psychogenic problems, some of which will be discussed later.

Psychotherapy, like all forms of treatment, has both advantages and disadvantages—as well as potential risks. One of the risks of psychotherapy is that the patient may compare himself or herself unfavorably with the therapist and this can lower feelings of self-worth. After all, a central element in the therapeutic process is the therapist's pointing out the patient's errors. No matter how sensitively this is done, and no matter how much benevolence there may be in the therapist's communication in this area, there is no question that a game of one-upmanship is being played. Accordingly, there is an intrinsic ego-debasing factor in the psychotherapeutic process, the benefits to be derived by the patient notwithstanding. In classical psychoanalysis especially there is this risk. The analyst strictly refrains from revealing his or her deficiencies to the patient and this cannot but ultimately be an ego-debasing factor in the treatment. Accordingly, when the therapist can reveal a deficiency in a noncontrived way in the course of treatment it can lessen the influence of this ego-lowering element in treatment. The way in which a therapist lost this opportunity, while playing a game of checkers with a child, is demonstrated well in the following illustration.

Case Illustration

The child made a poor move, to which the therapist responded: "Are you sure you want to do that?" The boy looked up slightly irritated, thought a moment and then replied: "I did it and don't want to change it." The child's manner and facial expression communicated his attitude: "I made the mistake and I'm man enough to accept the consequences." This was, indeed, a mature and healthy response on the boy's part but, unfortunately, the therapist did not take full advantage of the further therapeutic opportunities this incident provided. Had he said, "You're right. I'm sorry I treated you like a baby. Good for you for stopping me," he would have accomplished a number of things: Such a comment would have revealed that the therapist, too, is fallible and that would have helped the patient see him as a human being, with both assets and liabilities. It would have thereby served to lessen the chances of the unrealistic idolization of the therapist that so often occurs in treatment. It would have further communicated that the therapist was mature enough to admit his errors and that such admission enhances one's manliness rather than detracts from it. In the identification with the therapist that inevitably takes place in successful treatment, the child would have been exposed to these healthier attitudes for incorporation. Lastly, the suggested comment would have reinforced the patient's mature reaction, thereby increasing the likelihood that it would become ingrained in his personality and be utilized in the future.

The actual experience of having engaged in an activity which has been mutually enjoyable is ego-enhancing to the patient. This is not only related to the pleasure the child has derived from the game but because the child has been instrumental in providing the therapist with some pleasure as well. The child thereby feels needed, useful, and wanted. Such feelings are often minimal or even lacking in many children who are in treatment and experiencing them can be ego-enhancing. Furthermore, the child may have learned some better playing techniques from the therapist which have improved his or her game. The utilization of this knowledge in games with peers may be salutary, especially with regard to the enhanced feelings of self-worth that it provides.

Passive-Dependency

Passive-dependent children tend to be very compliant in many areas of their lives and this tendency is likely to reveal itself when playing checkers. Such children are likely to comply with the therapist's decisions with regard to the ground rules necessary prior to the game. For example, if asked which color checker he or she wants, the child may respond, "It doesn't matter, you take whichever one you want." Of course, the fear of engendering resentment in the therapist for insisting on a particular color may be operative in this response. Whether it be this or other psychodynamic factors that are operative in this response, the net result is that the patient is "anxious to please."

Although strict adherence to the rules of the game require jumping when one has the opportunity, many children do not follow this rule when playing with peers. Most play according to one of three rules pertaining to whether one has to jump: (1) a player must jump if he or she is in a position to do so, (2) the player himself or herself can decide when in such a position, and (3) if the player fails to jump and could have done so, the opponent may remove from the board the checker that has failed to make the jump. The therapist does well to discuss with the child before the beginning of the game exactly which rule he or she is used to playing with. To assume that the child has played with the traditional rule may result in an "argument" as the game gets under way. Accordingly, at the outset, I generally ask children which of the rules they follow and may inform them of the traditional rule if they are not familiar with it. In each case, we make a decision regarding which rule should be followed. This, of course, is dependent on the clinical situation. With passive children, however, the child is very reluctant to make the decision and prefers that the therapist decide which of the three rules to follow. Again, one often sees a fear element here with regard to stating the preference.

Egocentricism

Some children are egocentric in compensation for feelings of low self-worth. Others, however, are egocentric because they may have been indulged by overprotective parents. On the other hand, others may be egocentric on a neurodevelopmental level, and this is especially true for children with neurologically based learning disabilities (to be discussed in a later section). These children have little capacity for putting themselves in the position of other people and "want what they want when they want it." They often do not seem to be affected by the negative effects of their narcissim. Rejections and even punishments often do not get them to appreciate that their self-serving attitudes are alienating. When with friends, they are reluctant to share, even when their friends leave the home because of their selfishness.

When playing the game of checkers, such a child might insist that his or her version of the rules are the correct ones and be very unreceptive to playing even one game with another rule. Such children will often not wait their turn and become very impatient when the therapist pauses to think about his or her next move. Therapists do well not to allow themselves to be rushed by such children and may even feign contemplation in order to give them some lessons in self-restraint and respect for the rights of others. Of course, children playing with great levels of tension and anxiety may also exhibit impatience that may appear to be egocentricism. Impulsive children, as well, may also appear egocentric.

By careful observation of the egocentric child's play, one may observe other manifestations of their narcissism. The child may focus only on his or her own pieces without thinking about the opponent's position. Such a child then easily falls into traps. The mechanism by which the child focuses on his or her own pieces only, to the exclusion of the therapist's, is probably analogous to social situations in which the child does not place himself or herself in another person's position. Such a child might be helped to become more "socially aware" by such comments as, "Watch out for my king," "You fell right into my trap," and "If you had moved there, you could have had a double jump." These comments, of course, not only help the child improve his or her game but, more importantly for the purposes of this problem, can increase these children's motivation to project themselves into other people's positions.

Withdrawn, Autistic, and Schizophrenic Children

These children have little capacity for pleasure, whether it be while playing checkers or engaging in other activities in life. They have little joy in winning and little disappointment when they lose. In the course of the game they may be distracted by their fantasies. Schizoid children, or those who prefer their fantasy world to that of reality, may obsess at the end of the game about how it might have been otherwise, for example, "If I had moved there, then I would have gotten a double jump," or "If the checkers had been like this, then I would have won." To this, the therapist should respond in such a way that the child is directly confronted with reality: "Yes it's true that if your checkers had been that way, you might have won. But, they weren't. Maybe in the next game you'll be able to beat me by doing that."

Suspicious or paranoid children play cautiously and defensively. Paranoid children may project their anger onto their therapists and fear retaliation for its expression. Accordingly, such a child may be afraid to win in anticipation of the therapist's hostile reaction. This may be expressed in such comments as, "Don't be mad at me if I win." They may hug their pieces to the sides and rear of the board and may spend long periods of time deliberating in order to avoid being jumped or trapped.

The child whose schizoid behavior is the result of environmental more than constitutional/genetic factors is likely to have come from a chaotic and unpredictable home. In such households, there is little structure and the disorganization so engendered in the child may reveal itself in the game of checkers. They do not follow the rules and follow no plan of attack during play. The therapist's insistence that the rules be adhered to can be therapeutic in that it provides the child with the living experience that if the rules are not followed then he or she will be deprived of the

gratification of playing the game. Of course, if the child gets little pleasure from the game anyway, this deterrent will not prove significantly effective. In addition, the therapist's own commitment to an organized
lifestyle can serve as a model in contrast to that of the child's parents and
relatives.

Antisocial Behavior Disorder

Children with antisocial behavior may exhibit their symptoms in the
game. Such children will often play an aggressive and serious game with
great interest in winning. They will respond with glee at every advantage
and then rub salt into the therapist's wounds if they do win. Hostility displaced from other sources becomes vented on the therapist. When losing,
they may not hesitate to pick up the board and disrupt the whole game. Of
course, this can be seen in other children such as neurologically impaired
children with impulsivity or children with low self-esteem who cannot
tolerate losing. In the extreme, such children have no hesitation trying to
destroy the game itself—so great may be their rage.

Antisocial children often exhibit manifestations of associated impairments in superego development. This may manifest itself in their cheating
during the game. The therapist does well to point this out to the child and
not permit it. In such situations, I may make comments like, "Look, this
game is no fun if you're going to cheat. If you want to play with me,
you'll have to play it straight. I'm sure your friends feel the same way."
The child here is being provided with a living experience that the therapist will not tolerate the antisocial behavior. Of course, if the child is
willing to go further into the reasons why he or she is exhibiting such behavior, I am receptive to doing so. However, my experience has been that
these children (like most children in therapy) are not particularly interested in gaining insight into the unconscious roots of their problems, in
the hope that such revelations might bring about a reduction of their
symptoms. And antisocial children, especially, because their symptoms
are egosyntonic, are even less motivated for such self-inquiry.

Obsessive-Compulsivity

Obsessive-compulsive children may be so wrapped up in their doubting,
indecisiveness, and procrastination that they find it difficult to enjoy

themselves. They may become concerned with whether the checkers touch the marginal lines of the squares and are often concerned as to whether the crown side of the checker faces upward on the kings and the noncrown side of the checker faces downward for the unkinged checkers. Whereas Freud considered unresolved, oedipal, especially sexual, problems to be central to the development of obsessive-compulsive symptoms, my experience has been that repressed anger is more often involved in the development of such symptomatology. Accordingly, I make attempts to lessen guilt over anger in the course of my work with these children. If, for example, I suspect that the child may be angry over the fact that I have won a game and is too inhibited to express such anger, I will make comments designed to reduce such inhibition, for example, "I can't imagine that you're not even a little bit angry over the fact that I have now won three games in a row. Most kids certainly would be. I know that I would be." "I think the main difference between you and other kids is this. Other kids who get angry show it; you get angry and don't show it." "What do you think would happen if you told me how angry you were?"

Neurologically Based Learning Disabilities

Children with neurologically based learning disabilities may exhibit many manifestations of their disorder—both the primary organic and the secondary psychogenic—in the course of playing the game. Elsewhere (Gardner 1973a, 1973c, 1974, 1975b, 1975c, 1979a, 1979c) the author has described in detail both the organic and the psychogenic manifestations of children with this class of disorders. For the sake of brevity, I will refer to these children as NBLD (neurologically based learning disabilities) children.

Although in the age group when most children are well acquainted with the game, NBLD children may not know how to play. This may be due to either intellectual impairment or lack of exposure. Because they tend to withdraw from others in an attempt to hide their deficits, many of these children often deprive themselves of development in areas of basic physiologic and neurologic competence. Accordingly, such a child might intellectually be capable of playing the game but might not display aptitude because of withdrawal. Such children might be ashamed to admit their ignorance of the game when invited to play and may anxiously suggest another activity. When one attempts to teach such children the game, their difficulty in understanding and following the rules, in remembering what has been learned, and in appreciating many of the concepts can make such teaching an arduous task.

Prior to play, the author generally lets the child set up the board and the checkers. These children may place the board with the central fold at 90 degrees to its normal position or put the checkers in the wrong squares. They may try to set up four rows instead of three, then run out of checkers, and then become frustrated and confused.

Characteristically, NBLD children play a sloppy game. They do not place checkers in the centers of the squares due to coordination, motor, and/or perceptual deficiencies. They often forget whether it is their own or their opponent's turn, especially if there has been a long thinking lapse between moves. In such pauses, they may ask what the opponent's last move was or even who made the last move. Such children have to be repeatedly reminded of the rules because they tend to forget them, for example, only kings can go backwards or it was decided at the beginning that one must jump if one is in a position to. They may continue to move their checkers directly ahead rather than diagonally and jump over two instead of one checker. They may even jump over their own pieces. They may have trouble differentiating between the powers of kings and the regular checkers, although they usually understand that it is preferable to have kings.

These children, because of their marked feelings of inadequacy and hypersensitivity to defeat, will often react badly to losing. And because of their impulsivity they are often unable to restrain their disappointment and angry reactions. They may mess up the board, turn it over, and even fling the checkers at the therapist. The normal child, when putting away the checkers, usually places them in the box in a symmetrical fashion, forming piles of equal height. When these children attempt to do this, they often have difficulties. The piles are of different heights and they have trouble forming a symmetrical pattern.

The following game of checkers was the first one played with a 12-year-old NBLD child with an IQ of about 80. It illustrates both the neurophysiological as well as the psychogenic pathological reactions that can be observed when these children play checkers.

Case Illustration

The patient was first asked if he would like to play a game of checkers. He replied, "O.K., but I'm afraid I'll beat you." The comment revealed his feelings of inadequacy which he handled with compensatory bravado and projection onto the therapist of the retaliatory anger he would feel in himself if he were the loser. The author replied, "I usually don't take the game so seriously that I get angry if I lose. It's only a game, it doesn't mean the end of the world to me if I lose."

The patient chose red and tried to set up his checkers in four rows instead of three. Running out of checkers, he looked puzzled, removed them completely and tried again with the same results. I then set up mine, and after a few glances at my side of the board, he was successful on his third try. Suspecting that there might be much embarrassing tutoring later on, I let him learn this "without" me.

When asked about what rules he follows with regard to jumping, he said that the way he plays one doesn't have to jump. I agreed to play that way.

When I asked him who would go first, he replied, "Smoke before fire, so I go first." This comment, in the setting in which it was made, revealed many of his defects in conceptualization. The normal mnemonic that many children use to determine which color goes first is, "Fire before smoke." This refers to the colors red and black, and because fire precedes smoke, red goes first. The fact that the patient said, "Smoke before fire" revealed that he was not forming a visual image of the fire with the subsequent smoke, but was reiterating what he had heard. Furthermore, his rote repetition was also incorrectly recalled. Even if he were not thinking logically about the temporal sequence of smoke and fire, he still might have related smoke to black and fire to red. Had he done this, then by his statement "smoke before fire," blacks would have gone first. But because he had chosen red, it was obvious that his decision to go first had no relationship at all, on any level, to his comment.

Within a few moves, he was in a position to jump me and he asked if he had to jump. He had already forgotten the jumping rule we had agreed on. He made a number of errors commonly made by the NBLD child. He moved his own checkers backwards in the face of an attack and had to be reminded repeatedly that only kings can move backwards. He tried to jump his own checkers on a few occasions, did not see double jumps but only single ones, and often forgot to take my piece off the board after he had jumped it.

During play, he repeated, "If I beat you, I know you'll be a sore loser." Then he would reassure himself about his projected aggression: "You'll take it like a man," that is, "You'll repress your rage, you won't get angry at me the way I would with you if you won." The patient was again told that I didn't think the game so important that I judged myself or other people totally on whether or not they were good checker players.

At one point, the patient made an excellent blocking move. When I asked why he had so moved, he gave the wrong reason for the right move. He kept score by counting the number of checkers each of us had taken off the board and failed to take into account whether the pieces on the board were kings or not. When his checkers reached my side, he did not ask for a king, and when given kings, he did not move them to attack me from the rear.

In spite of all of this, the patient "won" the game, at which point he burst into gales of laughter. "I slaughtered you. . . . You can't win them all, old man . . . (guffaws). . . . Now, who's an expert at this game . . . (more cackling). . . . The expert beats them all . . . (further horse-laughs). . . . " Besides the compensatory ego enhancing mechanisms displayed here, the hostile element was also obvious. In this case, I represented his mother whom he unconsciously did wish to slaughter, because of her having sent him to a hospital for three years.

After some further chest thumping, the patient put the checkers back in the box. The piles were not of equal height and although this was finally accomplished, his attempts to form a symmetrical pattern of reds on one side and blacks on the other were unsuccessful.

SUMMARY AND CONCLUSIONS

When playing games with children, adults do far better for themselves and the children if they select a game that is enjoyable to both. When an adult finds a game tedious, but continues to play through obligation, the child is deprived of many of the benefits to be derived from the experience. The child usually senses the adult's boredom and lack of interest through the latter's impatience and easy irritability, and so the game can become a trying and oppressive ordeal. In child psychotherapy, it is especially important to make every attempt to engage in activities that are interesting and enjoyable to the therapist as well as the child. Checkers, which is a game that can be played with pleasure by both child and adult, is in this category.

After the first few games, however, much of the game's diagnostic value is gone but the therapeutic benefits can continue indefinitely. However, the therapist may find his or her enjoyment and interest lagging, especially after the game has exhausted its potential for diagnostic information. One way of stimulating ongoing interest in the therapist is to let the child get far ahead, then, when the therapist has only one or two checkers left, to the child's eight or nine, to play as diligently as one can. A variation that may also enhance the child's pleasure is to play "opposite checkers." In this variation one tries to get jumped and the "winner" is the one who is first depleted of all checkers.

Strupp (1975), one of the more sober evaluators of psychoanalytic psychotherapy, believes that a central element in the efficacy of psychoanalytic treatment is its capacity to teach individuals how to live more effectively and efficiently. When one handles life situations and problems in a better way, one is less likely to have to resort to neurotic adaptations. In a way, checkers can teach lessons in better living. One is responsible for one's fate and suffers the consequences of one's actions. Whether a person wins or loses is in part determined by one's own acts. If one plans ahead and is appropriately cautious, then one does better than if one sits back and leaves things to chance. The lesson of being master of one's fate is present in most skill games. However, one is not completely master; one must reckon too with others in the world with whom we must compromise, avert, deal with head on, and at times succumb to. All these lessons can be learned in microcosm in a relatively painless way in the game of checkers.

Checkers can also be used for decompression purposes at the end of a particularly tension-laden session. Although there may be little specific psychotherapeutic value derived from the game per se at that point, it does have the benefit of lessening tension. Finally, I consider it important to reiterate to the reader that checkers is a game of relatively low psychotherapeutic benefit. Accordingly, it should be used sparingly in the psychotherapeutic process. The author generally will use it only near the end of the session, after most of the time has been devoted to what he considers to be more highly efficient therapeutic activities. The reader who is interested in the author's views regarding what these are might refer to his publications in this area (1975a, 1979b). There are therapists who will spend many sessions completely devoted to playing checkers. I consider this to be a "cop out" for the therapist in that it is a relatively easy way to spend the session and it is a "rip off" for the patient and his or her family.

REFERENCES

Alexander, F., and French, T., et al. (1946). The principal of corrective emotional experience. In *Psychoanalytic therapy: Principles and application* (pp. 66–70). New York: Ronald.

Gardner, R.A. (1969). The game of checkers as a diagnostic and therapeutic tool in child psychotherapy. *Acta Paedopsychiatrica, 36*, 142–152.

Gardner, R.A. (1973a). *MBD: The family book about minimal brain disfunction.* New York: Aronson.

Gardner, R.A. (1973b). *Understanding children: A parents guide to child rearing.* Cresskill, NJ: Creative Therapeutics.

Gardner, R.A. (1973c). Psychotherapy of the psychogenic problems secondary to minimal brain disfunction. *International Journal of Child Psychotherapy, 2*, 224–256.

Gardner, R.A. (1974). Psychotherapy of minimal brain disfunction. In J. Masserman (Ed.), *Current Psychiatric Therapies* (Vol. 14, pp. 15–21). New York: Grune and Stratton.

Gardner, R.A. (1975a). *Psychotherapeutic approaches to the resistant child.* New York: Aronson.

Gardner, R.A. (1975b). Psychotherapy in minimal brain disfunction. In J. Masserman (Ed.), *Current psychiatric therapies* (Vol. 15, pp. 25–38). New York: Grune and Stratton.

Gardner, R.A. (1975c). Techniques for involving the child with MBD in meaningful psychotherapy. *Journal of Learning Disabilities, 8*, 16–26.

Gardner, R.A. (1979a). *The objective diagnosis of minimal brain disfunction.* Cresskill, NJ: Creative Therapeutics.

Gardner, R.A. (1979b). Helping children cooperate in therapy. In J. Noshpitz (Ed.), *Basic handbook of child psychiatry* (Vol. 3, pp. 414–433). New York: Basic Books.

Gardner, R.A. (1979c). Psychogenic difficulties secondary to MBD. In J. Noshpitz (Ed.), *Basic handbook of child psychiatry* (Vol. 3, pp. 614–628). New York: Basic Books.

Holmes, D.J. (1964). *The adolescent in psychotherapy.* Boston: Little, Brown.

Levinson, B.M. (1976). Use of checkers in therapy. In C. Schaefer (Ed.), *The therapeutic use of child's play* (pp. 283–284). New York: Aronson.

Loomis, E.A. (1964). The use of checkers in handling certain resistances in child therapy and child analysis. In M.R. Haworth (Ed.), *Child psychotherapy* (pp. 407–411). New York: Basic Books.

Loomis, E.A. (1976). Use of checkers in handling resistance. In C. Schaefer (Ed.), *The therapeutic use of child's play* (pp. 385–390). New York: Aronson.

Strupp, H.H. (1975). Psychoanalysis, "focal psychotherapy" and the nature of the therapeutic influence. *Archives of General Psychiatry, 32*, 127–135.

CHAPTER 12

Using Games to Improve Self-Control Deficits in Children

ARTHUR J. SWANSON

Self-control deficits in children are a common clinical problem. Estimates of the prevalence of this problem range from 1 to 15 percent of school-aged children, with most figures falling in the 5 to 12 percent range (Schrag and Divoky, 1975). A study by Kendall and Braswell (1985) revealed that second through sixth grade teachers rated approximately 10 percent of their students to have self-control difficulties sufficient to interfere with social and/or academic functioning. This suggests that, on the average, two to three children in a typical classroom experience significant problems in maintaining self-control.

According to the *Diagnostic and Statistical Manual of Mental Disorders* (Third Edition), children with self-control problems typically demonstrate both attentional deficits and impulsive responding in situations which require reflective thinking. Other characteristics of these children frequently include chronic under-achievement, poor self-esteem, emotional immaturity, and antisocial behavior (Weiss, Minde, Werry, Douglas, and Nemeth, 1971). Some children with self-control problems also exhibit hyperactive behavior. Among those children having hyperactive features, many show decreases in motor activity over time without demonstrating parallel improvement in their ability to attend to a task and/or to respond in a reflective manner (Hechtman, Weiss, Finkelstein, Wener, and Benn, 1976).

While both conventional analytic therapy and behavior therapy have met with some success in the treatment of children with self-control problems, each has also encountered troubling difficulties. Analytic therapists have found that the impulsive child's frequently underdeveloped recep-

233

tive and expressive communication skills make a "talking cure" a poor treatment of choice (Shapiro, 1981). Behavior therapy approaches, while often effective in changing behavior during treatment, have reported difficulties in achieving either generalization or maintenance of treatment effects (Kazdin, 1975). These difficulties may be due, in part, to the tendency of behavioral approaches to attend to the modification of specific behaviors rather than to the cognitions that mediate those behaviors.

The present approach is based on the assumption that children who exhibit self-control deficits are lacking in specific behavioral and cognitive skills. Behaviorally, these children are highly distractible and have difficulty remaining on-task. Cognitively, impulsive children tend to "fail to think before they act" (Kendall and Braswell, 1985). What follows are two games, the first focusing on the behavioral deficit, the second on the cognitive deficit, which can be played with impulsive children.

Games, such as the ones that will be described, have been found to be particularly effective with the impulsive child because they are enjoyable, they can be adapted to the child's needs, and they can be used in a variety of contexts by a number of people in the child's life. These games also offer the impulsive child an opportunity to succeed where he or she may have failed on previous academic and social tasks. In playing these games, impulsive children learn specific behavioral and cognitive strategies taught and modeled by the therapist.

BEAT THE CLOCK: A GAME TO IMPROVE ON-TASK BEHAVIOR

This game, adapted from a game described by Shapiro (1981), has a different goal from that of the one-time popular television show. The object of this game is for the child to outlast the clock so that he or she is actively engaged in the task at the time the clock strikes. Suitable tasks include reading, writing, or any other activity in which the child is frequently off-task. In the context of the game, behavior is defined as off-task when the child responds verbally or physically to off-task stimuli in the environment or when the child looks away from the task and fails to return to it within 10 seconds. The 10 second time period is intended to give the child an opportunity to stop and think while performing the task and/or to take brief, appropriate breaks as needed.

The child is given a set number of chips at the start of the activity. For example, if the goal is for the child to remain on-task for three minutes, he or she would be given three chips. A response cost procedure is used in which the child loses a chip each time he or she engages in off-task behavior. When the child engages in such behavior, the therapist briefly reminds the child of the contingency and takes away a chip. The therapist then redirects the child to the task without further discussion. At the end of the allotted time period, the therapist discusses these off-task incidents with the child and draws parallels between them and situations which may occur at home or at school.

The time period chosen should be appropriate to the developmental level of the child. It is important that a time period be selected in which the child can succeed. Gradually, this period can be increased as the child's ability to remain on-task improves.

A child has the opportunity to earn chips for each game that is played. Chips can be exchanged for a small prize—for example, a pretzel or baseball cards—at the end of each treatment session or accumulated over several sessions and exchanged for a larger prize, such as a game or a special outing. The specific prizes used should be ones both valued by the child and appropriate to the amount of work completed.

Case Illustration

T: Would you like to play some games today?

C: Yeah.

T: OK, in the first game we're going to do some reading. Go ahead and pick out a book you'd like to read. (Child chooses book). Got one?

C: Yeah.

T: Good, now, have you ever heard of the game *Beat the Clock*?

C: Yeah.

T: How do you play it?

C: You gotta hurry up and do something before the clock goes off.

T: Right, very good. Today we're going to play a different kind of *Beat the Clock*. In this game, I want you to work as hard as you can and still be working when the clock goes off. So, you're going to work harder and longer than the clock. Can you do that?

C: Yeah.

T: I think you can. In the first game, I want you to read for three minutes, okay?

C: Okay.

T: When I tell you to start, you begin reading and when the clock goes off, I want you to *still* be reading, okay?

C: Okay.

T: Now, I'm going to give you three chips. Every time you look away from your reading for a long time (10 seconds) or do something else instead of reading, I'm going to take a chip away.

C: What are the chips for?

T: Well, we're going to see how many chips you can get. At the end of the meeting you can trade your chips for a small prize or you can save your chips and trade them for a big prize later. (A discussion ensues about the available prizes). Would you like to earn a prize?

C: Yeah.

T: Now what are you going to do? (Child repeats his assignment). Good, are you ready to read?

C: Yeah.

T: I'll set the timer. Remember, pay real close attention. Ready? Go ahead. (Child begins to read. Therapist may wish to engage in a parallel activity while observing the child's ability to remain on-task).

C: (In response to distracting noise during minute two). What was that?

T: Somebody in the hall. I need to take a chip from you for talking. Go back to your reading. (Child reads for the rest of the time period). Time is up and you're *still* reading. Good for you. You have 2 chips. You lost a chip didn't you?

C: Yeah.

T: What happened?

C: I heard something. . . .

T: And what did you do?

C: I stopped reading.

T: Does that happen in school when someone makes a noise, you stop working?

C: Yeah.

T: What happens then?

C: Sometimes I get in trouble.

T: How?

C: I tell the kid to shut up.

T: What else could you do?

C: Mind my own business.

T: That's another thing you could do, what else?

C: Tell the teacher.

T: That's good. You were able to think of a lot of things to do when other kids make noise in class. So, you did really well. Lets play another game where you draw a picture, but this time for four-minutes. Do you think you can do that?

C: Yeah.

T: OK, I'll give you four chips. But remember, I'll take one away each time you look away for a long time or you talk, okay?

C: Okay. (Child proceeds with various activities using the same procedure).

In addition to creating contingencies which increase the child's ability to attend, this game helps the therapist identify the distractions in the child's environment. As described in the therapy session, a discussion can ensue regarding ways to cope with these specific distractions.

THE *STOP AND THINK* GAME: A GAME TO IMPROVE IMPULSIVE RESPONDING

Research reveals that a "coping" model is more effective than a "mastery" model in the treatment of a variety of clinical problems (Kazdin, 1974; Meichenbaum, 1971). That is, models who initially encounter difficulties which they eventually overcome are more likely to be emulated than those who consistently exhibit "perfect" performance. Presumably, coping models demonstrate behavior which more closely approximates the difficulties encountered by the individual, in this case, the child.

The primary purpose of this game, which has been adapted from the curriculum of Kendall and Braswell (1985), is to provide a vehicle by which a child can learn to use self-instructions to complete a task or to solve a problem. Through didactic instructions and exposure to a "coping" model, the child is taught a series of self-directed statements:

1.   What is the problem? (Task definition)

2.   What can I do about the problem? (Generation of alternatives)

3.   What is the "best" thing to do? (Selection of best alternative)

4.   How did I do? (Evaluation)

The child is encouraged to use his or her own words to describe each step. Once generated, the child's self-statements are written on a note card which becomes a reference tool for use in completing the assigned tasks.

In a typical session, the therapist models the use of self-instructions while performing the assigned task. The therapist verbalizes each of the self-statements and "thinks out loud" to solve each step of the process. The child then performs the same task, using his or her own self-statements taken from the reference card. Once the child is able to use the four steps consistently, the therapist performs the task while whispering the self-statements. The child is then instructed to whisper to himself or herself while solving subsequent problems. Once successful at this, the child is instructed to think through these steps without verbalizing them.

While numerous materials can be used to play the *Stop and Think* game, ones which are particularly suitable include matching familiar figures, mazes, and pick-up sticks. Once a child is successful using self-directed statements in the solution of impersonal tasks, tasks of a more personal or interpersonal nature can be assigned, that is, how to solve a problem with a friend.

In the *Stop and Think* game, one chip can be given for the appropriate use of self-statements and one chip for a successful solution to the given problem. As in the previous game, chips can be exchanged for a small prize at the end of each treatment session or saved and exchanged for a larger prize after several sessions.

Case Illustration

T: Do you like to do mazes?

C: Yeah.

T: Well, we're going to do some but maybe a little differently than usual, OK?

C: OK.

T: I'm going to tell you some steps that I use to solve a problem. I have written these steps on a card. First, I ask "What's the problem?" Then, "What can I do?" Then I ask "What's the best thing to do?" Finally, "How did I do?" When I try to solve a problem, I use these steps. What I would like you to do is to put these steps in your own words. How would you say this first step in your own words? (Child writes each step in her own words on a card.) What we're going to do is use these steps to solve these mazes. First, I'll do one, then you'll do one. Do you understand?

C: Yeah.

T: What are we going to do? (child repeats assignment) Good. Now for each problem you can earn two chips. One if you use the steps and one if you solve the problem. How many chips can you earn?

C: Two.

T: How do you get them?

C: Use the steps and solve the problem.

T: Good. Now I'll do the first problem, ready?

C: Yeah.

T: Okay, let's see "What's the problem?" Well I've got to get this guy out of here. "What can I do?" Well, I can go this way—no, that's a dead end—or I can go this way. "What's the best thing to do?" Go this way. (Draw line). "How did I do?" I got it right. Good work. Now you do one. (Child repeats process referring to steps on her own card.)

T: Good. You used all the steps and you got the mazes right. You get two chips. I find that when I use these steps, I do better in solving problems. Do you think they might help you?

C: Yeah, maybe.

T: Okay, let's try another maze. (Therapist repeats process. Child then does maze but begins drawing before deciding on the best route. Sequence went as follows:)

C: "What's the matter?" I've got to get this lady out of here. "What can I do?" Draw a line. (Child draws a line before considering alternative routes and proceeds to hit a dead end.)

T: How did you do?

C: I messed up.

T: What happened?

C: I went the wrong way.

T: Umh, how did that happen?

C: I don't know.

T: Did you stop and think before you started drawing the line?

C: No.

T: Okay. Well, let's try that next time, okay? I can't give you any points because you didn't use the steps and you didn't solve the problem. Sometimes we forget but let's work on that, okay?

C: Okay.

In the early stages of treatment, it is important that the therapist model a careful and reflective use of the steps, so that the child can see the effectiveness of good problem-solving behavior. The child will have lapses, however, in the use of these steps and the therapist's responses to these lapses is crucial to the child's willingness to continue using the procedure. Therapists, themselves, may wish to gain chips for their performance, may have their own lapses in the use of the procedure, and then stop themselves, returning to the appropriate step. Children appear to become more involved and learn more when they become both receivers and dispensers of reinforcement.

SUMMARY AND CONCLUSIONS

Two games found to be effective in the treatment of children with self-control deficits have been described. The requirements placed on the child in each game need to be appropriate to the child's developmental level. These requirements can be increased in difficulty as the child experiences success in the use of these games. In the *Beat the Clock* game, the therapist needs to attend to the distractions to which the child responds and to find ways to either reduce these distractions through isolating the child or help him or her respond more appropriately when they occur. In this light, it becomes important that the child begin to play *Beat the Clock* in his or her own classroom, under the supervision of the teacher or a teacher's aide so that the skills he or she has learned in individual treatment sessions can be generalized to the school setting.

In the *Stop and Think* game, children can be shifted from the solution of impersonal tasks, that is, mazes, puzzles, and so on to ones of a more personal nature. Practice in this game can help children use self-directed statements to guide both their academic and social behavior.

Each of the games that have been described attends to one of the deficits common to children with self-control problems. The games provide the context in which specific behavioral and cognitive skills are taught in the remediation of these deficits. Treatment is most effective in a well paced program which is sensitive to the developmental needs of the child, which combines game-playing with instruction in specific behavioral and cognitive strategies, which offers varied materials, and finally, which brings treatment into the settings for which it is intended.

REFERENCES

American Psychiatric Association (1980) Diagnostic and statistical manual of mental disorders, Third edition. Washington, D.C.: APA.

Hechtman, L., Weiss, G., Finkelstein, J., Wener, A. and Benn, R. (1976). Hyperactives as young adults: Preliminary report. *Canadian Medical Association Journal, 115*, 625–630.

Kazdin, A.E. (1974). Covert modeling, model similarity, and reduction of avoidance behavior. *Behavior Therapy, 5*, 325–340.

Kazdin, A.E. (1975). *Behavior modification in applied settings*. Homewood, IL: Dorsey.

Kendall, P.C. and Braswell, L. (1985). *Cognitive-behavioral therapy for impulsive children*. New York: Guilford.

Meichenbaum, D. (1971). Examination of model characteristics in reducing avoidance behavior. *Journal of Personality and Social Psychology, 17*, 298–307.

Schrag, P. and Divoky, D. (1975). *The myth of the hyperactive child*. New York: Pantheon.

Shapiro, L.E. (1981). *Games to grow on: Activities to help children learn self-control*. Englewood Cliffs, Prentice-Hall.

Weiss, G., Minde, K., Werry, J.S., Douglas, V.I., and Nemeth, E. (1971). Studies on the hyperactive child. VIII: Five year follow-up. *Archives of General Psychiatry, 24*, 409–414.

CHAPTER 13

Therapeutic Uses of Games with a Fine Motor Component

JAMES N. BOW and TERRY E. GOLDBERG

Even though games are frequently and widely used in child psychotherapy, their therapeutic value is often overlooked. Games are usually viewed as an effective way to engage children and establish rapport. However, in general games have not been closely analyzed to delineate those "active ingredients" that contribute to psychotherapeutic efficacy. Gardner (1969, 1971, 1975) is one of the few to devote effort to this area. His work has focused on boardgames (1969, 1975) and mutual storytelling techniques (1971). Goldberg (1980) has also reported on the use of a fine motor game, *Battling Tops*, as a psychotherapeutic tool. The following chapter will elaborate on the psychotherapeutic value of games, with special emphasis on those involving a fine motor component.

Utilizing games in a therapeutic setting has three main purposes: (1) it allows the therapist to assess social-emotional functioning, (2) it provides opportunities to analyze visual-spatial ability, and (3) it enhances the child's social and emotional growth through living experiences. Each of these will be reviewed.

SOCIAL-EMOTIONAL FUNCTIONING

Games provide a wide range of opportunities to assess a child's social-emotional functioning. Ego processing is indicated by the degree of competence, feelings of efficacy, defensiveness, impulse control, synthesis, reality testing, and general ego-strength (White, 1963). It is further reflected by the amount of self-directed behavior, the understanding of the relationship between action and consequences, and the ability to use what is learned as a design for future behavior. Each of these can be easily examined in a game setting. The drive for mastery is evident by the child's desire to practice and excel. It is reflected through the child's investment, persistence, expectations, and need for achievement. When a drive for mastery is lacking, it may suggest a fear of failure which commonly surfaces as self-doubt, anxiety, and avoidance. The range of alternative resources and coping skills can also be analyzed in a game setting because of the action orientation and numerous situations and roles created.

Cognitive strategies are important factors that reflect the degree of secondary process functioning. It is essential to assess whether the child's approach is logical and planned or impulsive and disorganized. The latter approach is commonly seen in children with attentional deficits. It is also pertinent to examine if the child learns from his or her mistakes. Does the child adapt or use the same strategy again and again? This may reflect the child's level of cognitive flexibility, problem-solving ability, and intellect. How the child responds to feedback is another critical area to assess. Does the child implement suggestions or ignore them? In addition, how does he or she react to praise? Praise is a motivator for some children, while other children (sometimes depressed) react with indifference.

Throughout the course of a game, it is important to monitor a child's attention, frustration tolerance, and ability to cope with pressure. These areas will further indicate the degree of control the child has over drives and impulses. Children with obvious or presumed brain damage often have great difficulty concentrating. They are easily distracted by extraneous stimuli and have difficulty focusing. Children with high levels of anxiety may experience similar problems. The degree to which a child can deal with disappointment, interference, delays, mishaps, and failure should also be noted. Children who are impulse-ridden commonly become very upset and unmanageable when faced with minor, often insignificant, problems. They may respond by refusing to continue the game, becoming destructive, and/or having a temper tantrum. Aggressive themes may also surface, along with a desire to retaliate. Pressure may involve a critical move, competing against time, and/or performing "in the clutch." Some children excel in these situations, while others deteriorate.

Some children attempt to avoid competitive situations (inherent in the games) by refusing to play, downplaying their significance, or attempting to terminate the game before it is completed. In contrast, other children become more motivated and intense in competitive situations. They continually challenge the therapist to another game or purchase the game for home practice. A preoccupation with the score, number of victories and defeats, and margin of victory are other ways competitive drive may surface. These situations also allow for examination of super-ego development as reflected by the child's willingness and desire to follow game rules and ability to accurately tally the score. Conduct disordered children will often attempt to take an extra turn, change or ignore rules, and/or delete or add points to players' scores. On the other hand, obsessive-compulsive children will rigidly follow the rules, often clearly stating how their actions are "in compliance."

Once success or failure has occurred, it is important to gauge the child's reaction. Success often brings forth feelings of omnipotence and grandiosity, along with increased motivation. Externalizing children will often make comments, such as "I'm the best," "You can never beat me," and "I'll beat you bad." In addition, they may belittle the performance of others, making comments, such as "You're no good" or "You'll never win." Failure may elicit feelings of anger, hostility, inferiority, and sadness. The therapist can play an important role in helping children manage affect by providing ego-level interpretations and a reality orientation.

The outcome of games also provides an excellent opportunity to analyze the child's locus of control. A simple question, such as "Why do you think you won (lost)?" will usually suffice. Children with an internal locus of control will express responsibility for their success or failure ("I failed because I did not try"; "I won because I am smarter"; or "I worked harder"). In contrast, children with an external locus of control will view their success or failure as being caused by external events ("I won because I am lucky" or "Your top is better than mine"). The causality attributed to one's performance greatly influences motivation. If a child feels a game has been "rigged" (external locus of control), he or she will have little motivation to continue. Motivation increases when a child feels he or she has control over the outcome.

VISUAL-SPATIAL ABILITY

Games provide an excellent opportunity for a therapist to assess a child's proficiency in the visual-spatial domain. Because children with psychiatric disorders have a higher rate of frank or presumed brain damage (Rutter, Tizard, and Whitmore, 1970), they may be presented as clumsy, inattentive, impulsive, and disorganized.

When analyzing visual-spatial ability, it is important to recognize that many components and subprocesses are involved. Specific analysis of discrete skill areas is not usually possible because games involve a combination of skills. However, a therapist should be able to identify the general proficiency of a child's visual-spatial ability, along with possible deficient areas. For example, when a child has difficulty matching shapes at an age appropriate level, this may suggest problems in the visual-spatial domain. However, it may be related to visual recognition, discrimination, closure, and/or figure ground deficits. It is difficult to tease apart the specific weakness(es) without psychological and educational testing.

THERAPEUTIC GROWTH

Games may be especially effective because the therapeutic boundaries are blurred (Goldberg, 1980): Is one playing, doing serious business, or learning in a didactic way? These ambiguities create what Redl (1959) called a "pressurized cabin" which promotes and fosters social-emotional growth. The development of the patient-therapist relationship that games tend to foster enhances the situation. Games are enjoyable and place the child at ease. They create a natural and informal setting for communicating. Games also provide for the child direct observations of the therapist as an active participant and role model. The therapist's reaction to pressure and frustration, ability to follow rules, and response to success and failure offer direct learning experiences for the child. In addition, the ability of the therapist to utilize reflective thought and cognitive techniques, such as the "Think Aloud" method (Camp and Bash, 1980), assists the child in learning ways of improving self-control by curbing impulsivity.

Games provide an opportunity for ego-level interpretations of a child's behavioral style. These interpretations help the child analyze his or her behavior. The willingness to accept such interpretations reflects the child's insight or resistance, perception of his or her behavior as ego-dystonic, and desire to change.

The therapist has a degree of control over the course and outcome of games, which adds to their therapeutic value. Stressful or pressured situations can be created, along with success and failure, depending on the nature of the child's problem(s) and stage of therapy, that is, the child's progress towards individual goals and the type of transference established. The therapist can also establish incremental inoculations against frustration. In addition, there is much opportunity for the therapist to provide support, encouragement, and reinforcement, which facilitates the treatment process.

To maximize social-emotional growth the therapist needs to be aware of counter-transference issues. Games are highly competitive. Hostility and anger may surface when defeat is experienced. These feelings become intensified when the child boasts about his or her performance ("You're no good. I'm the best.") In contrast, the therapist may feel sorrow and pity for a child who experiences an uneventful mishap. Rather than dealing with it therapeutically, the child may be encouraged to take another turn or violate other game rules.

DESCRIPTION OF GAMES

Games involving a fine motor component have certain advantages: Children are fascinated and intrigued by movement and it helps them channel and focus their energy. Second, they provide an avenue for learning to curb impulsive behavior, which is a common problem among children (Ross and Ross, 1976). Third, they allow an outlet for hostility and anger, thereby helping the child learn appropriate ways of discharging and ventilating feelings. Fourth, fine motor games increase arousal, and last, a variety of roles, such as the grandiose winner or angry loser, are created.

Numerous competitive fine motor games are available on the market. However, the games vary in therapeutic value, complexity, cost, and size. The selection of games depends on the patient's age, interests, dynamics, and stage of therapy. A series of competitive fine motor games used by the authors will be described in the following sections. These were selected for the following reasons: (1) they provide a wide range of therapeutic uses, (2) are usually available through local stores, (3) can be purchased at reasonable cost, that is, less than $20, (4) take up little office space and are easily set up, and (5) have instructions that are easily understood and learned. Although video games are popular and involve a fine motor component, they will not be reviewed because of the cost and accessibility factors.

Penny Hockey

Penny Hockey requires three coins and a table surface. Players position themselves across the length of the table top. One player is initially selected as the shooter, while the other player is the goalie. The goalie creates a three-sided goal by placing his or her hand at the edge of the table, with his or her index and little finger extended onto the table. The shooter, starting on his or her side of the table, slides the three coins together. This is called the "break." The object of the game is to score a goal by moving the three coins across the table by sliding one coin through the space created by the other two. A slide is created by flicking, not pushing, the coin with the index finger. The shooter may slide the coin in any direction, that is, sideways, backwards, or forwards, but he or she cannot slide the same coin consecutively. If the shooter eventually scores by flicking a coin into the goal, he or she is awarded one point and the shooter becomes the goalie and vice versa. A shooter loses his or her turn if (1) the coins touch each other after the break, (2) a shot is not possible, that is, three coins are parallel, or (3) any of the coins fall off the table. The winner is the first player to score 10 points. However, this score criteria can be varied depending on the age of the participants, time constraints, and skill level. The game is recommended for children aged eight years and older. Enjoyment of *Penny Hockey* is highly dependent on eye-hand coordination, ability to deal with pressure, and willingness to follow game rules. Cognitive strategies also play a role. The plan of attack should account for such factors as the number of flicks and distance of shots on goal.

Tiddly Winks (Pressman & Gabriel)

A common and widely used childhood game, *Tiddly Winks* consists of different colored and sized "winks" and a circular game board. The latter is divided into different sections according to point values, with the center section being assigned the highest value. The object of the game is to shoot the small winks onto the game board, aiming for the high point areas. This game is recommended for children aged six years and older. The therapeutic value lies in assessing eye-hand coordination, frustration tolerance, and persistence.

Battling Tops

Battling Tops is a commercially produced game consisting of a 12-inch plastic bowl, with spaces on the perimeter for two or more tops. By rapidly unwinding strings attached to the tops a whirling motion is created. The tops bump and knock each other in the common area until only one top remains—the winner. This game is recommended for children aged six years and older. The game can have two to four participants. As noted by Goldberg (1980), this game often elicits themes of aggression. It also creates opportunities to assess fine motor control, frustration tolerance, and ways of ventilating hostility.

Shoot-the-Moon (Wm. F. Drueke & Sons)

This game involves bilateral fine motor control, which makes it unique. It consists of two inclined rods that are supported by two wooden ends and a base. The rods can be manipulated (e.g., moved sideways) to cause a large steel ball to roll up the incline; the further up the incline the better. When the ball reaches the zenith, the rods are rapidly opened and the ball falls into one of the six holes below. The ball will also fall through anywhere along the incline if the rods are opened too far. The holes below the rods are assigned point values (e.g., −250, 250, 500, 1000, 2000, and 5000) depending on their position along the rods, with higher distances up the incline being assigned higher point values. The winner is the player with the most points, over one trial or a series of trials. This game has a high skill level and requires much practice. It is more appropriate for adolescents. As noted by Marten, Burwitz, and Zuckerman (1976), the game involves cognitive strategies, which they label the "creep" versus "shoot the moon." The "creep" strategy involves opening the rods slowly, thereby, causing the ball to inch up the incline. This strategy is low risk, but is inappropriate for obtaining high scores because the ball does not gain sufficient momentum. The "shoot the moon" strategy produces more extreme scores. It involves opening the two rods as far as possible and closing them just prior to the ball dropping. This quick motion causes the ball to "shoot" up the incline. It is the only strategy that will produce high scores. However, if the strategy fails low scores are obtained. Overall, the game provides good opportunities to analyze cognitive strategies, persistence, bilateral fine motor control, willingness to take risks, and frustration tolerance.

Perfection (Lakeside Games)

The object of *Perfection* is to match 25 geometric shapes with their analogous "cut outs" in a plastic tray as quickly as possible. After 60 seconds the tray pops up, scattering the pieces and no score is made. The winner is the person who completes the game in the shortest time period. The game is recommended for children five years or older. It provides good opportunities to assess organizational skills (reflective versus impulsive), cognitive strategies (matching geometric shape to "cut outs" versus matching "cut outs" to shapes from pile), and visual spatial skills. In addition, the game is time limited which increases psychological pressure. The game can be modified. For advanced levels less time can be allotted, while for beginners fewer shapes can be used.

Two other games, *Superfection* (Lakeside Games) and *Numbers Up* (Milton Bradley) are similar to *Perfection*, but involve matching pairs of designs and numbers, respectively.

Pic-Up Stix (Steven MFG)

Twenty-five sticks of assorted colors, including one black stick, are held in one hand and dropped, forming a pile of overlapping sticks. The object is to pick up the sticks, one at a time, moving only the stick being touched. If any other stick moves, the player's turn ends. A player may only remove sticks with his or her fingers. However, the player who obtains the black stick may use it to flip or tip other sticks. The game is finished when all sticks are picked up. Each player's score is calculated according to the number of sticks obtained, with different point values being assigned to each color. The highest score wins. The game is recommended for children five years and older. The game is highly dependent on eye-hand coordination and the child's willingness to follow and obey rules. In regard to the latter, the game provides ample opportunities for cheating, which can be dealt with therapeutically. Cognitive strategies are also involved. It is important to assess if the position of the stick or point value is more important to the child. In addition, it is worthwhile to note how the point value of different colored sticks and the special utility of the black stick effect the child's approach.

CASE ILLUSTRATIONS

Case 1

D.B. was intelligent, but impulsive. During *Penny Hockey*, he played quickly and carelessly. He displayed little foresight or logic. The therapist suggested D.B. use the "Think Aloud" cognitive strategy, which involves verbally rehearsing each move before it is made. D.B. utilized the strategy and his performance greatly improved. It helped him evaluate possible moves, along with their ramifications. This approach was used in other therapeutic activities as well, and D.B. was gradually able to generalize the strategy.

Case 2

T.S. was an average student, but very anxious. Her mother had long complained about her difficulty dealing with pressure and deadlines. The game *Perfection* was played to probe this area. When the game was introduced T.S. immediately expressed concern about the timer. While playing the game she was very efficient during the first 30 seconds, but as time ran out her anxiety greatly increased and her play became very disorganized. Two therapeutic approaches were used. First, T.S. was taught relaxation exercises to reduce her anxiety. Second, systematic desensitization was utilized. T.S. was given only 10 of the 25 shapes and allotted the full 60 seconds. Once she completed the task, which took her 20 seconds, she was asked to wait patiently until the timer was almost ready to ring before turning off the game. This was done to make her aware of the additional time, along with reducing her anxiety about the impending deadline. Gradually the number of shapes were increased until she was able to complete all 25 within a 60 second period.

Case 3

D.B. was a shy and quiet girl from a large family. She had great difficulty initiating activities, commonly expressing a fear of failure. She needed much encouragement to play *Tiddly Winks*. D.B. exhibited her fear of aggression by not wanting to press too hard on the winks, noting they might break. Reassurance was provided and she was told the winks were unbreakable. D.B. was very critical of each flip, noting it was either too hard or too soft. Again reassurance was provided. She also expressed feelings of inadequacy ("I'm no good." and "I'll never be any good.") which reflected her poor self-esteem and tendencies to internalize. D.B. slowly learned the proper technique and became quite competent. There was an increase in her assertiveness and confidence, which slowly generalized to other games and activities. She was also able to make positive comments about her performance.

Case 4

W.H. was an impulsive and excitable child. He was from a disorganized family and had a tension-discharge pattern of behavior. He displayed few controls, often screaming and banging the table during *Battling Tops*. The therapist said, "Hold on. It looks as if you're having a hard time controlling yourself." As a result, a long "countdown" procedure was instituted by the therapist. The tops could only be released after the therapist had counted backwards from 30 to "blastoff." There were also "hold" periods when W.H. became disruptive or impulsive. These techniques were generalized to other games and activities, with consequent improvement in his self-control.

Case 5

W.D. was a child from an achievement-oriented family who held high expectations for her. She was a below average student. During the intake the father described W.D. as "lazy" and "not motivated." W.D. presented as cooperative and pleasant. She said she enjoyed school, but found handwriting, spelling, and reading difficult. While playing the game *Shoot-the-Moon* and *Perfection* W.D. was persistent and displayed good strategies. However, her motor coordination was poor, especially with the left hand. In addition, while playing *Perfection* she had great difficulty matching shapes. This suggested problems with visual recognition and discrimination. As the result of these factors, W.D. was referred for academic and neuropsychological testing, which indicated she was learning disabled.

Case 6

M.S. was an impulse-ridden, omnipotent, 10-year-old male. He constantly boasted about his skills and how he was "going to beat the therapist bad." He selected the game *Pic-up Stix*, noting the therapist didn't have a chance. M.S. refused to listen to the directions, stating it was only a "dumb game and anyone with brains knew how to play it." After all the sticks were picked up, M.S. had 15 and the therapist 10. M.S. immediately noted he was the "winner." The therapist said the rules state that point values are assigned according to color. Final tabulations indicated the therapist had won. M.S. became angry, stating this was not fair and complaining he was unaware of this fact. It was pointed out to him why rules are reviewed at the beginning of the game. The rules were reviewed and the game commenced again. This time M.S. immediately attempted to pick up the black stick and in the process moved two other sticks. He continued to play. He was told his turn had ended because other sticks had moved. M.S. became upset, slamming his hand against the table. He stated the sticks had moved only slightly. It was emphasized that the rules of the game must be followed. The importance of strategy was also pointed out. M.S. was asked to watch the therapist. The therapist outlined each of his moves and the purpose behind it. M.S. was able to do likewise, which assisted in curbing his impulsivity. The therapist provided praise and encouragement, which M.S. returned during the therapist's next turn. M.S. gradually became highly successful at the game. It was emphasized that his success was attained through modeling, cognitive strategies, patience, and obeying rules.

These case illustrations demonstrate the therapeutic value of fine motor games. They also demonstrate the wide range of opportunities available for assessment and learning, which facilitate the treatment process.

SUMMARY AND CONCLUSIONS

Games with a fine motor component provide unique opportunities to assess social-emotional functioning and visual-spatial proficiency. In addition, games promote social-emotional growth by eliciting a variety of therapeutic issues (e.g., ego and super-ego development, locus of control, cognitive strategies, and impulse control) through living experiences. They also provide a direct opportunity for active role modeling.

The child observes how the therapist manages competition, pressure, mishaps, frustration, and failure. Additional therapeutic value is provided by the control the therapist has over the course and outcome of the game.

The fine motor games discussed in this chapter have a variety of applications. They may be used in many different settings with children having a wide range of psychopathological disorders. They can also be manipulated and adapted according to the child's dynamics and stage of therapy. Fine motor games are especially effective because movement fascinates and intrigues children and serves as a relaxant. They are also enjoyable. As a result, they engage children in the therapeutic process. In addition, fine motor games provide an outlet for anger and hostility and opportunities to learn to curb impulsive behavior. In comparison to other games (e.g., chess and checkers), the games discussed in this chapter have additional advantages, namely, allowing immediate feedback and not being over-engrossing or lengthy. Because the games are usually short, they allow for a greater number of learning experiences. However, fine motor games also have disadvantages, as chance plays a greater role and some children become overaroused.

Overall, games with a fine motor component are useful in child psychotherapy. They are more than "games," they are therapeutic tools.

REFERENCES

Camp, B. and Bash, M.A. (1980). Developing self control through training in problem solving: "The Think Aloud" program. In D.P. Rathjen and J.P. Foreyt (Eds.), *Social Competence* (pp. 24–53). Elmsford, NY: Pergamon.

Gardner, R.A. (1969). The game of checkers as a diagnostic and therapeutic tool in child psychotherapy. *Acta Paedopsychiatrica, 36*, 142–152.

Gardner, R.A. (1971). *Therapeutic communication with children: The mutual storytelling technique*. New York: Aronson.

Gardner, R.A. (1975). *Psychotherapeutic approaches to the resistant child*. New York: Aronson.

Goldberg, T.E. (1980). Battling tops: A modality in child psychotherapy. *Journal of Clinical Child Psychology, 9*, 206–209.

Marten, R., Burwitz, L., and Zuckerman, J. (1976). Modeling effects on motor performance. *Research Quarterly, 47*, 277–291.

Redl, R. (1959). Strategies and techniques of the life space interview. *American Journal of Orthopsychiatry, 28,* 1–18.

Ross, D.M. and Ross, S.A. (1976). *Hyperactivity: Current issues, research, and strategy.* New York: Wiley.

Rutter, M., Tizard, J., and Whitmore, K. (1970). *Education, health, and behavior: Psychological and medical study of childhood development.* New York: Wiley.

White, R.W. (1963). Ego and reality in psychoanalytic theory. *Psychological Issues, 3* (24–43).

CHAPTER 14

Therapeutic Use of Card Games with Learning-Disabled Children

STEVEN E. REID

Learning-disabled children are those who demonstrate marked academic underachievement whose cause cannot be traced to intellectual limitations, sensory deficits, motor impairments, socioeconomic disadvantage, inadequate instruction, or emotional disturbance (Rourke, 1985a). These children not only present problems in terms of designing adequate educational programs, but also are likely to constitute a significant proportion of mental health problems. Many of these children go on to develop difficulties in conduct, self-esteem, and depression as a result of years of frustration and failure in school. A substantial percentage of learning-disabled children drop out of school, thereby contributing substantially to the population of juvenile delinquents in this country (Brown, 1978).

Despite the significance of the problem of learning disabilities, it remains one of the most confusing areas in the literature of child psychology. For example, as many as six different diagnostic labels have been used to describe this problem, including "minimal brain dysfunction" (Millichap, 1977), "dyslexia" (Benton and Pearl, 1978), and "brain-injured" (Strauss and Lehtinen, 1947). Only recently has the term "learning disabilities" gained widespread usage. Accordingly, estimates of the prevalence of this disorder have varied, ranging from as low as 3 percent (Ross, 1976) to a high of 10 percent (Millichap, 1977) of the school-age population.

For many years, the inability of children to learn despite adequate educational opportunities and intellectual ability was believed to result from underlying emotional conflict. While this notion has fallen into disrepute, there remains considerable debate in regard to the causes of specific

257

learning disabilities. The etiological theories encompassing genetic factors (Boder, 1973), social-environmental influences (Denckla, 1979), attentional problems (Ross, 1976), and visual-perceptual deficits (Orton, 1937) have not received much empirical support. Support has been growing for the notion that neuropsychological immaturity and/or dysfunction is the cause of the learning problems of a large number of these children (Barkley, 1981; Rourke, 1978, 1985a). Central nervous system dysfunction may take two general forms: diffuse brain damage, resulting in widespread cognitive and behavioral deficits, or highly focal lesions resulting in highly specific disruptions in cognitive functioning. The term *learning disabilities*, in its current usage, refers to those children whose learning problems are attributable to neurogenic origins.

The literature on identification and classification of subtypes of learning disabilities easily exceeds other related research in terms of general confusion, disorganization, and controversy. Recent research (see Rourke, 1985b, for a review) has at least made it possible to coherently summarize existing knowledge about learning disability subtypes, as follows: (1) children with learning disabilities represent an extremely heterogeneous group with regard to their pattern of cognitive skills and level of academic achievement (2) specific disorders of reading, spelling, mathematics, or written expression are also not homogeneous subtypes of learning disorders, (3) the various subtypes of learning disorders do not result from simply a critical deficit in any one cognitive skill, and (4) at least four general areas of cognitive development appear to be important to adequate achievement skills: linguistic-conceptual, visuospatial-constructive, sequential-analytic, and motor planning, execution, and regulation. Where these skills develop out of synchrony from one another, problems with achievement are likely to occur.

To appreciate the complexity and breadth of the conceptual and research issues regarding learning disabilities, the reader must understand that the above constitutes only the briefest of overviews of the literature on these disorders. Familiarity with these issues is a first step toward greater understanding of the psychological world of the learning-disabled child. Interest in the psychological functioning of these children remains high. It is widely held that socioemotional difficulties often occur in conjunction with childhood learning disorders. Inefficient learners are commonly referred for psychological counseling and represent a substantial proportion of referrals to mental health clinics (Adams, 1975). Early investigations into the secondary emotional problems of learning disorders were poorly designed and yielded little reliable information. However, recent well-controlled research has brought the psychological functioning of learning-disabled children into clearer focus. The research can be divided into three general areas: the behavior of learning-disabled children, their interpersonal environment, and their emotional and personality functioning.

AREAS OF RESEARCH

Behavior

A number of studies have documented the greater frequency of behavioral problems of learning-disabled children in and out of the classroom. Conduct problems, such as aggression, hyperactivity, social withdrawal, anxiety, and school phobias, are more commonly found among learning-disabled children than those achieving at a normal rate (Douglas and Peters, 1979; Klinsbourne and Caplan, 1979; Peter and Spreen, 1979; Rutter, 1978). Cunningham and Barkley (1978) have demonstrated how academic failure can come to create classroom behavior problems, inattentiveness, off-task behavior, and aggression in children. Although these behaviors may occur simultaneously with learning disabilities, they may also develop in response to extended failure in the classroom. A number of learning-disabled children also suffer from hyperactivity. Children whose primary diagnosis is hyperactivity, or Attention Deficit Disorder (DSM III, 1980), typically are underachievers and manifest behaviors, such as distractibility, that interfere with classroom learning.

Interpersonal Environment

In general, the literature indicates that learning-disabled children must deal with an environment that differs significantly from that of their normally achieving peers. In contrast to normal achievers, learning-disabled children tend: (1) to be perceived as less pleasant and desirable by parents, teachers, and peers, (2) to be ignored and rejected more often by their teachers, (3) to be the recipients of more negative communications from their parents, teachers, and peers, (4) to be treated in a notably more punitive and derogatory manner by their parents, and (5) to live in families that resemble in certain crucial ways those of emotionally disturbed children (see Porter, 1980, for a review of this literature).

Socioemotional Functioning

Considering the apparently negative environment facing learning-disabled children, one would certainly expect to find that they have difficulty functioning emotionally and socially. Researchers have consistently identified secondary emotional problems—such as low self-esteem, lack of drive for mastery, helplessness, and depression—among these children (e.g., Black, 1974; Bryan and Pearl, 1979; Zimmerman and Allebrand, 1965). However, some studies (e.g., Connolly, 1969; Silverman, 1968) found no significant differences in levels of emotional adjustment and self-esteem between learning-disabled children and their normally achieving peers. Ribner (1978) found that underachieving children in regular classrooms were likely to have low self-esteem, but that those segregated in a learning-disabled classroom were not likely to have a negative self-view. In their summary of the literature in this area, Porter and Rourke (1985) suggest that a substantial proportion of children with learning disorders do not experience emotional difficulties.

While this notion certainly goes against established opinion, it is nevertheless plausible. Since learning-disabled children are an extremely heterogeneous group with regard to their pattern of cognitive deficits, it seems likely that these children are also not homogeneous in terms of their emotional functioning. Some may have adapted to their limitations, while others clearly suffer a great deal from the loss of social status. A number of factors, in addition to pattern of cognitive deficits, probably impact on the overall emotional adjustment of the learning-disabled child. Unfortunately, investigators are only beginning to identify relationships between socioemotional functioning and such factors as subtype of learning disorder and educational placement. One consistent finding is that children with language-based disorders tend to be more socially responsive and emotionally flexible, but, predictably, less verbally expressive, compared to children with visuospatial-based disorders. The latter group tends to exhibit stereotyped and constricted emotional responses (Ozols and Rourke, 1985). Clearly, there is a need for more research into the nature and patterns of emotional disturbance among learning-disabled children.

TREATMENT

The neurological impairments that presumably underly many children's learning difficulties are not easily detected by existing neurodiagnostic methods. Damage to the brain and spinal cord cannot be directly treated or cured. Thus, treatment approaches to learning-disabled children have necessarily focused on the overt academic, behavioral, and emotional manifestations of the neurological deficits. Treatment of the academic problems includes both retraining through use of the child's cognitive strengths and a frontal assault on the deficient areas (Rourke, 1976). Modification of related behaviors, such as attention span and impulse control have also been a part of efforts to improve academic performance.

The question of treatment of the secondary, emotional and behavioral problems that occur simultaneously with learning problems has not received much attention in the literature, largely because of the relative recency of the learning disabilities diagnosis. Only play therapy has any sort of established history of use with this population. The goals of play therapy are broader than those interventions designed to modify specific behaviors. Play therapy is designed to relieve the child's emotional distress and engender a more positive attitude about achievement in general. This approach involves, essentially, permitting a child to play freely with a variety of expressive and imaginative play materials, such as dolls, puppets, art materials, miniature objects, sand, and clay. The therapist responds empathetically to the child, and sets limits on his or her behavior, but otherwise does not actively intervene during the child's play. The assumption here is that children will express and work through emotional conflicts on their own within the metaphor of play.

In their books on play therapy, both Axline (1947) and Ginott (1961) describe the application of nondirective play therapy with learning-disabled children. Guerney (1983) elaborates on the curative aspects of play therapy with this population. She states that the "special physical and interpersonal environment can permit learning disabled children to succeed and develop a feeling of satisfaction with themselves and their competences" (p. 424). The atmosphere of the playroom is one of playfulness and permissiveness, in which fantasy expression is encouraged. As a result, a special environment is created which allows for expression of feelings and experimentation with situations that in "real life" are experienced as threatening. The repetition inherent in play permits the child to work through and master uncomfortable feelings.

One assumption inherent in the play therapy approach is that a child's feelings and attitudes about learning and academic achievement will surface in his or her play. Therefore, no attempts are made by the therapist to elicit expression by the child of particular emotions or concerns. The open-ended quality of this approach may have its drawbacks with learning-disabled children. Primary is the problem of generalization. Play therapy may help children strengthen their general sense of self, but this feeling of competence may evaporate in the school setting. For many children with learning impairments, the very concepts of school and learning are strongly associated with failure and with feelings of inferiority compared to "normal" children.

Game playing is an activity that appears to have potential to more directly address the learning-based emotional and behavioral problems of learning-disabled children. Game therapy is a form of play therapy that utilizes formal, organized games, such as checkers and *Monopoly*. Common boardgames, fine motor games (e.g., *Tiddly Winks, Pic-Up Stix*), and card games are among those that have been brought into the therapy situation. It is only recently that games have gained recognition and acceptance as psychotherapeutic tools. Games, like free play, are separate from reality, and thus provide a context for fantasy experience. Games are seen as a natural medium for expression (Nickerson and O'Laughlin, 1983) and the preferred play activity of school-age children (Piaget, 1962). Thus, a playful and open atmosphere similar to that strived for in play therapy can be generated using games. Throughout history games have been created and played, not only for leisure, but as a vehicle for dealing with specific anxieties. For instance, *Monopoly* was created during the Great Depression of the 1930s, when many dreamed of escaping the economic hardships of the times.

It follows, then, that the primary advantage of games for learning-disabled children is their focusing potential. Games are structured, rule-bound, task-focused, and goal-directed activities. However, they do not possess the same evaluative quality as other task-focused activities, such as schoolwork. Games provide an opportunity to learn basic skills necessary to attend to and complete a task, such as concentration, impulse control, and persistence. Additionally, games are more "cognitive" than free play. Most games require logical thinking and strategy (the exceptions being pure chance games, such as adult gambling and *Candyland*, among others). Others tap motor dexterity (e.g., target games) and visual skills (e.g., many card games, such as Concentration). Games are structurally analogous to academic tasks. Unlike schoolwork, however, games are inherently pleasurable, and children will learn more readily from activities that are enjoyable.

A second advantage of games is therapist control. The therapist can control the outcome of the game to provide the learning-disabled child with a success or failure experience, depending on the child's particular therapeutic needs at the time. During game play, the therapist can encourage and reinforce experimentation, attempts at mastery of skills, and actual successful responses. The therapist can stop the play temporarily to explore issues that may come up during the game. The child's sense of competence, feelings of trust toward adults, and defenses are likely to be revealed by the competition involved in playing the game. The therapist can thus formulate diagnostic impressions during game play and make ego-level interventions within the framework of the game.

The number of publications on the therapeutic potential of games has increased dramatically in recent years, but there has been little evaluative research to date, and only a few reports on game play with learning-disabled children. Gardner (1973) discussed the use of his *Talking, Feeling, and Doing Game* with underachievers. Goldberg (1980) has used the *Battling Tops* game with children who have "cerebral dysfunction." He argues that the game, in which tops are spun and collide in a bowl-shaped area, is useful to promote success experiences and curb the impulsive behavior exhibited by many learning-disabled children. The game is also thought by Goldberg to have value in rehabilitation of fine motor deficits, attention problems, and in providing a sense of mastery, since small increments of improved performance are highly visible. Goldberg cautions, however, that *Battling Tops* or other fine motor games must be used only as a limited therapeutic modality and not as a complete therapeutic program per se.

CARD GAMES

An important consideration in game therapy is choosing a game or set of games which maximize therapeutic efficiency for the individual client. For the learning-disabled child referred for therapy, the game(s) selected should: (1) provide opportunities for intellectual as well as emotional growth, (2) require of the players a wide range of neuropsychological abilities, and (3) have varying levels of difficulty so that children can start at their own level and experience increasing increments of success. One set of games, those which use a regular set of playing cards, has been found by the author to meet these requirements and to be of particular therapeutic value with learning-disabled children.

Card games are an extremely flexible therapeutic tool. Scores of different games exist and new ones are easily created, all from a finite and fixed set of stimuli: the 52 playing cards. The advantage of using the same props over and over is that children gain a sense of comfort and safety with what is familiar. Later, the repetition involved in card playing enables children to acquire a sense of mastery and competence which will generalize to other task-focused activities. Most card games can be played more than once during a therapy hour, thus increasing the likelihood of the child learning from the previous game. Card games vary widely in terms of intellectual ability required. Therefore, they can be used with children of all ages and of various intellectual capacity. The most simple games can be used with younger children or those with more severe intellectual impairment. More complex games can be introduced as children master the easier games. Older children and adolescents may be more motivated to participate in card games than in traditional play activities, as the latter are often viewed as being childish forms of amusement.

With card games, learning is "painless" because games are intriguing, challenging, and fun. They are not usually resisted when offered as a part of therapy. Card games are intrinsically motivating and are not usually viewed as hard work by children, despite the fact that they require a variety of cognitive abilities and real intellectual effort from the participants. The following is a brief discussion of the cognitive skills that card games can help develop. Specific card games that can be used for developing different skills are also named, but a description of each game is prohibited by considerations of space. The reader may wish to consult Golick (1973) for a complete description of the specific card games that are mentioned.

Motor Skills

Handling, shuffling, dealing, and learning to form a "hand" of cards all offer practice in an extensive range of hand and finger movements. Fine motor skills are essential to handwriting, drawing, painting, crafts, and other school activities. Some games, such as Stinker, Slap Jack, Bow to the King, and Spit, require quick reflexes and fine motor speed and agility.

Rhythm

Some children with learning disabilities exhibit little awareness of the orderly timing that is needed in physical activities, that underlies fluid speech, and that is essential to the appreciation of music and poetry. Card playing exposes children to a variety of simple rhythms. Efficient dealing of cards involves a steady rhythm pattern. Having a child close his or her eyes can help him or her learn to *hear* these rhythms, and with practice to develop a good sense of rhythm. Games which proceed in rhythmic patterns include War, Pisha Paysha, and Earl of Coventry.

Sequence

Sequencing problems are common among learning-disabled children. Many seem unable to understand the order or arrangement in time or space of a series of sounds, movements, or ideas. Card games provide opportunities for learning sequence concepts. Orderly dealing and turn-taking teach temporal sequencing. Some games, such as Stop and Go, Rummy, Poker, Kings in the Corner, Up and Down, Cribbage, and Spit involve number sequencing.

Number concepts

Card games offer opportunities to learn a wide range of number concepts. Simpler games such as Go Fish and War help with identification of numbers as well as the concept of greater/lesser. A variety of sensory modalities are invoked during game play. Seeing numbers, hearing them called out during dealing, and feeling the number of separate movements as one deals the cards all help the child form associations between numbers and tangible phenomena. The finite and intriguing properties of a deck of cards—52 cards, 4 suits, 13 cards in each, 2 pairs of every denomination, and so forth—also entice children to use numbers. Sharing a group of objects between several individuals is a precursor to understanding the concept of division. Handing the cards out two or three at a time (e.g., as with Manville or Euchre) or counting up pairs after a game of Go Fish provides beginning counting exercises. Addition is practiced in keeping score, especially in games where cards have different values (e.g., Casino, Yukon, and Rummy). In games such as Blackjack, adding numbers is a part of the game. A final mathematical concept that can be practiced is categorization, which helps a child learn about sets. Go Fish, Old Maid, and Hearts involve categorization.

Visual Skills

All card games require visual discrimination. Simple matching games (e.g., Go Fish) give practice with color and form discrimination. Visual tracking is involved every time a player scans his or her fan-shaped hand to select a card. In Slap Jack, Bow to the King, and Spit, the players are rewarded for speed and accuracy of visual recognition and response. Concentration is a game that requires good visual memory.

Verbal Skills

In a card game, verbal stimuli are reduced, and particular verbal responses are practiced over and over again. A new vocabulary is often created during card play. The experience of learning a new word and using it meaningfully has a stimulating effect on overall vocabulary growth. Receptive language skills are also practiced in processing verbal instructions and comments made by the therapist.

General Intellectual Skills

Logical thinking, planning, and organization of ideas are all rewarded in card playing. Another intellectual asset fostered by playing cards is the ability to hold many factors in mind at once. Mental flexibility is also tapped in card games, in that a player must be ready to change his or her mental set during a game or from game to game.

It is clear, then, that card games provide many opportunities for learning and practicing of a wide range of intellectual and neuropsychological abilities. Card games also strengthen nonintellective factors that impact on learning and academic performance. Card games demand attention, mental alertness, concentration, self-control, and active participation. All these factors are important for learning of any sort.

Card games can also stimulate emotional growth. As mentioned previously, card playing within a therapeutic framework can enhance children's self-esteem, build a sense of mastery and self-confidence, and increase their motivation toward academic achievement. Other therapeutic ingredients of game play have been identified, including the following:

Therapeutic Alliance

The enjoyable and familiar aspects of games lure children into therapy. As children become more comfortable, they also become more willing to discuss uncomfortable topics. Children also experience a sense of trust and safety in the therapist who plays fairly but is not overly competitive.

Pleasure

Pleasure in moderation has the power to soothe and to reduce an individual's overall level of distress. Games are, above all, fun to play and are meant to be enjoyed.

Self-Expression

Games are not "for real," so players are more likely to express feelings and attitudes in this context. To prove this point, one need only observe how emotional some usually reserved children become during the course of a game. Games entice children to relax their defenses and become affectively involved with their immediate environment.

Socialization

There are many opportunities for social learning through game play. Games are thought to parallel many real life social situations. Games, like life, require obedience to a fixed set of rules for behavior, recognition of and compliance with group norms and expectations, self-control, acceptance of authority, and controlled expression of aggression and competitive feelings. During game play, players must communicate with each other about the rules and procedures of the game, and are expected to compete with a friendly and respectful attitude.

GENERAL THERAPY CONSIDERATIONS

Repetition and practice are crucial for developing the cognitive skills described previously and for engendering a feeling of special competence. The therapist should encourage repeated use once the child starts playing cards. I have found that children do not become bored during prolonged intervals of card playing; rather, they tend to become more confident and interested in mastering new games.

An atmosphere of fun and joy must be maintained if children are to challenge themselves to improve. With many learning-disabled children, a sense of inadequacy and defeat pervades their thinking and prevents them from risking failure in many endeavors. These children are likely to view any competitive situation as threatening. Others may express their fears in the form of chronic cheating or testing of the rules. The therapist can downplay the competitive aspects of the game to entice children to play. Success can be built into the child's performance by creating handicaps for the therapist. The therapist may need to let the child win during the initial stages to help him or her gain confidence. The therapist can also structure the game play so that children "graduate" to games of higher complexity and challenge, thereby building their self-esteem. Cheating is thought to be a manifestation of a child's urges toward fantasy gratification and antisocial adaptation (Meeks, 1970). Cheating should not be permitted, but the therapist must be open to exploring the child's need to cheat.

The therapist must keep in mind that the game is not an end in itself; it is only a vehicle for learning and emotional expression. The basic receptive and understanding stance of the therapist should not be compromised for the sake of continuing the game. The therapist should encourage temporary departures from the game for discussion. If the therapist's own need to win becomes primary, then the original goals of the game therapy are lost.

Card games are not a panacea. They should be used only as one intervention tool within a broader context of psychological therapy. Some learning-disabled children are not ready to engage in game play. A number of these children are so convinced of their own incompetence that they refuse to enter into any competitive situation. Others are so emotionally distressed or impulse ridden that they cannot engage in structured, organized play. Still others have specific cognitive deficits which are more efficiently addressed with specific games or learning devices. For instance, children with isolated motor difficulties might benefit from playing several fine motor games, which would offer a wider range of hand and finger movements than card games. A final limitation of card games in therapy is that there are some children who simply do not like to play cards.

CASE ILLUSTRATION

Robert (fictitious name), a 10-year-old boy of average build, height, and general appearance, had a history of learning problems. Educational testing done when Robert was six revealed a broad range of deficits, including: underdeveloped expressive skills, poor comprehension and concept formation, visual-motor problems, and difficulty processing auditory stimuli despite intact hearing. On the Weschler Intelligence Scale for Children-Revised (WISC-R), Robert obtained the following scores: Verbal IQ 80, Performance IQ 74, Full Scale IQ 78. A number of "soft" neurological signs were evident in Robert's overall output. Projective testing found a good deal of internal emotional turmoil, an active fantasy life dominated by aggressive themes, and a poor self-concept. Robert was seen as being "at high risk for future academic problems." He was placed in special education classes in a public school where he remained for three years.

Robert made little academic progress during these three years; in fact, his records suggest that his overall functioning deteriorated. His classroom behavior usually consisted of fluctuations between extreme social withdrawal and provocative, attention-seeking behaviors, such as teasing others and defiantly refusing to comply with teacher requests. Aggressive behavior gradually increased over the three years. These behaviors seriously interfered with learning, and prompted his being transferred to a private school for children with emotional and learning problems.

On entering this school, Robert was retested. His math skills were at the 1.9 grade level, while his reading was at the kindergarten level. He knew basic adding and subtracting skills. He recognized primary numbers but not all the letters of the alphabet. His new Verbal WISC-R score was 15 points lower than his score of two years earlier. While Robert's behavior stabilized at his new school, he remained highly distractible and had a very short attention span. His teachers remarked that he had no desire at all to learn and did everything he could to avoid schoolwork. On the other hand, Robert attached much importance to working with his hands. He prided himself on being a "fix-it" man.

During the initial stage of therapy, it became apparent that Robert was a very well-defended young man with a very strong denial system. Although he related to the therapist, he would not self-disclose or otherwise examine himself for fear of compromising his "macho" image. Initially he spent much time building castles and houses with a Lego building set. He became interested in cards after watching the therapist shuffle the deck. Robert wanted to learn how to create the "bridge" while shuffling.

The only game Robert knew how to play was War. His style of play was revealing. He attributed success in this game to skill; when he won, he couldn't control his glee; when he lost, he accused the therapist of taking advantage of a child. Repeated reminders that the game involved nothing but chance and luck finally got through to Robert. His more realistic outlook was followed by less extreme emotional reactions to the outcome and by him giving up his rather transparent attempts to cheat. I attempted to draw analogies from the luck-skill concept of the game to real life situations. These attempts met with only limited success. Robert seemed to absorb the notion that some things in life result from nothing more than chance, and that one cannot blame oneself or others for chance events. However, he quickly backed off when direct references were made to his life.

Robert sharpened his visual and number skills during the course of play. At first he had trouble distinguishing sixes and nines, was unsure of many greater/less/than pairs, and didn't understand how the picture cards fit in. He mastered these concepts rather quickly. He also learned how to count to 52 by doing his share of dealing. After about two months of playing War, it was clear that Robert was more affectively involved with the therapist. He began to relate stories about his home life. He identified strongly with his father, who in Robert's eyes embodied all the qualities of a macho superhero. Robert made few references to his mother, but they were thematically consistent; he disappoints her often, and somehow must redeem himself to win back her favor.

Robert became so comfortable with War that he refused to try new games. Finally he agreed to a game of Crazy Eights because he believed it to be a pure chance game like War. He needed a good deal of support to finish the game. The concepts of a wild card, of different suits, and of following suit during play did not come easy to Robert. For the first few games the therapist spent much time helping Robert arrange the cards by suits and hold the hand in fan style. With a little help from the therapist, he won his first game after several defeats, and seemed ecstatic. I pointed out his improvement and suggested that he must be getting very good since I do not get beat in this game very often. This seemed to heighten Robert's sense of accomplishment. As time passed, he became more aware of the different strategies involved, such as holding a wild card (an eight) until it is really needed, or anticipating a change of suit several turns ahead. Robert's improvement was rather striking: This normally scattered and impulsive child would spend up to 40 minutes in quiet and relaxed concentration during card play, all the while exhibiting the kind of cognitive organization and flexibility in his play that was nowhere to be found during his four-plus years of school.

Robert's teacher observed that he had particular difficulty remembering visually presented material. Auditory cues had to be used often to aid his learning of basic reading skills. The teacher felt the auditory processing problem identified by a previous psycholinguistic examination was an artifact of Robert's motivational and emotional problems, which resulted in his blocking and resisting of the verbal commands of others, especially adults. The teacher also thought that Robert's distractibility contributed to his problem with visual tasks.

Since his visual memory was not tapped to any great extent by the two card games Robert and I had been playing, I decided to introduce the game of Concentration to Robert. Interestingly, Robert was much less resistant to changing games than previously, perhaps reflecting his growing sense of competence and willingness to risk failure. However, he felt that there were too many cards to remember, so I suggested we play a modified game using only the picture cards and those numbered four to seven (28 cards). Robert also felt he could not beat me, so I handicapped myself by halving the value of my tricks won. Robert made noticable gains in his ability to remember cards he had seen. These gains were reflected in the classroom; he exhibited improved attention during reading, and his sight vocabulary subsequently increased.

Robert began to discuss himself more in therapy. He confessed that he never believed that he would be able to play cards so well. Robert also offered that he would never be good at schoolwork, however. I reminded him that he had trouble learning card games at first, but that he mastered all the games by sticking with them, and that it never hurts to at least try to do your best. This was a message that I imparted from the beginning of therapy; that Robert was a capable student who only needed to give learning a better shot.

By the end of Robert's first year at the private school, he had shown considerable growth. His teacher observed that he no longer anxiously avoided schoolwork. He was able to work for an entire period without distracting himself or putting his head down in defiant noncompliance. Robert's reading and math scores improved almost two grade levels. He seemed more "connected" and less hostile in his interactions with other people. He also seemed more self-confident and did not rely on his "macho" defenses as frequently. Most significantly, Robert's mother reported that he really appeared to enjoy school, whereas previously he found it boring.

Of course, there were factors other than game therapy that were helpful to Robert. The classroom teaching focused on engendering positive attitudes and on individualized learning rather than on performance *per se*. Family dynamics also contributed to Robert's problems. His mother had unrealistic expectations for his academic achievement and seemingly had not yet dealt with the narcissistic injury involved in having a handicapped child. These issues were addressed in family therapy and some progress was made.

This case illustrates how card playing within a therapeutic environment can help children gain a sense of competence and mastery with task-focused activities. The parallels between card playing and academic tasks facilitate generalization of attitudes about learning, feelings about the self, and actual cognitive skills from the play situation to the classroom.

SUMMARY AND CONCLUSIONS

It is only recently that children who do not learn, despite adequate educational opportunities and intellectual capacity, have been identified and labeled as a distinct clinical entity. Our knowledge about and understanding of learning disabilities have greatly increased over the last 20 years. The current thinking is that a large group of children with learning difficulties have neurological deficits which interfere with normal cognitive processes. At least four general areas of cognitive development are important to acquiring achievement skills: linguistic-conceptual skills, visuospatial-constructive skills, sequential-analytic skills, and motor planning and execution.

It has been empirically demonstrated that many learning-disabled children also suffer from emotional, interpersonal, and behavioral problems. Although these problems may develop simultaneously with the learning disorders, they are more easily explained as responses to extended failure in the classroom. The loss of social status and negative feedback from the environment exacerbate the adjustment problems of learning-disabled children. Many of these children begin school as highly motivated students only to lose interest in—as well as develop aversive associations to—academic material after several years of classroom failure. When emotional difficulties appear to dominate the clinical picture, they are often mistakenly viewed as the cause, rather than the result, of academic failure.

Treatment of learning disabilities is limited by the fact that neurological impairment is, with our present state of knowledge, for the most part permanent and incurable. Treatment has instead been directed toward the cognitive, behavioral, and emotional manifestations of the neurological deficits. Cognitive training has generally been the domain of educators, while behavioral psychologists have developed programs to modify specific learning-related behaviors, such as attention span. Treatment of the emotional problems of learning-disabled children has been left to mental health personnel, and has tended to focus on relieving emotional distress and enhancing children's self-esteem. Traditional forms of therapy with these children, including play therapy, typically do not directly address their specific cognitive and behavioral problems.

In this chapter a specific therapeutic medium—card games—for use with learning disabled children is presented. Card playing appears to have considerable potential for helping these children deal with their specific learning-related emotional and motivational concerns. Card games present children with "mini-learning" situations in which they can experience success, experiment with new roles and behaviors, and develop a sense of mastery and competence. Card games tap a wide range of neuropsychological processes and cognitive abilities which are also important to academic learning. Playing card games requires persistence, attention-to-task, impulse control, and concentration, all of which are crucial to classroom learning. Children are likely to actively engage in card play because it is intrinsically enjoyable and carries none of the pressure or evaluative qualities of school tasks. Children will be more willing to risk failure and attempt to learn something new in therapy because of the sense of trust and safety that is provided by the therapeutic relationship. Generalization of new learning to the classroom situation is facilitated by the similarity between card playing and other task-focused activities.

Card playing does not constitute a self-contained therapeutic program. Rather, it is a specific intervention to be used within the broader context of psychological therapy and educational remediation. The value of card play is its potential to simultaneously address children's problems across the areas of academic, emotional, and behavioral functioning.

REFERENCES

Adams, P.L. (1975). Children and para-services of the Community Mental Health Centers. *Journal of the American Academy of Child Psychiatry, 14*, 18–31.

Axline, V. (1947). *Play therapy*. Boston: Houghton Mifflin.

Barkley, R.A. (1981). Learning disabilities. In E.J. Mash and L.G. Terdal (Eds.), *Behavioral assessment of childhood disorders*. New York: Guilford.

Benton, A. and Pearl, D. (Eds.). (1978). *Dyslexia: An appraisal of current knowledge*. New York: Oxford University Press.

Black, F.W. (1974). Self-concept as related to achievement and age in learning-disabled children. *Child Development, 45*, 1137–1140.

Boder, E. (1973). Developmental dyslexia: A diagnostic approach based on three atypical reading-spelling patterns. *Developmental Medicine and Child Neurology, 15*, 683–687.

Brown, B.S. (1978). Foreword. In A. Benton and D. Pearl (Eds.), *Dyslexia: An appraisal of current knowledge*. New York: Oxford University Press.

Bryan, T. and Pearl, R. (1979). Self-concepts and locus of control of learning disabled children. *Journal of Clinical Child Psychology, 3*, 223–226.

Connolly, C. (1969). The psychosocial adjustment of children with dyslexia. *Exceptional Children, 46*, 126–127.

Cunningham, C.E. and Barkley, R.A. (1978). The role of academic failure in hyperactive behavior. *Journal of Learning Disabilities, 11*, 15–21.

Denckla, M.B. (1979). Childhood learning disabilities. In K.M. Heilman and E. Valenstein (Eds.), *Clinical neuropsychology*. New York: Oxford University Press.

Douglas, V.I. and Peters, K.G. (1979). Toward a clearer definition of the attentional deficit of hyperactive children. In G.A. Hale and M. Lewis (Eds.), *Attention and the development of cognitive skills*. New York: Plenum.

DSM-III. (1980). R. Spitzer, and J. Williams (Eds.), *Diagnostic and statistical manual of mental disorders*. Washington, D.C.: American Psychiatric Association.

Gardner, R.A. (1973). *The talking, feeling, and doing game*. Cresskill, NJ: Creative Therapeutics.

Ginott, H. (1961). *Group psychotherapy with children*. New York: McGraw-Hill.

Goldberg, T. (1980). Battling tops: A modality in child psychotherapy. *Journal of Clinical Child Psychology, 9*, 206–209.

Golick, M. (1973). *Deal me in! The use of playing cards in learning and teaching*. New York: Norton.

Guerney, L.F. (1983). Play therapy with learning disabled children. In C.E. Schaefer & K.J. O'Connor (Eds.), *Handbook of play therapy*. New York: Wiley.

Klinsbourne, M. and Kaplan, P.J. (1979). *Children's learning and attention problems*. Boston: Little, Brown.

Meeks, J. (1970). Children who cheat at games. *Journal of Child Psychiatry, 9*, 157–174.

Millichap, J.G. (Ed.). (1977). *Learning disabilities and related disorders*. Chicago: Year Book Medical Publishers.

Nickerson, E.T. and O'Laughlin, K.S. (1983). The therapeutic use of games. In C.E. Schaefer and K.J. O'Connor (Eds.), *Handbook of play therapy*. New York: Wiley.

Orton, S.T. (1937). *Reading, writing and speech problems in children*. New York: Norton.

Ozols, E.J. and Rourke, B.P. (1985). Dimensions of social sensitivity in two types of learning-disabled children. In B.P. Rourke (Ed.), *Neuropsychology of learning disabilities: Essentials of subtype analysis*. New York: Guilford.

Peter, B.M. and Spreen, O. (1979). Behavior rating and personal adjustment scales of neurologically and learning handicapped children during adolescence and early adulthood: Results of a follow-up study. *Journal of Clinical Neuropsychology, 1*, 75–92.

Piaget, J. (1962). *Play, dreams, and imitation in childhood*. New York: Norton.

Porter, J.E. (1980). Identification of subtypes of learning-disabled children: A multivariate analysis of patterns of personality functioning. *Dissertation Abstracts International, 41*, 1125B.

Porter, J.E. and Rourke, B.P. (1985). Socioemotional functioning of learning-disabled children: A subtypal analysis of personality patterns. In B.P. Rourke, (Ed.), *Neuropsychology of learning disabilities: Essentials of subtype analysis*. New York: Guilford.

Ribner, S. (1978). The effects of special class placement on the self-concept of exceptional children. *Journal of Learning Disabilities, 11*, 319–323.

Ross, A.O. (1976). *Psychological aspects of learning disabilities and reading disorders*. New York: McGraw-Hill.

Rourke, B.P. (1976). Issues in the neuropsychological assessment of children with learning disabilities. *Canadian Psychological Review, 17*, 89–102.

Rourke, B.P. (1978). Reading, spelling, and arithmetic disabilities: A neuropsychological perspective. In H.R. Myklebust (Ed.), *Progress in learning disabilities* (Vol. 4). New York: Grune and Stratton.

Rourke, B.P. (1985a). Overview of learning disabilities subtypes. In B.P. Rourke (Ed.), *Neuropsychology of learning disabilities: Essentials of subtype analysis*. New York: Guilford.

Rourke, B.P. (Ed.). (1985b). *Neuropsychology of learning disabilities: Essentials of subtype analysis*. New York: Guilford.

Rutter, M. (1978). Prevalence and types of dyslexia. In A. Benton and D. Pearl (Eds.), *Dyslexia: An appraisal of current knowledge*. New York: Oxford University Press.

Silverman, R.G. (1978). An investigation of self concept in urban, suburban, and rural students with learning disabilities. *Dissertation Abstracts International, 38*, 5398A. (University Microfilms No. 78-01, 877)

Strauss, A. and Lehtinen, L.S. (1947). *Psychopathology and education of the brain-injured child*. New York: Grune and Stratton.

Zimmerman, I.L. and Allebrand, G.N. (1965). Personality characteristics and attitudes toward achievement of good and poor readers. *Journal of Educational Research, 57*, 28–30.

FOUR

Socialization Games

The final section of this book contains three chapters that describe the use of games for modifying the social behavior of children and adolescents. Socialization games take advantage of the inherent social-interactive nature of games, as well as the developmental readiness of older children and adolescents to engage in social play. As would be expected, socialization games are usually played in a group therapy setting. The chapters cover a wide range of uses of games, illustrating their flexibility for therapeutic applications. Socialization games can be used as a part of a highly structured, behavioral-based program to shape and reinforce the practice of a variety of social behaviors, from simple ones, such as eye contact and attention, to more complex ones, such as group cooperation, sharing, and empathic responding.

Since games provide important socialization experiences in normal human development, and also are analogous to many real life social situations, they have great potential for providing therapeutic or corrective socialization experiences. Shraga Serok's chapter explores the therapeutic possibilities of games with juvenile delinquents—those young people who exhibit chronic destructive and antisocial behavior patterns. What is suggested in Serok's chapter is that by "simply" playing familiar childhood games with a therapist who provides guidance and limit-setting, conduct-disordered children can relearn and practice socialized behavior, attitudes, and values. The implications of this concept are obvious, and further suggest that we have only begun to tap the therapeutic possibilities of game playing.

CHAPTER 15

Therapeutic Games in Group Therapy with Adolescents

BILLIE F. CORDER

Many researchers in the field of adolescent group psychotherapy describe the critical differences between adult and adolescent groups as consisting of the adolescents' intense focus on peer interaction, along with their greater difficulty with impulse control, lower tolerance for anxiety or ego-dystonic feelings, and intermittent periods of regressive behavior (Kraft, 1961; Masterson, 1958; Sugar, 1975). In a previous paper comparing therapists' functioning in adult and adolescent groups, experienced therapists described themselves as more verbally active, employing more structured techniques, and as making fewer analytically oriented interpretations in adolescent groups (Corder, Haizlip, and Walker, 1980). Modifications of traditional approaches to adolescent group psychotherapy fostered by these critical differences include the use of informal discussion aids and materials to structure groups (MacLennan and Felsenfeld, 1968), modified encounter techniques (Rachman, 1971), therapeutic activities, such as an "insults game" for discharge of aggressive drives in adolescent boys' groups (Dyck, 1969), and video taped feedback of group behavior in alternate group sessions (Corder, Whiteside, McNeill, Brown, and Corder, 1981).

The majority of the modifications described in the current literature provides additional structure within adolescent groups, such as using video tapes to model social skills (Savin, 1976), or specific training in areas, such as decision-making processes (Larsen and Mitchell, 1980), and may include specific pretherapy training in group participation (Corder, Haizlip, Whiteside, and Vogel, 1980). These modifications of traditional treatment techniques tend to share a common focus: the facilitation of movement from activity to verbally oriented behavior and an emphasis on building skills related to the developmental tasks of adolescence. This chapter describes a structured therapeutic game which attempts to facilitate this movement and skill development, as well as providing group interactions characterized by related research as "curative factors" in adolescent group psychotherapy (Corder, Whiteside, and Haizlip, 1981). A brief review of some similar therapeutic games follows the discussion of applied uses of the game.

BACKGROUND FOR DEVELOPMENT OF GAME MATERIALS

Schaefer, Johnson, and Wherry (1982) summarize typical difficulties in adolescent therapy groups reported by a number of authors as involuntary attendance by members and lack of self-motivation in groups (Godenne, 1965), high resistance to experiencing threatening emotions, and difficulty in handling high group anxiety levels (Rosenthal, 1971). Adding to these general problem areas for therapists, Naylor and Corder (1976) have described patients referred to adolescent groups in many state residential treatment facilities as typically demonstrating low verbal expressive and social interaction skills, limited experience with any therapeutic interventions, and histories of some impulsive, acting out or antisocial behavior. Materials for the therapeutic game were developed with similar patient groups in a variety of treatment settings, and were also based on research in techniques for optimizing opportunities for development of "curative factors" in adolescent groups. Another report (Corder, Whiteside, & Haizlip, 1981) summarizes results of research in which Yalom's (1975) descriptions of curative factors in adult groups were sorted by adolescent group members into rankings of "most helpful" to "least helpful." Descriptions of curative factors judged as "most helpful" by adolescent group members from therapy groups in a wide range of treatment settings were: (1) being able to say what was bothering me instead of holding it in, (2) learning how to express my feelings, (3) learning that I must take ultimate responsibility for the way I live my life, no matter how much guidance and support I get from others, (4) other members honestly telling me what they think of me, (5) being in the group was, in a sense, like being in a big family, only this time, a more accepting and understanding family, (6) belonging to a group of people who understood and accepted me, (7) the group's giving me an opportunity to learn to approach others,

(8) seeing I was just as well off as others, and (9) helping others and being important in their lives.

These descriptions correspond to Yalom's categories of catharsis, existential factors, interpersonal learning (input), family reenactment, group cohesiveness, interpersonal learning (output), universality, and altruism (Yalom, 1975).

The stimulus items for the game (individual questions for sharing with the group, suggested group verbal exercises, role playing, etc.) were developed from an original pool of items based on tasks perceived as highly related to these curative factors, and from modifications of concepts suggested by items from a number of other group facilitation activities (Jongeward and James, 1973; Simon, Howe, and Kirchenbrum, 1972; Frye and Rockness, 1974; and Gardner, 1973). Game items were focused on the general developmental tasks of adolescence, and were varied in the degree of intimacy and self-disclosure required.

Three judges (two psychologists and one social worker) first separated the initial item pool into three separate categories labeled as follows: "knowing youself"—items aimed at practicing and encouraging verbalization of feelings and feeling states; "understanding each other"—items designed for practice in group interaction and discussion along with developing understanding of basic communication skills; and "problem solving"—items requiring role playing and discussion of problems related to specific developmental tasks of adolescence.

Then each of the items in these categories were ranked by judges into five graduated levels of "difficulty" which were operationally defined as the perceived level of intimacy, self-disclosure, or group cohesion required for responding to the item. These difficulty items were labeled A through E for each of the three categories as shown:

Level A   Items requiring fairly neutral, nonthreatening statements about self, representing "warm-up" activities for the group to encourage verbalization and ensure participation.

Level B   Fairly general statements about one's goals and ideas are required, and some problems with mildly difficult social problems are introduced.

Level C   These items require both positive self-disclosure and positive feedback to others in the group, along with the introduction of items containing progressively more difficult and ambiguous social problem situations for group discussion.

Level D   Items at this level require some self-disclosure of negative perceptions of self and negative feedback to others, requiring that the group members demonstrate group trust and a higher level of group cohesion.

Level E   Highest level of group cohesion and trust required for dealing with intimate self-disclosure and discussion of difficult moral and social issues and problems.

Examples of items for each of the three categories and levels of items are shown.

Understanding Each Other

Level A, Item 4	Pick two people in the group and tell them something about themselves that you would like to copy.
Level B, Item 4	Tell what kinds of clothes you usually wear—describe your usual outfit. What do you want those clothes to say about you? To boys? To girls? Ask a group member of the opposite sex to answer this same question.
Level C, Item 2	If you have a bad reputation and decide to change, how can you get across to other people that you are different now. Have the person on your right answer this also.
Level D, Item 6	Who in this group seems maddest most of the time? Ask a person of the opposite sex if they agree with your choice. Do you think this group can help this person with their feelings? How?
Level E, Item 2	Do you know anyone who committed or attempted suicide? Why do you think people do this? What do you think about them? Ask the person on your right the same question.

Problem Solving

Level A, Item 2	Should you tell other people outside the group that you come to group therapy? Ask each member of the group what they plan to do about this.
Level B, Item 4	How do you think teenagers should be punished by their parents? What do you think is a fair punish-

ment? Tell about a fair and unfair punishment you have had from your parents. Have each person in the group do the same thing.

Level C, Item 1	Act out: With the person on your left, act out a scene in which you try to persuade them to do something which would probably get them in trouble (stealing, skipping school, etc.). Then let the person decide what they would do in real life and act it out. Each of you should then tell how you felt. Have the group talk about how each of you might have handled this situation differently, to keep out of trouble.
Level D, Item 4	Have you ever been afraid you were on your way to being hooked on alcohol or drugs? How can a person know when this is happening? Discuss this with the group.
Level E, Item 8	What is a boy's responsibility if his girlfriend gets pregnant? Have the whole group discuss this question.

Knowing Yourself

Level A, Item 6	If your house were on fire (and all the people and pets were out) and you could only carry two things out with you for yourself, what would you carry out and why?
Level B, Item 1	What are some of the "nicknames" you have had? What did you feel about them? Pick another person and have them answer this question also.
Level C, Item 8	What is the most recent criticism that you gave someone else? Is it hard for you to criticize someone? When and how do you usually do it?
Level D, Item 10	Tell about a time when you felt really lonely. What did you do about it? How do you usually handle your lonely feelings? Have a person on your right (of the opposite sex) answer the same question.
Level E, Item 5	Have you ever deliberately tried to hurt yourself? What was going on and what did you finally do? Ask the person on your right the same question.

In addition, a group of items were developed for optional inclusion in the game which contained questions and suggestions for group discussion regarding progressively more complex transactional analysis concepts. These items were added to the game at the discretion of the group therapists.

GAME DESCRIPTION AND PROCEDURES

The therapeutic game includes a brightly colored game board labeled with equally spaced numbers of squares along the sides, which are labeled with the three item categories (knowing yourself, understanding each other, and problem solving). The item cards for the squares are placed in a labeled area in the middle of the gameboard, along with a space for transactional analysis cards, if they are used. Each player is given a game piece (usually a checker or poker chip with a gummed label for each name) which they move along the board for the number of places indicated by a dice roll, and then draw an item card from the stack corresponding with the square on which they land. The auxiliary "learning cards" with transactional analysis concepts may be read by the therapist or group members in sequence, after each member has had a turn at rolling the dice. After an item is completed by the group, it is placed at the bottom of the pile of items and the game may continue until all items have been completed.

It should be emphasized that the purpose of the game is to provide structure for ensuring opportunities for development of group interaction and other curative factors in the group process, and time spent on each item should be extensive. At times, the group may focus on one item for an entire session, since the items often require extensive responses from each member of the group. Therapists generally join the game as a player, providing opportunities for modeling appropriate verbal and communication skills.

DISCUSSION OF GAME APPLICATIONS

The game was initially used in a variety of outpatient mental health centers and residential treatment settings for adolescents, along with several special education classroom settings. Since publication of the materials

(Corder, Whiteside, and Vogel, 1977), they have been utilized in most states in specialized group homes, public classrooms for emotionally handicapped youth, juvenile detention centers, residential treatment centers within correctional systems, and a wide variety of public and private psychiatric treatment settings. Feedback from questionnaires and other communications with the author have indicated that therapists tend to use the game in a variety of creative ways. Some therapists reported use of the game as a therapy "training tool," concentrating on the materials to structure the first six or eight sessions, and gradually abandoning the materials as group cohesion and verbal interaction levels increase. Others scheduled one half of the group session for continuing use of the structured materials and used the other half of the sessions for unstructured interactions among group members. The author and coworkers developed a structured format for collaboration in cotherapy sessions to review group process, which requires a formal count of the number of "curative factors" operating within each group session. Especially in earlier stages of group process within the first two to three months of weekly sessions, the materials invariably resulted in higher counts of perceived curative factors (catharsis, interpersonal feedback, etc.) operating within the group.

Therapists in both long- and short-term psychotherapy groups report positive experiences with the materials, and most describe them as a valuable tool for groups where members show a wide range of intellectual, social, and verbal skills. Some therapists reported that they were able to successfully include more acting out, aggressive adolescents in groups when using the materials to structure group process.

At times, therapists reported that they found it useful to "stack the deck" of item cards prior to sessions to ensure dealing with a specific issue which was highly relevant to current group issues. Others indicated they might begin by using the higher levels of intimacy game card items for groups which were already formed, such as those in a group home setting. Use of transactional analysis cards varied according to therapists' orientation, but inclusion or deletion of these cards did not appear to affect group results in a significant manner. Therapists familiar with transactional analysis concepts did report finding the vocabulary "prompts" and information contained in the cards useful in dealing with other game materials.

Adolescent group members who were interviewed found the materials interesting and engaging. Some of the less verbal adolescents reported that they, "liked knowing I would have something to talk about," since they found it difficult to initiate spontaneous statements in early group sessions. Some described an advantage of the materials as, "This way there can't be times when the group is over, when somebody didn't get a chance to talk at all." In addition to helping therapists ensure participation by withdrawn or passive members, the structure of the game appeared to offer a useful tool for helping the group deal initially with members who monopolize sessions.

Several therapists reported using the materials in individual therapy sessions with very passive or nonverbal adolescents, and perceived the materials as a helpful tool for encouraging verbalization in early individual therapy sessions.

OTHER GAMES AND MATERIALS

The author has used some portions of Gardner's (1973) *The Talking, Feeling, and Doing Game* with some very socially immature or intellectually limited adolescents. While the item cards in the game are aimed at younger children, many cards with open-ended questions can be used with lower functioning adolescent and preadolescent groups to facilitate interaction and to model verbal communication skills. In this game, players roll dice, move about a colorful game board, and respond to a variety of tasks and questions described on cards corresponding to the squares on which they land.

A widely available game, *The Ungame* (Zakich, 1975) has been used by the author with some positive results to facilitate group interaction in early stages of adolescent groups. Difficulties with these materials appeared to be a lack of focus on specific tasks of adolescent development as well as variability in levels of intimacy and self-disclosure required by task items within the various game "sets."

Quinsey and Varney (1977) have developed a social skills game for adolescents which combines didactic social skills training with role playing and feedback from peers. Players roll dice, move about a game board, and accumulate points through tasks indicated on game board squares. An additional feature of this game is a group decision process involving group judgment of player performance for accumulations of points and "fines."

A somewhat similar approach was used by the author and co-workers in an *Etiquette Olympics* game which may be incorporated in group therapy sessions or more didactically oriented social skills training programs (Corder, Whiteside, and Wall, 1981). After structured "training" with role modeling and didactic materials, each group member role plays a specific social task (making introductions, admitting a mistake, making an apology, etc.). Then in the manner of an olympics sports competition, large cards showing "points" or ratings for task performance are held up by group members functioning as judges. In addition, members are assigned "homework" for practice of these social skills which must be completed between group sessions, and for which they may accumulate "points" in facilities functioning on a token reward system.

The features which seem appealing to group therapists in all the materials described, appear to be the intrinsic appeal of the game materials to resistive, nonverbal adolescents who have difficulty tolerating anxiety levels generated by more traditional less structured sessions, and the effectiveness with which the games facilitate development of communication and interaction skills. Use of these materials appears to allow therapists to successfully deal with a difficult "group mix" of adolescents who show a wide range of intellectual and social functioning, and to include larger numbers of aggressive, acting out members in a group. It should be emphasized that most therapists perceive game materials as an adjunct tool for development of effective group process, and as most useful in earlier stages of group development.

REFERENCES

Corder, B.F., Haizlip, T., and Walker, P. (1980). Critical areas of therapists' functioning in adolescent group psychotherapy: A comparison with self perception of functioning in adult groups by experienced and inexperienced therapists. *Adolescence, 15,* 435–442.

Corder, B.F., Haizlip, T., Whiteside, R., and Vogel, M. (1980). Pre-therapy training for adolescents in group psychotherapy: Contracts, guidelines and pre-therapy preparation. *Adolescence, 59,* 699–705.

Corder, B.F., Whiteside, L., and Haizlip, T. (1981). A study of curative factors in group psychotherapy with adolescents. *International Journal of Group Psychotherapy, 3,* 345–354.

Corder, B.F., Whiteside, R., McNeill, M., Brown, T., and Corder, R. (1981). An experimental study of the effect of structured videotape feedback on adolescent group therapy process. *Journal of Youth and Adolescence, 4*, 225–263.

Corder, B.F., Whiteside, R., and Vogel, M. (1977). A therapeutic game for structuring and facilitating group psychotherapy with adolescents. *Adolescence, 46*, 261–268.

Corder, B.F., Whiteside, R., and Wall, S. (1981). *A structured social skills learning program for adolescents.* Chapel Hill: University of North Carolina Press.

Dyck, G. (1969). Talking the dozens: A game of insults played in a group of adolescent boys. *Bulletin of the Menninger Clinic, 33*, 108–116.

Frye, R. and Rockness, P. (1974). *Life skills for health.* Raleigh: North Carolina Department of Public Instruction.

Gardner, R. (1973). *The talking, feeling, and doing game.* Cresskill, NJ. Creative Therapeutics.

Godenne, G. (1965). Outpatient adolescent group psychotherapy. *American Journal of Psychotherapy, 19*, 40–53.

Jongeward, D. and James, M. (1973). *Winning with people.* Reading, MA: Addison-Wesley.

Kraft, I. (1961). Some special considerations in adolescent group psychotherapy. *International Journal of Group Psychotherapy, 11*, 196–203.

Larson, J. and Mitchell, C. (1980). Task-centered, strength-oriented group work with delinquents. *Social Casework, 61*, 154–163.

MacLennon, B. and Felsenfeld, M. (1968). *Group counseling and psychotherapy with adolescents.* New York: Columbia University Press.

Masterson, J.F. (1958). Psychotherapy of adolescents contrasted with psychotherapy of adults. *Journal of Nervous and Mental Diseases, 27*, 511–517.

Naylor, K. and Corder, B.F. (1976). Evaluation of adolescent treatment needs and assessment of service deficiencies in treatment and follow-up of hospitalized adolescents. *North Carolina Journal of Mental Health, 4*, 51–61.

Quinsey, V. and Varney, G.W. (1977). Social skills game: A general method for the modeling and practice of adaptive behaviors. *Behavior Therapy, 8*, 279–281.

Rachman, A. (1971). Encounter techniques in analytic group psychotherapy. *International Journal of Group Psychotherapy, 21*, 319–329.

Rosenthal, L. (1971). Some dynamics of resistance and therapeutic management in adolescent group therapy. *Psychoanalytic Review, 58*, 353–366.

Savin, H.A. (1976). Multi-media group treatment with socially inept adolescents. *Clinical Psychologist, 29*, 30–39.

Schaefer, C., Johnson, L., and Wherry, J. (Eds.). (1982). *Group therapies for children and youth.* San Francisco: Jossey-Bass.

Simon, S., Howe, L., and Kirchenbrum, H. (1972). *Values clarification.* New York: Hart.

Sugar, M. (Ed.). (1975). *The adolescent in group and family therapy.* New York: Brunner Mazel.

Yalom, I. (1975). *The theory and practice of group psychotherapy* (2nd ed.). New York: Basic Books.

Zakich, R. (1975). *The ungame.* Anaheim: The Ungame Company.

CHAPTER 16

Socialization Games for the Mentally Retarded

BARBARA EDMONSON and NEVALYN NEVIL

We first describe the situation that led to the need for a habilitative program for a "worst ward" in an institution for the mentally retarded. Then, as the context for the 70 socialization games we devised, we will sketch the scope of the overall program; describe the games and the rationale; explain how they were employed, and give the outcome of the program. The use of games in group homes, special eduation classes, sheltered workshops, and by parents is then discussed. We conclude with a brief discussion of some of the requirements of social development and a summary.

HISTORY AND INTRODUCTION

It was widely believed during most of the last 100 years that mental retardation resulted from bad living and progressively degenerate heredity. To protect society and to provide shelter for these "unfortunates," strenuous efforts were made to remove the mentally retarded and persons with epilepsy from society. Large numbers were placed in state institutions, typically located at some distance from urban activity. The trend toward institutionalization included young children. Until the 1960s, and in some cases, even later, physicians often urged a family to place a newborn anomalous infant in a private "home" for such babies and to forget about "it." In such settings and in most state institutions, even in those where the children may have received some affection with their nourishment and hygiene, play was not a part of the day. Caretakers and institutional

291

aides were not hired for skill or interest in developmental interaction with children, and few of them would try to encourage communication, let alone tactile or spatial exploration or social interactions. Most "residents" would expend their lives in a simple daily routine of assisted self-care, meals, occasional sessions of recreation and, if physically mobile, performing various chores. For some, there were educational programs, but it was assumed that many were uneducable. As it was expected that few would leave the institutions, education was not provided to all, and teachers were rarely state-certified or supervised. In such settings, the "good" children grew up to be plasticly acquiescent to the schedule. Residents not employed at institutional work would spend much of their time merely sitting in their wards or walking on the grounds. One would often see adult men or women sitting side-by-side with no intercommunication.

In the custodial setting, some of the children who did not grow up "good" became, behaviorally, very bad indeed. The most difficult of them would not be permitted to leave their locked wards unescorted. Because they were aggressive and hard to deal with, teachers would exclude them from classrooms, and they could be restricted to their ward for meals. The ward would be barren because they were destructive. Many were aggressive toward one another, or toward themselves; and, if they felt they could get away with it, toward aides. Thus would develop a battle-scarred "back ward" where visitors were not encouraged. Such a setting is self-perpetuating. With the barrenness, the uproars and screams, and need for physical intervention, it is a noxious place in which to be employed, and aides who are stuck with it would understandably spend as much time as they could in their ward office, as far from the residents as they could get. If they were on the ward, it would be more rewarding to chat with one another or watch television than to interact with residents. With the minimal training they were provided, which emphasized record keeping, they would respond to a serious incident with threats, restraints, or whatever punishment they felt they could get away with. Punishment has been, of course, taboo for at least 10 years, but the alternatives were not often provided. At the time of our involvement in a "worst ward," punishment was regularly occurring, more or less covertly. The residents, with no other opportunities to be rewarded for competence, became asocially competent at creating damage and producing hurts and screams. Some garnered attention by weird and unpleasant behavior of various kinds—smearing feces, having tantrums, making strange movements, or unpleasant sounds. Some gained attention by eating or drinking nonedible or even toxic substances. A few in such settings, became expert at invisibility, squatting in a corner or covering themselves in bed. The most socially competent were probably those who tried to escape.

The current shift in thinking—from getting the mentally retarded away from the community to placing them back into the community, into least restrictive, most normal situations—began in the late 1960s and 1970s (Nirje 1970; Wolfensberger, 1972). In 1975, Public Law 94-142, "the education for all children act," mandated education to all children aged 3 to 18 (later 3 to 21), including residents of institutions.

In many institutions as late as the 1970s, however, there was a locked, battle-scarred ward. When it no longer became permissible to maintain residents in restraints or in a locked room for long periods of time, the institutional staff would typically feel unable to cope with the behavior, and would term such residents "emotionally disturbed" in an attempt to have them moved to a psychiatric facility. The occasional transfers would be termporary as psychiatric facilities rarely felt that their programs were appropriate for the mentally retarded. Ohio was one of the states where, finally, a suit was brought against the State Department of Mental Health and Mental Retardation by the Association for Retarded Citizens to force some treatment for "emotionally disturbed retarded persons." In its consent decree, the State agreed to establish a special program for a small number of residents in each of several institutions. The funding that was appropriated for the special programs allowed for the recruitment and training of staff, special furnishings, and modifications to the physical space, and, where the proposals requested it, funds for token economies and other special programs. The selection of eight to ten residents for these special programs, unfortunately, left others with seriously maladaptive behavior just as they were.

We proposed in 1979 to 1980 the development of a program for the worst ward residents who were not selected as the official "dual diagnosis" group. The senior author half-time with three part-time graduate student assistants would work with the institutional staff to devise a program that the staff could continue at the end of our involvement.

The initial group were 16 women (ultimately 20) aged 18 to 32, averaging 13.2 years of institutional residence. All were ambulatory, but most were poorly coordinated, and overweight. They ranged from severely to mildly retarded, but most were in the moderate range. There was little academic skill. One could print a few words, interspersed with nonsense clusters; several could read a few words and use numerals appropriately. Several could copy and match letters or numbers. One had been taught to make potholders. Several were heavily medicated at the beginning, and one or two talked to themselves, at times appearing to hallucinate. There were biters, kickers, pinchers, hitters, destroyers of furniture and clothing, whiners, criers, and screamers. One sat immobile on the ward and responded to questions with whispers. Another spent her time covered up in bed when she was not being aggressive.

The first task was to get aides to notice and respond to some of the positive things—the self care and routine chores—that the residents were capable of accomplishing. This was initially approached by use of a pictorial behavioral chart on each resident's locker. The behaviors were 10 simple daily activities of getting up, showering, brushing teeth, dressing, combing hair, making beds, and so on. An aide would go with each resident in turn to the chart to mark an OK or a smiling face, and offer praise for what had been accomplished. Once a week one of us, or the cottage administrator or supervisor, would call residents and aides together in groups to review the charts. Some techniques and suggestions for "holding" and working with such groups are illustrated and discussed in Moxley, Nevil, and Edmonson (1980). The review group leader would solicit positive comments about each person's achievements. When a chart showed the attainment of certain (initially very low) criteria, there was much praise, and the resident would be offered a choice of privileges that were graphically visible on the wall of the ward. Although a possible choice was something from the goodie box (that was purposely not visible during the meetings), such as a soft drink, trinket, potato chips, cigarette, or what-not, we frankly emphasized the other possibilities—to receive a letter from one of the aides or ourselves, a shampoo or a beauty treatment, special time alone with a member of the staff, a visit to someone's home, or a meal at a fast food place off grounds. Although we did participate in the rewards, all could be handled by the existing staff. As behavior improved, privilege choices were added.

A description of the full program as it evolved over a two year period is reported in Edmonson, Nevil, and Moxley (1982). It included our efforts to involve aides in planning, to make positive comments on their contributions, occasionally to model a way of dealing with a difficult resident, to improve communication between the aides and the administration, and to arrange for sessions of in-service training. For the residents, we also worked to improve communication; at times helping them to formulate the words they lacked in order to make a complaint or a request; at times accompanying them as an advocate for a problem or a need. Our objectives, of course, were to demonstrate and shape "other ways" of getting attention and being competent.

After the first year, the program was facilitated by a move to a physically better ward, and by an exchange of several old-timer aides for new ones whose interaction with the residents was usually positive.

To develop the residents' pride and responsibility, in addition to their discrimination of socially approved behavior, we inaugurated a system of merit badges. A resident who met certain criteria — good grooming, good housekeeping, being friendly, being responsible — based on her behavior chart — would receive a special T-shirt with an iron-on pictorial badge. As additional criteria were met, badges would be ceremoniously presented. Although this system was not problem free, the merit badges had the effect of generating attention and positive comments from people when residents wore them on outings, and they were a tangible reminder to the residents of their social competence.

The program resulted in a vastly improved ambience on the ward. There were fewer incidents of aggression, virtually no physical destruction, some communication, opportunities for schooling for the several residents under 21, vocational training for several others, and improved staff morale. By mid-year of the program's second year, all of the residents had earned grounds privileges based on good marks on their behavior charts.

It was apparent, however, that the absence of hostile behavior was not the equivalent of *friendly* behavior. The years of aversive interaction had made almost every resident a negative stimulus for every other. They still competed for attention, avoided proximity, and rarely interacted with one another in a spontaneously friendly way. Their experiences had perpetuated egocentricity and poor self-awareness — they could characterize one another in terms of disagreeable behavior or in terms of some possession they might envy, but were uncaring about the likes and dislikes of others, and actually knew very little about themselves.

SOCIALIZATION GAMES

To counter this social isolation and egocentricity we developed socialization games (Moxley, Nevil, and Edmonson, 1981). The technique had to be simple enough for use by aides or volunteers after demonstration or simple written instruction. The activities had to be interesting and rewarding to the residents, easy to explain or demonstrate, move at a quick pace, and be of short duration to retain their attention, require little in the way of props, be adaptable for residents at different levels of attentiveness and skill, and be designed for several different socialization goals.

Rationale

Our program was built on White's (1959) contention that competence (effectance) is motivating. Because we wanted to develop a sense of competence and pride in being competent, we used the behavior charts, merit badges, recognition, privileges, and praise. We felt this procedure would make residents more inner-directed and responsible; less dependent on rewards and punishments from others, a goal that it is difficult to attain from a token economy. With the games, we wanted, first, to develop tolerance of closeness; then, awareness of themselves and others—their appearance, behavior, likes, and dislikes; then, peer reciprocity—responsiveness toward one another's interests and needs. Later, we would use the game procedure for other goals, such as simple problem solving.

Rules and Procedures

The rules were explained to the groups: No hitting, biting, pinching, or hostile teasing was permitted during the games. A violator was not punished, but would have to move a little away from the group. A further incident would require the violator to leave the group for a brief time. He or she could return when ready to play.

Group size and make-up would vary with the number of group leaders. When one starts out with behaviorally deviant persons, two leaders are important for a group of any size, in order that one leader can keep the game going while the other deals with a member who tests the limits. Two leaders were also helpful when members were especially handicapped physically or intellectually; although in time, group members helped the less able. With our institutional population with whom we were well acquainted, two of us, or one of us assisted by an aide, could work with from 8 to 10 residents at a time.

Each week two of us would spend an hour conducting one or more games in some relatively quiet part of the cottage. They were used with both male and female groups. At first, we had to shape basic behaviors such as sitting, listening, and taking turns. An effective device was a timer we set to go off at variable intervals. At the signal, pretzel sticks would be given to group members who were sitting quietly. Initially, of course, members clamored to be chosen for an activity. As one device for turn-taking, we used a spinner on a circle of cardboard. The person to whom the arrow pointed had the first turn. That person could then draw blindly from a set of photographs the picture of the next person to have a turn. Sometimes, turns simply followed one another around the seated group. After several sessions, the groups grasped and accepted the rules. Soon, most residents became interested enough to organize themselves, sometimes to ask for certain games, and take turns at leading various games.

Because of the occasional resistance of individuals in our wards, we conceived of two zones of participation. The core group were the members who would sit in a circle and be involved in face-to-face interaction. The second zone, the "outfield," were individuals who would approach, but resist invitations to join and would remain sitting or standing on the fringe to watch. The group leader from time to time would address these individuals to try to get them to respond and to participate in some way. Over a period of time, these would join the groups.

It is difficult to sustain group cohesion when members differ widely in developmental level. To prevent unusually capable persons from being satiated or bored, we would introduce variations on a game and would involve the more able as coaches for the less able.

Some additional procedures, suggestions for managing groups, the process of "warm up" and termination, duration of games, props, and other topics are included in Moxley, et al, (1981).

Closeness

For the first goal, tolerance of closeness, the principle followed was desensitization. Although the residents had been assembled in groups, weekly, to have their charts reviewed and to receive their badges, propinquity was still a stimulus for wariness and sometimes for aggression. To desensitize them to these reactions, we provided an activity in which the participants would function closely together while being relaxed and having a good time. One example, a propinquity game with the title *Blow Round* calls for a table, enough chairs for the participants, a ping-pong ball and a timer. The participants sit as closely as possible around the table while the group leader places the ball on the table and tells the members to try to blow it off the table on the opposite side. If the group can maintain the ball on the table until the timer goes off, everyone is given a pretzel stick. The activity was exciting and rewarding enough to most players to make them forget that the person next to them was known as a biter or a hitter.

Another game that does not require waiting to take turns is *Do This*. In the manner of "Simon Says . . ." members are instructed to "Do what I do when I say 'Do this.'"

Another game that reduces wariness is *Don't Drop the Can*. This requires a few pieces of masking tape, an empty can, and a piece of wood about three feet long and four inches wide. Two members are shown the starting point that is marked on the floor with tape. Each holds an end of the board with the coffee can placed in the center. They must walk together to get the can to the stopping line, also marked with tape, without knocking it off. Other members encourage them as the whole group earns a pretzel stick if each of the pairs succeeds. In a variation, the can may contain a small amount of water, and the spills that result can be wiped up by a pair who volunteer, while the rest of the group cheer them on.

Another propinquity game is called *Trading T-Shirts*. The props are two large pull-over shirts and a timer. In this game, two members at a time face one another in the center of the circle. Each is given a T-shirt and told to put it on his or her partner. If they succeed before the timer rings, everyone in the group receives a pretzel stick. Moxley, et al (1981) describe 16 propinquity games.

Knowing About Yourself

A second group of 11 games was designed to make participants more conscious of what they liked, how they felt about various things, and their activities. One of these games is *Finish the Sentence*. The group leader provides unfinished sentences. The published version of the game

gives 10 examples such as "On my hamburger I like . . . ," "I like pictures of . . . ," "When I need help I can go to . . . ," "When I have free
time I like to . . . ," and so on. The group leader goes around the group
giving members a chance to respond to a question. If a member is nonverbal, other members can be asked to reply, and that reply responded to
by the nonverbal person with an affirmative or negative signal.

A more exciting version of the game is called *Honk If You Know*. We
used a bicycle horn. In this version, the leader asks a question and group
members were told that if they knew the answer, one at a time they could
come up to honk the horn and answer the question. Some examples of
questions: "Who is your favorite friend?" "What color is your favorite
shirt?" In another game in this series, *I Feel Really Good About* . . . " the
group leader asked each member in turn "Do you feel good or bad when
. . . " and described a situation. Some examples are "Your clothes are
torn." "You help your friend go shopping." "Someone teases you." "You
can sleep late." After the member responded the leader would then ask
the group "Who else feels good (or bad) when this happens?"

Knowing About Others

The next games focused attention on other people. The published version
describes 23 games in this series. A very simple one is *Clothing Color
Match*. The props are a set of cards each marked with a different color,
placed in a box. Group members take turns drawing a card and are asked
to walk around the group and try to find someone who is wearing something that is the chosen color.

Somewhat more difficult is *Pick a Friend*. A group member is selected
to sit in the center with hands out, palms up. The group leader places a
snack in each hand and the member is asked to look around the group and
to pick out a person, but not say his or her name. Instead, the member
must give some clues, for example, "I am thinking of someone wearing
blue shoes." The others try to identify the person. When correctly identified, that individual gets one of the snacks, the seated member gets the
other and may be replaced by the person who made the correct identification.

Another game is *The Blindfold Game*. A member seated in the center is
blindfolded. Another member is quietly chosen to sit beside the blindfolded person. The leader guides the blindfolded person in touching the

other person's hair, nose, glasses, wristwatch, clothing, or whatever, while the blindfolded person tries to guess the identify from the tactual clues. Variations may include suggestive questions, or hints, from other members or from the leader—"Do you think this person is a girl or a boy?" "Is the hair curly or straight?" "Do you think he or she is big or small?" And so on.

Prosocial Behavior

A third series of eight games is for sharing or helping behavior. A very simple game, *The Magic Box I* makes use of a photograph of each group member and small wrapped candies or pennies. Before the game, the leader tapes two candies or pennies to the back of each picture and puts them in a box. "The magic box" is passed around for members to draw out a picture, identify the person, and share the prize with that person.

In a higher level game, *Helping My Neighbor II*, the leader provides a hypothetical situation about a member of the group; for example, "Here's (Betty). She is really angry. What can someone do to make her feel better?" A member who volunteers can demonstrate his or her idea.

Social Competence

The fourth series consists of the social competence games. An example is *Being Responsible I*. This requires a 3×5 card for each member on which there is a picture of an adult-appearing individual and the word "responsible." The leader explains the picture and word, and then enacts or describes a situation. Group members must decide whether the behavior is responsible or not. If they think it is responsible, they hold up their picture card. If not, the card remains in their lap.

A variant entitled *Don't Lose Your Cool*, has members evaluating behavior in terms of "He or she was cool," or "He or she lost his or her cool!"

The publication describes 70 games, together with an assessment scheme which shows the degree of verbal, motor, and cognitive ability required for each; states whether individuals or the group are to be rewarded; whether materials or advance preparation are required; whether the game is appropriate for a warm-up period, the major game phase, or the termination phase; and whether group involvement will be high or low. In addition there is an assessment of "psychological risk" as either low or high. This refers to the possibility that in certain games a group member might be exposed to embarrassment or ridicule by disclosing his or her feelings, preferences, or fantasies.

EVALUATIVE RESEARCH

Our report on effectiveness will concern the women, the only group on which we collected data; however, the overall program resulted in a marked decrease in social isolation and an increase in friendly and generally prosocial behavior among both sexes. As previously mentioned, all of the women became able to earn grounds privileges, the freedom to come and go from the ward whenever it did not conflict with their schedule, by meeting behavioral criteria. Over the project's two year duration, 10 women were transferred. Of these, one was released to her mother at the parent's request after a trial period at home. Seven were transferred to other buildings and two to group homes in the community. Three others had had trial visits to group homes, returning to the institution at their request. Five referrals for vocational training had been made to the Bureau of Vocational Rehabilitation. Of these, one who had been a frequent inhabitant of an isolation room was now proud of her grounds privilege and her job in the institution. One who had been excluded from classes because of terrible tantrums, feces smearing, destruction of clothing, and aggression, was doing well in school. Another who had been noncommunicative and withdrawn was attending school, had earned a socialization badge, and was one of four who had earned the badge for responsibility. One, a woman who had sought attention by eating or drinking noxious or toxic substances, had earned the responsibility badge and was to be referred to the sheltered workshop. Another, whose tantrums and destruction of clothing had been routine, had settled down, was proud to have a badge and was working in a workshop without serious incident. A woman who had once been immobilized on the ward by restraints for long periods of time had earned three badges, including responsibility, and had been offered the opportunity to move into a group home. One who had spent most of her life in the institution and feared the idea of leaving, had earned a trial period in a group home, but chose to return to the institution.

Of the original residents in our ward, 10 were still there when our project terminated. Four had earned a responsibility merit badge, and others had earned other badges. Although all had earned grounds privileges, one would frequently lose this privilege. The behavior charts and system of reviewing them was continued under the leadership of several members of the cottage professional staff. Although the badges were discontinued, they remained desirable and meaningful to those who had earned them. During the year after the project termination, eight of the women were transferred into the preplacement unit, a unit for special preparation in living in the community. The cottage was then converted for use with a different population.

The effect of socialization games was examined by Han (Edmonson & Han, 1983). She compared the effect of 12 games with the effect of 12 "placebo" sessions of arts and crafts or stories that were presented in random order to two small groups of the maladaptively behaving women residents over an eight-week period. She looked at the effect of time of day by scheduling half of the sessions in the morning and half in the afternoon before supper. Her procedure consisted of 30 minutes of game or placebo activity, followed by a 10-minute period of behavior observation, and then by a 15 to 20-minute period for refreshments. A videotape recorder system was employed for observations during the 10-minute free time period after the games and placebo sessions, in a room in which the floor was marked off into large squares. The tapes were analyzed by coding the first behavior of each subject during the first three seconds of each 30-second interval as either friendly, unfriendly, or inactive; and also by measuring the distance of each woman from each other woman at intervals of 30 seconds.

Results of analysis of variance showed that the two groups responded similarly, with significantly more friendly behavior after the socialization games than after the alternative activities, and with significantly more friendly behavior in the afternoons than in the mornings. Unfriendly behavior occurred more frequently after the alternative activities than after the games with no difference attributable to time of day. The anlaysis of interpersonal distance data demonstrated that members were closer to one another after the games than after the placebo activities.

Han also devised a peer knowledge questionnaire that she presented to her two experimental groups and to members of a third group who were not exposed to the activity sessions. The mean scores, indicating correct answers to questions about characteristics and preferences of the residents, of 63.6 (SD = 17.5) and 60.3 (SD = 14.1) of the two experimental groups were higher than the 43.1 mean score (SD = 21.9) of the control group, but the difference failed to achieve significance at the .05 level. By chance, one member of the control group was one of the most accurate women, her score causing the large standard deviation for that group. A more extended trial and/or larger groups would have demonstrated significant gains in awareness of others by the women who participated in the games.

USE OF THE GAMES WITH NONINSTITUTIONAL GROUPS

Residents of Group Homes

The trend of trying to maintain mentally retarded persons in a "normal" community environment has led, of course, to group homes, where relatively small groups of individuals have opportunities for social interaction and recreation, and are provided whatever supervision is necessary. Typically, the residents, whether mildly, moderately or severely retarded, go to work each weekday, some to regular jobs, others to sheltered workshops. Most members of group homes are moderately or severely retarded, as the mildly retarded are more apt to reside with their families, or with a friend or a spouse. Group home residents share in the chores of their home. Until recently, many were residents of an institution and the transition from that restricted life to living in the community reveals many deficits in social knowledge and skills.

As a remedial device, the second author has introduced the socialization game procedure into many group homes and has collaborated with the staffs in creating games. One home started off a new group with the *Introduction Game*, in which the house rules were reviewed, and a picture taken of each member. This was followed by a *Self Description* game and rehearsal of one another's names. Members were to look in a mirror and describe themselves—hair color, color of eyes, height, type of clothing, whatever, and give their name. Then they would have an opportunity to describe another member and try to apply the correct name. Additional games for acquaintanceship included *What I Like*. Members referred to their favorite event of the week. Other members, each holding a 3×5 card, would hold up their cards if they shared a liking for this event. In a variation, each member would model or role play an activity he or she liked, and the others would try to identify the activity and indicate how they felt about it. An orientation game for the newly arrived, *Learning About Our House*, helps them with features of the new residence. In this game, new members take turns trying to locate the various necessities—coffee, cups, pans, tableware, washing machine, detergent, mailbox, and so on. In another orientation game, *Learning About the Neighborhood*, participants explain or demonstrate where they can cash a paycheck, buy something, play ball, entertain their date or friends. The involvement of the more experienced together with newcomers can lead to informative and friendly interaction. Other games for group homes have included *Getting to Know Others, How I Can Help, Sharing with Others, How I Help Others Feel,* and *When I Am Angry.* . . . Once the procedure is established by the home staff, many useful variations will spring to mind. Buchan (1972), suggests many situations that can be helpfully clarified through his role playing procedures (for the most able) or through our simpler game procedures for the less able. A discrimination activity perhaps invented by Fudell (1982) calls on group members to identify what they do in the community that is the same as what they did when they lived in an institution, and what is different now in the community. Fudell emphasized the more painful consequences of failures, in the community, to meet the social criteria such as being slovenly, being late to work without notice to the employer, goofing off on the job, poor response to criticism, and so on. Situational examples of a given behavior can be modeled to a group for their evaluation as to whether the behavior is appropriate. A curriculum that Rosen and Hoffman (1975) developed to teach appropriate behavior does something similar. In their program, a group counselor or a member of a counseling group models a behavior that is presumed to fit a situation. The group then discusses and evaluates the behavior in terms of "weird" or "OK." These terms are useful, as they seem to be enjoyed and remembered by persons with whom we have worked. For additional suggestions, see Rosen, Clark, and Kivitz (1977).

A major current concern is exploitation of the retarded. With their need for recognition and affection, they are very vulnerable. Group homes have used games to identify the enticing tactics that people sometimes employ, such as offering them cigarettes, a meal, a drink, a ride, and so on. This is a topic, however, that we would prefer to see addressed through a long-range program in sociosexual education.

Games in School Settings

The second author, under a contract with a local mental health board, introduced the game procedures and techniques of working with groups of retarded persons to a number of special education teachers. Typically, after identifying several desired goals, the teacher would be assisted by someone who was experienced with the game procedures in presenting 10 to 15 weeks of hour-long or 90-minute sessions to the pupils. Teacher aides were phased into the sessions so the process could be continued through the year. Teachers reported that pupils enjoyed the games so much that they were sometimes used as a contingent reward; that is, "After you have finished . . . we will have a game."

A number of parents of the special education children were sufficiently impressed to attend a workshop where they learned to conduct a summer socialization program for their children, using games.

Some topics that are listed in Palomares and Ball (1974, who developed "magic circle" activities for levels from preschool through grade six, are similar to some of our original games, and they describe many others that would be valuable as part of a school curriculum. Among their goals are improved self-concept (through awareness of growing abilities), respect for others, skill in interpersonal relationships, being aware of emotions, taking responsibility for one's behavior. Suggestions can also be drawn from Fischer (1972), whose curriculum is for nonretarded children.

Vocational Settings

A workshop involved all of its prevocational level workers in daily socialization games with a series of goals, such as appropriate and inappropriate clothing, work behavior, clocking in and out, responding to criticism, identifying and correcting errors, improving listening skills, following directions, and so on.

Some workshops have made use of down-time, when work was not available, to present games to further competence in areas, such as human sexuality, nutrition, community safety, and assertiveness training. Buchan (1972) suggests a number of role-play situations for vocational preparedness and independent living that would be appropriate for some moderately and mildly retarded persons.

Games with Sensorily Impaired Persons

Many of the games in Moxley, et al (1981) can be used with persons who are nonverbal or who have impaired hearing, as they rely on visual props and demonstration, and can be responded to by gestures or signals. As an example, persons with impaired hearing can signal or sign "yes" or "no," "right" or "wrong" when playing *What's Wrong with These Clothes?* Games can also be used to teach basic signs to people. In one group, which consisted of six persons with hearing and one who was deaf, each session introduced a basic sign and the chaining of several signs. The group members had opportunities to respond with the appropriate movements, and to request other members to use them. The leader would frequently make an error so the group could demonstrate the correct response. The deaf member seemed especially to enjoy this, and began to interact more with the nonimpaired.

For the visually impaired, many games must be modified in order to provide auditory cues. To do this, information from the leader can be used for guidance; or, other members of the group can be shown how to assist.

Profound Retardation

For use with multiply handicapped and profoundly retarded persons, the goals must be realistically attainable. Leaders must be prepared at times to physically "mold" a desired movement, and to provide edible incentives when attentiveness lags. Appropriate goals are self-awareness, attending, simple object identification, functional communication, and self-care skills, such as dressing and feeding oneself. *Finding the Ball* can facilitate attending. In this game members take turns finding the ball (or a small edible) that the leader has openly (or secretly) placed under one of several boxes. For object identification, members take turns identifying from a tray of objects the particular item that the leader has named or has demonstrated the use of. *Picking Out My Clothes* requires members to select a complete outfit (shirt, pants, underwear, and socks) from a collection of clothing. The further discrimination of clothing for cold weather and clothing for warm weather can be similarly taught. One way of addressing eating skills is to have group members indicate "yes" or "no" to table behavior, such as eating food with hands, grabbing or taking another's food, throwing things on the floor, and so on. All of these sessions, of course, are presented with humor and "hamming it up."

DISCUSSION AND SUMMARY

Many persons with mental retardation, and certainly those who have resided for many years in custodial institutions, have been deprived of the developmental experiences that foster self-awareness, interest in and knowledge about other people, and the responsible self-directed behaviors that are the hallmark of normal development. This is a situation that should not occur. Insofar as possible, from early years retarded children should have play opportunities, such as those provided in "infant stimulation classes," (Infant Stimulation Curriculum (1978)) and quality preschools, from which to develop coordination, locomotion, competence at handling objects, spatial exploration, language, self-awareness, a sense of competence, and numerous social skills. All caretakers and teachers of the retarded should become aware of developmental goals, and should have access to techniques and materials that facilitate development, such as those by Hankerson, Meddaugh, Strausbaugh, and Wood (1975), Pizzi and Paul (1981a; 1981b), Frankenfield (1981), and Horstmeier, MacDonald and Gillette (1975). But these should be supplemented by activities that focus more on self-knowledge and other awareness.

Unfortunately, many mentally retarded persons are very ego-centered, and lack the social skills that would enable them to function well in community settings, while others acquire socially maladaptive behavior. The socialization games that we developed, because of the extreme needs of a behaviorally disturbed institutional population, are useful adjuncts to an educational program, and are equally useful as therapy. We described a number of games that we developed, but the possibilities are infinite. They can be adapted to a group's attention span, and to levels of physical, sensory, and intellectual ability. To be most successful, the games require a leader (sometimes a coleader, also) who can convey a sense of pleasure in the activity, and who enjoys the developmental process. Leaders who work with difficult individuals should be experienced in techniques for dealing with maladaptive behavior.

We briefly described a treatment program we designed for a "worst ward" of young retarded women in a state institution, which was eventually also used with men whose behavior was comparably maladaptive. Although this program used principles of operant conditioning, it differed in some ways from typical programs. It was designed to foster a sense of pleasure and pride in social competence (rather than on earning "goodies"). The most immediate reward for accomplishments was praise. The back-up reward of a choice of privileges was from several days to a week delayed. Merit badges that were awarded for less ephemeral achievement were reminders of worth, and brought intermittent recognition from other people. Our program was successfully carried on by others at the expiration of our project, with the result, after two years, of getting all of the women out of a barren, locked ward, and preparing all of them for the rewards of social activity.

REFERENCES

Buchan, L.G. (1972). *Roleplaying and the educable mentally retarded.* Belmont, CA: Fearon.

Edmonson, B. and Han, S.S. (1983). Effects of socialization games on proximity and prosocial behavior of aggressive mentally retarded institutionalized women. *American Journal of Mental Deficiency, 87* (4), 435–440.

Edmonson, B., Nevil, N., and Moxley, D. (1982). *Promoting prosocial behavior: A residential program for retarded adults.* Columbus: The Nisonger Center Publication Department, Ohio State University.

Fischer, C. (1972). *What about me?: Dimensions of personality.* Dayton, OH: Pflaum/Standard.

Frankenfield, B. (1981). *Teachers: Instructional modules to assist teachers in generalization programming for moderate, severe, and profound mentally retarded students.* Columbus: The Nisonger Center Publication Department, Ohio State University.

Fudell, S.E. (1982). *How to hold your job.* Austin, TX.. Pro-Ed.

Hankerson, H.E., Meddaugh, G., Strausbaugh, L., and Wood, J.M. (Eds.) *Parent involvement: For the sake of all children.* Columbus: The Nisonger Center Publication Department, Ohio State University, 1975.

Horstmeier, D., MacDonald, J.D., and Gillette, Y. (1975). *Ready, set, go—talk to me: Prescriptive training programs for pre-language and early language skills.* Columbus: The Nisonger Center Publication Department, Ohio State University.

Infant stimulation curriculum. (1978). 2nd edition. Columbus: Nisonger Center Publication Department. Ohio State University.

Moxley, D., Nevil, N., and Edmonson, B. (1980). Meeting time: Structured group activities with the mentally retarded. 27 minute videocassette. Columbus: Nisonger Center Publication Department, Ohio State University.

Moxley, D., Nevil, N., and Edmonson, B. (1981). *Socialization games for mentally retarded adolescents and adults.* Springfield, IL: Thomas.

Nirje, B. (1970). The normalizational principle—Implications & comments. *Journal of Mental Subnormality, 16* (31), 62–70.

Palomares, U.H. and Ball, G. (1974). *Human developmental program: "Magic Circle."* La Mesa, CA: Human Development Training Institute.

Pizzi, M. and Paul, L. (1981a). *Parents: A guide for teaching persons with moderate, severe, and profound mental retardation in home and community settings.* Columbus: Nisonger Center Publication Department, Ohio State University.

Pizzi, M. and Paul, L. (1981b). *Working with parents: A guide for helping parents of persons with moderate, severe, and profound mental retardation in home and community settings.* Columbus: Nisonger Center Publications Department, Ohio State University.

Rosen, M., Clark, G.R., and Kivitz, M.S. (1977). *Habilitation of the handicapped: New dimensions in programs for the developmentally disabled.* Baltimore: University Park Press.

Rosen, M. and Hoffman, M. (1975). *Personal adjustment training: A group counseling manual for the mentally handicapped.* Elwyn, PA: Elwyn Institute.

White, R.W. (1959). Motivation reconsidered: The concept of competence. *Psychological Review, 66,* 297–333.

Wolfensberger, W. (1972). *The principle of normalization in human services.* Downsview, Canada: National Institute on Mental Retardation.

CHAPTER   17

Therapeutic Implications of Games with Juvenile Delinquents

SHRAGA SEROK

Games are a natural expression of a child's energy. Game play is a pleasant, joyful activity that does not have to be imposed on the players. If one observes children playing, he or she will see excitement, involvement, concentration, consistency, obedience to the rules and norms of the game, interpersonal interaction, and group cohesiveness. Games serve many purposes, such as recreation, development of skills, leisure, and psychotherapy.

The readiness to play games is most visible in older children and adolescents. They look constantly for the opportunity to play. This is true even with juvenile delinquents, who show a high level of readiness for social play. The implication here is that games, which are so easily adapted and modified for different uses, have therapeutic potential for work with juvenile delinquents. In order to elaborate on the potential of games for therapy with delinquents, it is first necessary to review the theoretical concepts of socialization, delinquency, and game play.

THEORETICAL CONCEPTS

Social life in any society is based on a set of social rules established by its majority. The purpose of these rules is to guide the individual's behavior. The process of learning to adapt to societal rules and norms is called socialization. Zigler and Child (1956) define socialization as:

The whole process by which an individual, born with behavioral potentialities of an enormously wide range, is led to develop actual behavior which is confined within a much narrower range—the range of what is customary and acceptable for him according to the standards of his group.

Socialization is generally understood as the process by which individuals acquire the knowledge, skills, and dispositions that enable them to conform to a set of shared behavioral norms in a particular society.

Delinquency, on the other hand, is defined as a deviation from societal rules. It is a socially ascribed label, not a psychiatric syndrome, that adolescents acquire after repeatedly violating well-established codes and rules for conduct. Thus, delinquent behavior is unsocialized behavior. Conversely, nondelinquent behavior is socialized behavior. Occasional deviant acts do not fit the definition of delinquency; only a pattern of chronic, flagrant violation of societal rules is labeled delinquency.

The similarities between the concepts of socialization and delinquency do not end here; delinquency has been further conceptualized as a failure in the socialization process. Most socialization theories deal with two basic factors: (1) the process of learning the elements of socialization, and (2) the product, what behaviors could be expected from as a result of this learning process. Some delinquency theorists have turned to research on the socialization process to explain the development of delinquency. Learning-based theorists assume that delinquency is a learned behavior; that is, a result of a failure to learn socialized behavior.

In a review of the literature on socialization and delinquency, Cressy and Ward (1969) describe the theories of Sutherland, Burgess, Akers, and Glaser. Sutherland's Differential Association Theory (DAT) states that a person's criminal behavior is a result of learning criminal behavior patterns, principally through interaction with others as a member of one or more groups. The individual's adoption of the motives, drives, and values underlying deviant behavior, rather than the learning of the actual behavior, is what explains the individual's criminal behavior, according to this theory. The "differential" part of the theory can be interpreted as follows: Everyone learns social as well as antisocial attitudes and values. The relative influence of these attitudes that are operating at a given time is what determines whether or not a person will commit a deviant act. With DAT, one could expect such factors as social class, exposure to criminal behavior, or attitudes of significant others during childhood, and peer group pressure to be important in the development of delinquency.

Burgess and Akers attempted to add precision to the DAT. They believed the theory lacked specificity regarding the actual process of learning of delinquent behavior. Their basic contribution was to more clearly define independent variables and reinforcements to make the theory more amenable to research. Glaser emphasized the process of identification with delinquent models in development in his reformulation of the DAT.

The common factor in the three theories is that delinquency is learned, whether through exposure to a criminal environment, reinforcement of criminal behavior, or identification with a criminal person. Indeed, these three formulations are not mutually exclusive; rather, they are probably complementary and represent different aspects of the learning process.

The implication of a learning perspective of delinquency, of course, is that delinquency can be unlearned. Game playing may have value to that end. Games are universal contexts for learning of social rules and norms. Games require that children conform to the norms of the collective. Many theorists have emphasized the role of games in the socialization process.

Piaget (1962) suggests that games give children practice with the rules which compose a social order. The function of play according to Piaget is, "exclusively an assimilation of reality to the self." Erikson (1964) emphasizes the importance of play in the development of the child and his or her physical growth by the combining of bodily and social processes. Boyd and Simon (1971) described play as:

> A social discipline, partially because it provides a constructive release of potentialities and partly because it affords children a more varied and more intensive experience than do other forms of human activity. By shaping the child to the social pattern in its own field, play makes a unique contribution to social discipline. . . . A game, then, is a situation set up imaginatively and defined by rules which together with the prescribed roles, is accepted by the players . . . just as mathematics is a way of thinking, so play is a way of social behaving.

The most dramatic finding about the importance of play and its effect in later life is Harlow's research on young monkeys (Harlow, 1964). He found that monkeys raised on cloth mothers, yet given the opportunity to form infant-infant affectional patterns through play, develop normal sexual responses in adulthood. Conversely, monkeys deprived of infant-infant play opportunities failed to develop normal sexual responses in adulthood.

In view of these theories concerning the importance of play, we may state that playing and the processes of play have far reaching consequences for maturation, development, and socialization. Play in childhood is a vital necessity for the development of all human beings, and serves the individual in many ways, one of the most critical of these is in the learning of social skills, rules, and social adaptation. Most of the theories of game play agree that game playing is a learning experience for social adjustment. The process of this learning can take place through practice and training in the necessary skills, through assimilation of new schemes (structures), or through exploring new situations and relationships. Games offer the child mini-life, controlled situations which he or she can master and learn according to his or her needs. What is unique in game play as a learning method is its internal motivational system, the joy and the pleasure of playing a game that motivates the child to continue playing. This internal motivation differentiates to a certain extent play from work and real-life social situations. The difference is that while in work the reward is frequently at the end of the process, in completing the product or receiving payment (except perhaps for artists), in game play the process itself is the reward.

We conclude that game play is a fundamental necessity for the child's development and a determinative factor in the socialization process. Game play is a learning experience and at the same time it also reinforces itself. The areas of conformity in socialized behavior can be specified according to Zigler and Child (1956), as follows: conformity to rules, controlling aggression, and adaptation to social norms. Delinquent behavior is the opposite of these behaviors. Playing games requires one to follow rules, control aggression and adapt to defined social norms. Therefore, a major context within which these behaviors are learned is games, and games should be considered as a therapeutic method for intervention with juvenile delinquents and for the prevention of delinquency. Our assumption is that delinquency is a learned behavior. The learning of delinquency is similar to the learning process in socialization. Games, because of their nature, are a unique learning method in socialization.

RESEARCH

If delinquency is a result of failure in the socialization process, it would follow that delinquents and nondelinquents differ in terms of their own behavior during games and their preference for types of games. Differences in these areas would provide a measure of the success or failure of the socialization process. Studies by Serok and Blum (1980, 1982) examined these questions, and a brief description follows.

The research project conducted contained two parts: (1) an analysis of game preferences as reported by delinquent and nondelinquent children, spontaneously and on a structured instrument, and (2) youth counselors' observations of the children's actual behavior in games. Fifty delinquent and 50 nondelinquent white, working-class boys aged 13- to 16-years-old, residing in an inner-city, low income area, comprised the sample. These 100 boys were grouped systematically to form 10 neighborhood after-school treatment groups. Data on game preferences were collected directly from the boys through individual interviews using a pretested game list, as well as the boys' rankings of games chosen to reflect particular characteristics of rules, competition, and aggressiveness.

For the first part of the study, three categories of games were defined following Roberts and Sutton-Smith (1962):

1. *Games of Physical Skill.* Games where the outcome is determined by the players' physical and motor activity and in which the physical attribute is the dominant one in the game. This category includes games of pure physical skill, for example, tug-of-war, dodge-ball, and so on.

2. *Games of Strategy.* Games in which the outcome is determined by rational choices among possible courses of action, and in which the attribute of choice is the dominant one in the game, for example, checkers, 20 questions, and so on.

3. *Games of Chance.* Games in which the outcome is determined by guesses or by uncontrolled artifact, and in which the attribute of guess or accident is the dominant one in the game, for example, matching coins, dollar poker, and so on.

Within each of the three game categories, the games were classified further as to the number and specificity of rules, the degree to which the direct expression of aggression is part of play, and the level of competitiveness. All subjects ranked in terms of personal preference a preselected list of games chosen to reflect these particular characteristics.

The second part of the study was concerned with the behavior of children in actual game situations. Six areas of behavior were identified, namely: (1) peer interaction, (2) socialization characteristics of rules, competition, and aggressiveness, (3) tolerance for mistakes or errors (his own or others), (4) tolerance for cheating (self and others), (5) reaction to winning and losing situations, and (6) motivation for games. The objective of the research was to obtain ratings on the boys' behavior over time within the natural setting of their groups as it occurred in the normal course of play. The group workers rated each of the following items, which were randomly distributed on a questionnaire, on a six-step Likert scale for each child in his or her group.

Peer Interaction

1.   Does the child's behavior conform to what his or her peers expect of him or her in playing games?

2.   Does the child try to be the focus of peers' attention during games?

3.   How often is the child willing to be an active participant in games?

Socialization Characteristics of the Game

4.   Does the child follow the rules of the game?

5.   Does the child play games in an aggressive manner?

6.   Does the child choose to play competitive games?

Tolerance for Mistakes or Errors (His or Her Own and Others)

7.   Is the child accepting of others who make mistakes or errors in a game?

8.   Does the child accuse others who make mistakes or errors in a game of cheating, rather than accepting their behavior as a mistake or error?

9.   Does the child deny his or her own mistakes or errors in a game?

Tolerance for Cheating (Self and Others)

10.   Does the child cheat in games?

11.   Although the child may be angry, does he or she permit some-one caught cheating to apologize and remain in the game?

12.   Does the child physically or verbally attack others who he or she catches cheating in a game?

13.   When the child gets caught cheating in a game, does he or she deny it in any way?

Reactions to Winning and Losing

14.   When the child is in a winning situation, does he or she want the game to continue as long as possible?

15.   When the child is in a losing situation, does he or she try to break up the game before it should normally end?

16.   If the child is on a losing team, does he or she blame others and deny his or her share of the responsibility?

Motivation

The question here was handled in a different way. The workers were asked to rank the five motivations indicated below for each of the children.

17.   Does the child like to take part in games because they provide opportunities to:
_____ Make friends
_____ Exert his leadership
_____ Gain recognition for his ability
_____ Just kill time
_____ Experience real enjoyment or pleasure

The study found that delinquents showed less preference for games of strategy like *Battleship*, chess, and more preference for games of chance such as poker, and Slot machine. Strategy games and chance games do have different characteristics. While games of strategy call for rational choice and evaluation of alternative courses of action, games of chance do not require this behavior. In games of chance, the player is less in control of the consequences, which leads to a reduction of responsibility for the outcome. There are fewer decisions to be made by the player and leaves the determination of the outcome more to accidental happenings. The fact that juvenile delinquents preferred more games of chance and less of strategy reflects a choice pattern of games which is characterized by less need for assessment of behavioral consequences, the making of fewer decisions, and less need to understand and behave within the norms which dictate strategy. According to the socialization literature, socialized behavior is characterized by rational thinking in the decision-making processes, responsibility for consequences of behavior and a realistic, planned approach as compared to allowing things to happen by chance. Juvenile delinquents demonstrated in their preference for games of chance, a low level and demand for socialized behavior.

Another finding in the study is that delinquent children prefer games with fewer rules like slot machine which reflects a desire to be in a situation which demands only a low level of socialization. Games with fewer and less specific rules require less conformity or obedience from the players. Moreover, one may speculate that in such situations deviation from the rules is less noticeable and, therefore, easier to get away with.

On the surface, this may look as if delinquents avoid problem situations by passive withdrawal; namely, they choose situations with fewer rules, but when we add their preference for more aggressive games, we get the active aspect of delinquency. It is not just a matter of omission, but also commission. By preferring more aggressive games with few rules, juvenile delinquents put themselves into situations in which the situation offers little control of their aggression. If we assume that aggression exists in all human beings and there is a need to express it, it is the adaptation and conformity to the social norms and standards (rules) which controls and channels the expression of aggression.

From the youth counselor's observations of the childrens' behaviors in games, we obtained additional important information. These findings can be presented as a profile of the juvenile delinquents' behavior in games as compared to nondelinquents. Juvenile delinquents try more to be the focus of their peers' attention, follow less the rules of the game, play in a more aggressive manner, are less tolerant of others' mistakes and cheating and are more ready to attack cheaters, while they deny more their own mistakes and cheating. Juvenile delinquents cheat more in games, more often want to continue games while they are winning, and frequently try to break up a game when they are losing. This profile is consistent with an unsocialized pattern of behavior, a lack of conformity to shared social norms.

IMPLICATIONS

Games appear to provide a simplified social situation with clearly defined social rules and expectations and a context within which therapeutic intervention can take place. Games also provide a minilife situation within which youths chose those games which are consistent with and reflect their general behavioral inclinations. There are major therapeutic implications resulting from the theories and the study presented in this chapter. We have developed a model which can be applied with delinquent youth as follows:

Contact and Motivation

In any therapeutic interaction, contact and motivation for therapy are of major importance and essential for the therapeutic process to begin. In working with groups of juvenile delinquents, the therapist often faces difficulties in getting their attention, in engaging them in group discussions, and in helping them change their behaviors. The resistance often encountered in involving delinquents in therapy is not found in involving them in games. Knowing juvenile delinquents' choice patterns in games and their style of behavior in games, the therapist can predict in advance where and when they will have difficulties in playing games and which games they like most. Knowing also the importance of games as a motivational factor, the worker can initiate a game planfully as an introductory activity which will provide content for later verbalization. For example, starting an activity with a game could provide enjoyment for the parties involved and at the same time provide for better functioning in the discussion. Moreover, such a start may decrease aggression and increase positive interpersonal behavior.

Differential Diagnostic Observation

By observing youth's behavior during the game and the games they prefer to play, a personal behavioral profile can be developed. In other words, having them play and relate to the others involved in the game will display their behaviors which are real, relevant, and reflect personal behavior. For example, game behaviors may display difficulties in conforming to rules, controlling aggressions, being intolerant of errors made by others, cheating, projecting on others their misdeeds and so forth. These behaviors are not unusual among adolescents; it is the prevalance and the intensity of these reactions that are more typical for delinquents. Developing a behavioral profile for each individual will provide a diagnostic tool for optimal intervention.

Planned Therapeutic Intervention

Another way to utilize the findings in developing programs for delinquents would involve designing a planned program of games in which the therapist would gradually introduce games with increasing levels of rules and diminishing levels of aggression. This requires systematic introduction of games and careful observation, in order to see whether the child himself or herself is able to adapt his or her behavior to the expectations of the games. Using learning principles, we could observe whether the child was able to handle his or her aggression and to conform to the rules of the game as he or she is given some rewards for achievement, and slowly introduce new games which have higher levels of expectations. We have identified the following dimensions of games which include values of socialized behavior and can be utilized systematically as a therapeutic intervention.

Self-Discipline

In order for a game to proceed smoothly, players must learn and perform within the role expectations of the game. Rules require conformity to the norms of the game and these are reinforced by the other players and the authority of the rules. Adult authority is not central to most games, but the depersonalized authority of the rules and the group norms serve to assist the player in learning and establishing self-discipline in order to perform successfully in the game.

Games vary greatly as to the number and rigidity of rules and the clarify of role definitions. Contrast, for instance, the low-level rules and the lack of differentiation of roles in a game, such as king-of-the-mountain, with the numerous rules and more clearly differentiated roles in a game, such as football, which gives a name to each position, requires a different behavior of each player, and the self-discipline of performing the role within the limits of the rules. Even in less structured games, such as relay races, there is a demand for each player to restrain his or her enthusiasm until his or her turn comes and not to start an activity until the previous player has completed the required task. Therapists too, can modify games so as to increase the demand for self-discipline. For instance, in basketball, a player who commits a foul can be required to call the foul on himself or herself rather than leaving this to an adult referee. Card and table games, too, vary greatly in the level of rules and the requirement to await one's turn.

Cooperation

Beginning with two-person games and increasingly in team games, the game itself requires the players to enter into cooperative efforts. The players must give up some of their own styles of behavior and immediate gratification for the good of the team. They must adapt to the demands of cooperative efforts. Included in cooperation is the encouragement and support which players give to other members of the team.

It is obvious that team games require more cooperative effort than do games where players participate as individuals, such as king-of-the-mountain or many relay races. Less obvious, perhaps, are differences among team games, such as football and baseball. Wherein football requires on every play a coordinated team effort, baseball only in rare instances, such as hit-and-run play or relay throw, requires team coordination. Therapists too, can, through rule changes or emphasis, increase the need for cooperation by, for instance, developing special recognition and scoring for assists in basketball in addition to making the basket, or requiring that there be at least two passes before a basket can count or, even in a less organized game like dodgeball, requiring two or three passes before the ball can be thrown at the "it" player. Even in such solitary activities as model building, the worker can encourage or discourage cooperation by giving a tube of glue to each individual, or forcing the sharing of a single tube of glue by two, three or more participants. Thus, the game, variations in the game, and therapist activity can increase or decrease the cooperative requirement.

"Socialized" Competition

Many games are competitive in nature and the outcome designates a winner and a loser. The rules set the parameters of the competitive effort and require that the players compete within certain limited boundaries, play fair, and accept responsibility for the outcome. Unless these rules are maintained, the game cannot proceed. Youth spend a considerable amount of time arguing the interpretation of the rules, the "fairness" of the decisions, and are continually alert to cheating. This provides an exercise in how to handle competition.

Although most of us ascribe to the old saying that what is more important is "how you play the game than who wins the game," we often do not behave consistently with this maxim. We are often negligent in giving thought to giving recognition and reward for effort and improved performance unless it ends in victory. For youth who are unable to tolerate loss or quickly lose motivation when losing, the choice of games and the development of an alternate reward system based on effort and/or improvement in performance is crucial. Emphasis must also be given to how should winners behave in relation to the losers. Youth who adapt the belief that winning by any means is acceptable should be engaged either individually, in the groups, or through a behavioral reward system to modify this attitude. Competition per se is not the issue, but recognition of feelings of others, fairness, the importance of rules, and the importance of effort and improvement of performance, however marginal it may be, are critical.

Concentration

To play games well requires concentration. Many games require a relatively long span of interest, patience, and persistence, even when losing. A short span of interest for many youth prevents them from successfully performing in many games and is a common symptom among disturbed youth. The demand for concentration is obviously different among games, such as flip-the coin, checkers, chess, and *Monopoly*. Even in a game, such as baseball, it is important to assess whether a 3, 5, 7, or 9 inning game can best maintain the youth's interest and concentration. One of the most difficult tasks for therapists is to sense the point at which the players are beginning to lose their interest and concentration in a game and the play is beginning to deteriorate as a consequence. Too often, we permit games to go on too long and a game which starts out with players enthusiastic, involved, and enjoying the play, ends up in disorganization and with conflicts among the players. Poor timing as to when to end a game because players are losing concentration is one of the most frequent self-inflicted problems faced by therapists. As therapists introduce a game, they should be alert as to when to end it and should have previously considered an alternative activity. Ideally, games should be ended before the players lose interest. Reward systems can be developed which reinforce the efforts of youth to stick with a game for longer periods of time.

Socioflexibility

Role demands within and among games differ. As players move from game to game or assume different roles within a game, there is a demand that they establish flexibility in how they relate to the other players and in assuming the appropriate role in the game. Games require players to learn how to assess the expectations for social interaction and to adapt to the demands of the different game situations.

Within the course of a game, many game players are required to change roles which move them into different social relations, such as being the dealer in a poker game, going from the ball carrier to a lineperson in football, and so on. Often, we observe that youth act up, resist, or show off when these role changes occur. In some instances, poor players must assume the limelight and experience the anxiety of failure, as in baseball when a poor player is placed in right field but must also assume his or her turn at bat. Therapists must be sensitive to the demands of changes in role during the game and to how they can use the group to support and encourage a player, to reduce the sense of inadequacy or failure, or to control inappropriate behavior which angers or upsets the group. Individual counseling, group discussions, and behavior plans can be utilized to assist those youth who have difficulty or display inappropriate behavior in particular roles.

Since a considerable amount of the stimulus in such situations is provided by the reactions of the other players, attempts to modify such behavior should take into consideration the reactions of the other players, and even the spectators.

Leadership-Followership

Team games require decision making and complimentary role assumption. Often, there is a requirement that a leader be designated and that other players follow the leader. Social learning is possible in relation to the choice of leader, the feelings involved in being or not being chosen leader, the behavioral expectations of leadership, and the appropriate behavior and expectations of followership.

Follow-the-leader type games, of course, provide the clearest examples of games which designate specific leadership and followership roles. Other games, such as football, require a play caller to initiate the activity, but the leader cannot control the behavior of the players. Whereas in baseball, the leader is the provider of inspiration, but has little control over the game and the players. Youth need to perform as both leaders and followers. This requires a sensitivity to the behavior requirements of leadership in specific games. Leadership can be rotated among players in games in which the performance demand is such that even poor players can assume a leadership role. Being captain of a relay team game in which each player performs individually requires less skilled leaders. Too often, it is easier to go along with the "natural" leader of the group, and the leadership role becomes reserved for only a few youth. This limits the opportunity for these youth to learn a followership role which includes listening to others, modifying one's own wishes to conform to the leader's decision, dealing with peer authority, and so on, and does not provide opportunities for all youth to learn to function in a leadership position.

Emotional Control and Tolerance

In playing games, players experience emotional excitement, the need to be aggressive, the emotional tolerance related to winning and losing, and the recognition or lack of recognition associated with skill and success. The rules and norms of the game provide the boundaries within which the players' emotions can be expressed and the response expectations of other players to emotional expression can be experienced. These expressions of emotions must be controlled and remain within the acceptable boundaries of the game.

Games which permit the direct expression of aggression are numerous, that is, king-of-the-mountain, football, boxing, arm wrestling, tug-of-war, and so on, and it becomes the task of the therapist to choose among these games based on what the youth can handle in relation to the limitations of the activity and the rules. Unstructured aggressive games such as king-of-the-mountain, when played by youth who have trouble controlling their aggressiveness, can be a disaster. Placing fearful youth into games which require direct, aggressive play without protection and support can be destructive. For youth who are less able to express aggression in physical skill games, one can choose among such games as War (cards), *Battleship*, chess, and so on. The activity required in the game and the rules of the game can serve to limit or encourage the expression of aggression; the choice of games must be related to an assessment of what the youth needs and can tolerate constructively. When making choices among games which permit the direct expression of aggression, a critical factor is the degree to which the game is susceptible to group contagion. Often, we find that each individual in the game is able to behave appropriately until the excitement, enthusiasm, and degree of aggressive behavior builds to a point where group contagion sets in and overwhelms the control of the individual players. Since the appropriate expression of aggression is a problem for so many delinquent youth, aggressive behavior in games can provide an extremely important focus for individual, group, and behavioral intervention.

Problem Solving

Games require a player to understand the task, establish goals, assess alternative paths to a goal and their consequences, follow through with the appropriate behavior, assess the outcome as to the choices made, and use this assessment as feedback as the game proceeds. The problem-solving process is essential for success and each step provides an opportunity for learning to approach problems thoughtfully and systematically.

Games can be differentiated as to the degree of strategy and problem solving they require. Games of chance, such as dollar poker, flip-the-coin, slap jack, require little problem solving as compared to checkers, chess, 20 questions, *Battleship*, and so on. One of the tasks of therapists is to help youth who treat games which require thought and strategy as if they were games of chance to recognize the need to enter into a problem-solving process. Poker can be played as a game of chance, or the players can be taught how to analyze the odds, how to assess the face cards, when to "fold" the hand, and so on. A therapist sitting with a group of youth watching football on TV can engage them in a discussion of why a play was successful or not, why the play was called, what play they would call next and why, as a means of involving those youth in a problem-solving process. A game-like treasure hunt can be initiated by first developing a plan of action. Youth who tend to react impulsively and without consideration of consequences should be helped to recognize and learn to develop a plan of action based on information, assessment, choice of alternatives, and possible consequences. Choices among games which encourage problem solving and worker emphasis on the problem-solving process are important supports to assist in this learning.

These dimensions of games reflect aspects of socialization which all youth must learn to function successfully in daily life. Although the previously mentioned dimensions are inherent in games themselves, they must be learned and can be used to assess the degree of learning which has taken place and where youth need assistance in the learning process.

Adding here our own research, we found that delinquent youth prefer games of chance, and did not prefer games of strategy. As we analyzed these games, we found that games of strategy required decisions based on a rational problem-solving process, awareness of alternative courses of action, evaluation of consequences, delay in immediate reaction in favor of longer-term strategies, and acceptance of personal responsibility for failure in the game. Games of chance, on the other hand, were dependent on accident for the outcome, did not require rational planning, do not make the player responsible for success or failure, and the consequences of choices could be blamed on things outside the players span of control, such as "luck." The dynamics of games of chance, which were preferred by delinquent youth, were consistent with descriptions delinquents give of the "chance" events which they say are responsible for the acts they commit—it was just "bad luck" that I got caught; I did not think about the consequences or what would happen, I wasn't responsible for what happened; if the other person hadn't behaved as he did, I wouldn't have done anything, and so on. The consistency between the characteristics of the preferred games and the behavior of delinquents is striking.

Our research also demonstrated that delinquent youth preferred within each category of games—physical skill, strategy, and chance—those games which had low numbers and specificity of rules and in which there was greater opportunity for the direct expression of aggression as compared to nondelinquents (Serok, & Blum 1980). These findings, too, are consistent with the rule-breaking behavior of delinquents and their inability to control their aggressiveness. We present these research findings as illustrative of the difference among youth in their preference for games and the consistency of the dynamics of their game preferences with their behavior in the community. An understanding of the games each player prefers and the dynamics of the preference provide us with potential insights into their general behavior. Although our research analysis was limited, it does give evidence of the importance of games and their potential use as a diagnostic device. Combined with the eight dimensions of games and how they relate to the needs and game performance of delinquent youth, this information provides us with areas for therapeutic intervention.

The theoretical orientation of the therapist, however, will determine the use that will be made of each game situation. For example, those who are more behaviorally oriented may want to develop a program of games for a youth having difficulty with cooperation, beginning with games which, for instance, require minimal cooperation. As the youth learns to cooperate in the initial game, he would be rewarded. The next game would require a greater degree of cooperation and a reward system could be developed in relation to each new level of mastery. This type of planning could be done in relation to each of the eight game dimensions. Therapists whose orientations are psychodynamic and who prefer the use of verbalization could, likewise, plan a program of games. For the youth who is having difficulty in cooperation, his or her inability to cooperate in the game would become the basis for discussion and analysis. If individual therapy is preferred, his or her game behavior could be discussed during the therapy session. For those therapists who prefer the use of the group and the milieu, the game could be halted and the behavior discussed with the player, or the group could discuss what occurred in the game after its completion. Each game, before it is chosen, should be analyzed in relation to the eight dimensions of games identified earlier. The game assessment should include the degree to which the rules, norms, and the form of the game require cooperation, "socialized" competition, concentration, emotional control, and so on. The point we are trying to make is that the minilife situation which constitutes the game situation provides the context in which various therapeutic approaches can be utilized. Games in themselves have learning value, but they also provide the content and context for treatment. Therefore, introducing the games according to the personal behavioral profile of a delinquent child, individually or in a group, helping him or her joyfully practice the game and to incorporate its characteristics and values is the essence of the therapy presented in this chapter.

SUMMARY AND CONCLUSIONS

Games represent a potentially useful vehicle for therapy. Social learning and socialization can also be enhanced through the systematic use of games. The therapeutic advantages that are associated with games include: games are a natural, enjoyable activity and even the most resistant youth will participate in games; the rules and norms of games represent a depersonalized source of authority in the socialization process; they provide an opportunity for channeling aggressive feelings into constructive activity; they offer opportunities to utilize the peer group in the therapeutic process; the characteristics of different games provide a wide range of choices and learning opportunities; and success and the enjoyment of play serves to reinforce the therapeutic process and change. To utilize these advantages, however, requires the analysis of each game and its dimensions, an assessment of each of the players, and a therapeutic plan as to how games are to be utilized to meet the needs of the players. In some instances, the choice of the game itself and the inherent learning which is built into the game will be of help. In other instances, games provide the context within which therapists can intervene and provide the content which can be utilized by the therapist and the youth to bring about changes in behavior. Games as context and content can be utilized differentially by therapists with different theoretical orientations and adapted to meet a variety of needs of youth. In our opinion, games constitute an untapped resource which can be used systematically as a therapeutic tool. Since games are a minilife situation of a recurring nature, the participants can practice what they have learned in the therapeutic program. The natural enjoyment of playing games and the satisfaction resulting from good performance also act to reinforce their achievement.

REFERENCES

Boyd, N.L. and Simon, P. (eds.) (1971). *Play and game theory in group work*. Chicago: University of Illinois at Chicago Circle.

Cressy, R.D. and Ward, A.D. (1969). *Delinquency, crime and social process*, New York: Harper & Row.

Erickson, Erik H. (1964). *Childhood and society*, 2nd ed. New York: Norton.

Harlow, H.F. (1964). The heterosexual affectional system in monkeys. In W.R. Bennis et al. (Eds.), *Interpersonal Dynamics* (pp. 36–51). Homeward IL: Dorsey.

Piaget, J. (1962). *Play, dreams and imitation in childhood*, New York: Norton.

Roberts, J.M. and Sutton-Smith, B. (1962). Child training and game involvement. *Ethnology*.

Serok, S. and Blum, A. (1980, March). Game preferences of delinquent and non-delinquent boys. *Journal of Sociology and Social Welfare*.

Serok, S. and Blum, A. (1982). Rule violating behavior of delinquent and non-delinquent youth in games. *Adolescence*.

Zigler, E. and Child, I.L. (1956). Socialization. In G. Lindzey and E. Aronson (Eds.), *Handbook of social psychology*. Reading, MA: Addison-Wesley.

Author Index

Van Cura, L. J., 138, 144
Van Sickle, R., 136, 145
Varenhorst, B. B., 6, 17, 137, 145
Varney, G. W., 286, 288
Vogel, M., 137, 143, 279, 283, 287–288

Walker, P., 279, 287
Wall, S., 287–288
Wallace, K. M., 140, 144
Ward, A. D., 312, 329
Watrous, Peter, 73
Watslawick, P. W., 78, 92, 94
Weakland, J. H., 78, 92, 94
Weiss, G., 233, 241–242
Wener, A., 233, 241
Werry, J. S., 233, 242
Wheeler, E., 130, 144
Wherry, J., 280, 289
White, R. W., 243, 255, 296, 309

Whiteside, M., 137, 143
Whiteside, R., 279–280, 283, 287–288
Whitmore, K., 246, 255
Wicks-Nelson, R., 86, 94
William F. Drueke & Sons, 249–251
Wineman, D., 8, 13, 16
Winnicott, D., 198, 214
Wolfensberger, W., 309
Wood, J. M., 307–308

Yalom, I., 162–164, 167, 185, 280, 289
Yuschak, M., 137, 142

Zakich, R., 22, 39, 286, 289
Zigler, E., 7–8, 13, 17, 311, 314, 329
Zimmerman, I. L., 260, 276
Zitsman, S., 22, 39
Zuckerman, J., 249, 254
Zweban, J., 137, 145

Subject Index